Normal Binocular Vision

Theory, Investigation and Practical Aspects

David Stidwill, F.C.Optom., Dip.C.L.P.
Sessional Lecturer/Visiting Clinician, Aston University, Birmingham, UK
Honorary Secretary, The Orthoptic and Binocular Vision Association
Examiner, The College of Optometrists

and

Robert Fletcher, F.C.Optom., D.Orth.
Professor Emeritus in Optometry and Visual Science, City University, London
Sometime Dosent, H.i.B.U. Kongsberg, Norway

A John s, Ltd., Publication

Registered office
John Wiley & Sons Ltd, The Atrium, Southern Gate, Chichester, West Sussex, PO19 8SQ, United Kingdom

Editorial offices
9600 Garsington Road, Oxford, OX4 2DQ, United Kingdom
350 Main Street, Malden, MA 02148-5020, USA

For details of our global editorial offices, for customer services and for information about how to apply for permission to reuse the copyright material in this book please see our website at www.wiley.com/wiley-blackwell.

Library of Congress Cataloging-in-Publication Data

Stidwill, David.
  Normal binocular vision : theory, investigation, and practical aspects /
David Stidwill and Robert Fletcher.
      p. ; cm.
  Includes bibliographical references and index.
  ISBN 978-1-4051-9250-7 (pbk. : alk. paper) 1. Binocular vision. I.
Fletcher, Robert. II. Title.
  [DNLM: 1. Vision, Binocular–physiology. 2. Vision Tests. WW 400 S854n
2011]
  QP487.S75 2011
  612.8′4–dc22

                                                                    2010018329

A catalogue record for this book is available from the British Library.

Set in 10 on 12.5 pt Sabon by Toppan Best-set Premedia Limited
Printed and bound in Singapore by Fabulous Printers Pte Ltd

1 2011

CONTENTS

Colour plate section follows page 88

PREFACE

This book is intended to be an introduction to the study of human binocular vision. It is intended for preclinical optometry students and also for students of psychology. The development and normal characteristics of binocular vision are described; also the effects of errors in binocular motor control, and in sensory fusion of the right and left eyes' images. The assessment of binocular vision parameters is included, but the management of anomalies is left to textbooks on abnormal binocularity. The contents are presented in sequence, but as different aspects of binocular vision interact with each other, references are made early in the text to fuller explanations later. For this reason, it may be helpful to read through the book quickly before returning to the first chapter. As scientific papers are produced in large quantities each year on binocular vision research, this text should be regarded as a basis for understanding the concepts of normal binocular vision. To review recent changes in specific topics, the relevant reference should be entered into an Internet browser.

ACKNOWLEDGEMENTS

The authors would like to thank their families for their support. Andrew Stidwill helped with research, input and copy-editing. The Librarian at the BOA Library of the College of Optometrists assisted with source material. Katrina Hulme-Cross and the staff in various parts of the Publisher have given much guidance and aid.

ABBREVIATIONS

These abbreviations are also introduced in the unabbreviated form at their first occurrence in the text.

°	Degree of arc (angular measurement)
Δ	Prism dioptre (angular measurement)
AC	Accommodation-induced convergence
AC/A ratio	Accommodation-induced convergence to accommodation ratio
ARC	Anomalous retinal correspondence
Areas 17, 18, 19	Brodmann anatomical visual areas
BSR	Binocular summation ratio
CA	Convergence-induced accommodation
CA/C ratio	Convergence-induced accommodation to convergence ratio
Cardiff PL	Cardiff preferential looking test (for visual acuity)
CFF	Critical flicker fusion frequency
cm	Centimetres
cpd	Cycles per degree
CS	Contrast sensitivity
D	Dioptre
D/MA	Dioptres/metre angle
DOG	Difference of Gaussians
DS	Dioptre sphere
EMG	Electromyography
EOG	Electro-oculograph
EOM	Extra-ocular muscle
FEF	Frontal eye (movement) field
GT	Golgi tendon
HARC	Harmonious anomalous retinal correspondence
Keeler PL	Keeler preferential looking test (for visual acuity)
LGN	Lateral geniculate nucleus
LIO	Left inferior oblique extra-ocular muscle
LIR	Left inferior rectus extra-ocular muscle
LLR	Left lateral rectus extra-ocular muscle
LMR	Left medial rectus extra-ocular muscle

logMAR	Logarithmic minimum angle of resolution (visual acuity measure)
LSO	Left superior oblique extra-ocular muscle
LSR	Left superior rectus extra-ocular muscle
mm	Millimetres
MRI	Magnetic resonance imaging
ms	Milliseconds
M visual pathway	Magnocellular visual pathway
MST	Middle superior temporal cortical area
NPC	Near point of convergence
NRC	Normal retinal correspondence
OKN	Optokinetic nystagmus
P visual pathway	Parvocellular visual pathway
PAT	Prism adaptation test
PL	Preferential looking (visual acuity measurement)
PPRF	Paramedian pontine reticular formation
REM	Rapid eye movement
RIO	Right inferior oblique extra-ocular muscle
RIR	Right inferior rectus extra-ocular muscle
RLR	Right lateral rectus extra-ocular muscle
RMR	Right medial rectus extra-ocular muscle
RSO	Right superior oblique extra-ocular muscle
RSR	Right superior rectus extra-ocular muscle
r-VOR	Rotational vestibulo-ocular reflex
Teller PL	Teller preferential looking test (for visual acuity)
t-VOR	Translational vestibulo-ocular reflex
UARC	Unharmonious anomalous retinal correspondence
V1, V2, V3, V4, V5/MST	Cortical functional visual areas
VA	Visual acuity
VEP	Visually evoked potential
VIP	Ventral inter-parietal area
VMC	Vieth–Müller circle
VOR	Vestibulo-ocular reflex

Chapter 1

INTRODUCTION TO NORMAL BINOCULAR VISION

1.1 The end product of binocular vision

Normal binocular vision is defined as the integration of monocular sensory and motor visual information into a combined percept of the surrounding physical space. This visual percept is heavily edited by the brain. It is affected by visual memory, and we sometimes react to visual stimuli before they pass into consciousness. This book sets out the processes and equipment involved in that editing.

Human binocular vision has several advantages over monocular vision. The obvious advantage is **single vision** rather than double vision, or vision alternating between each eye. Next, the subtle difference between the right and left viewpoints allows the most accurate form of depth perception, **stereopsis**. It is possible to see the effect of the different viewpoints in binocular vision by holding a hand edge in front of the eyes, and then closing each eye in turn. Stereopsis assists primates in hand–eye coordination and in precise interception of mobile food sources. Stereopsis helps to identify threats – adversaries may be spotted moving across the visual field with monocular vision, but when stationary, three-dimensional vision helps to identify a specific threat from background visual information. This is known as **figure–ground separation**, or breaking camouflage. With binocular vision, the amount of **binocular convergence** used to fixate a target with each eye allows an approximate assessment of the target distance by triangulation. Binocular vision also helps with **spatial localisation**: visual attention can be concentrated on objects situated in the plane of the binocular fixation point, allowing distracting stimuli nearer or farther away to be ignored. Binocular perception has advantages over monocular vision in assessing **surface curvature**. It also allows enhanced **surface material perception** using lustre perception.

At a higher level of visual performance, fine stereopsis allows very precise detailed tasks, e.g. using binocular operating microscopes, or mapping the apparent height of terrain using stereoscopic photographs. The brain also averages the visual input when combining right and left eye images, so that an individual with early cataract, who sees a letter 'O' as a 'Q' with one eye and as an inverted 'Q' with the other eye, correctly perceives 'O' in binocular vision. This process, binocular **visual summation**, improves binocular performance over monocular for:

Normal Binocular Vision: theory, investigation and practical aspects. By David Stidwill and Robert Fletcher. © 2011 Blackwell Publishing Ltd

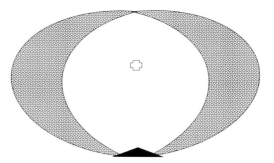

Figure 1.1 The human visual fields. With both eyes open and fixation on the central cross, binocular vision is possible where the right and left fields overlap. The lower triangle represents the highly variable influence of the nose. The grey areas show the monocular extensions of the binocular visual field on each side.

- high-contrast visual acuity, and the upper spatial frequencies of contrast sensitivity;
- absolute light detection at threshold of perception;
- threshold contrast sensitivity function;
- reaction time to flashing visual stimuli, e.g. sine-wave bar gratings. This can be important in several occupational situations.

Two eyes and binocular vision supply a paired and therefore **spare organ**, true for many of the body's functions as insurance against injury and disease. Two eyes also give a **wider field of vision**. In animals that are subject to predators, the horizontal visual field may extend to 360 degrees, i.e. **panoramic vision**. In humans, the horizontal binocular visual field is 120 degrees, with a further monocular field of about 45 degrees (the temporal crescents) on each side of the binocular field, on the horizontal (medial-lateral) axis passing through the eyes, but reducing to zero superiorly and inferiorly (Fig. 1.1). The nose reduces binocular field inferiorly. In animals the monocular and binocular visual fields vary according to the species (Fig. 1.2).

1.2 The requirements for binocular vision

The requirements for binocular vision are as follows.

- **Two eyes**, and a separation between the eyes called the **interocular distance**, generally about 65 mm in adult humans.
- A **neural pathway** to transfer the two images to the brain (Fig. 1.3).
- **Neural processing systems** to integrate the different types of raw visual information, such as luminosity, size, movement relative to the eye, colour and contrast. These systems also analyse and produce further percepts, such as distance, shape, movement relative to the body and stereopsis.

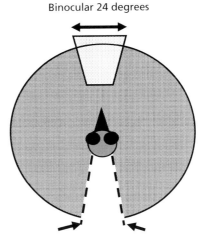

Figure 1.2 The visual fields of the pigeon, showing a 24-degree binocular field, and a total field of 340 degrees, mainly monocular (after Walls, 1942).

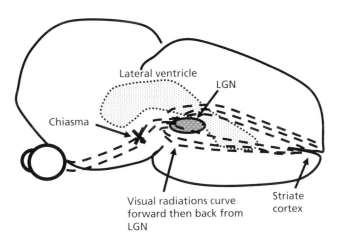

Figure 1.3 The human neural pathway for vision, from the retina to the visual cortex. LGN, lateral geniculate nucleus.

- **Extra-ocular muscles** to allow the object fixated to be imaged on appropriate retinal areas of each eye (Fig. 1.4).
- **Motor control systems** to govern voluntary and reflex eye movements – e.g. to maintain or vary fixation. Also there has to be a method of correlating binocular sensory input and binocular motor function: **motor correspondence**.
- Further enhancement of binocular perception is obtained by the **triangulation of objects** observed using head and body movements and the addition of other, monocular, clues to the total visual perception.

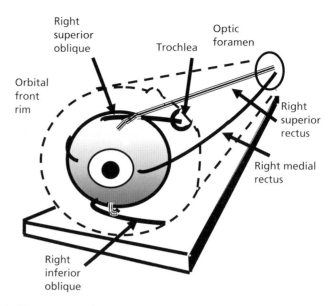

Figure 1.4 The extra-ocular muscles and the right orbit in outline. The orbit is represented as a cone extending backwards to the optic foramen. Only the superior rectus and the medial rectus are shown, with the two oblique muscles. While the recti pull backwards towards their origins at the rear of the orbit, the obliques pull towards the medial wall of the orbit. For clarity, the inferior and lateral rectus muscles are indicated but not labelled.

1.3   Monocular visual direction

Spatial sense is the body's recognition of the location of external objects, involving the tactile sense, hearing and vision. The determination of external locations by visual means involves the relationship between the external location, the eyes and the head position. **Visual direction** describes the visual position of an object in a two-dimensional plane, i.e. its vertical and horizontal location. To move from **physical space**, which exists without our presence, to **visual space** (the visual representation of physical space) involves initially the use of visual direction to build up the perceived picture. Complications in building up visual space may be illustrated by an experiment with inverted vision. It is possible to adapt to inverted vision (which can be produced by an optical system) so that after 2 weeks' wear, vision becomes upright. Upon removing the lenses it takes about 30 minutes of alternating upright and inverted vision before normal vision is stable.

The recognition of monocular visual direction is attained by the association of a visual receptor in the retina with the external position of an object imaged on that visual receptor. The line passing through the centre of the entrance pupil, to any object of regard is called a **line of sight** (Alpern, 1969). For an object fixated by the fovea, this line is known as the **primary line of sight** or, in clinical practice, the **visual axis** (Ogle, 1950). The entrance pupil is the image of the actual pupil formed by the cornea, as seen by an observer.

The visual axis is more strictly defined as the external light ray that, after refraction by the optical system of the eye, will fall on the fovea (Freedman and Brown, 2008). The fovea is the retinal area that receives images from objects observed straight ahead. Visual acuity and colour perception are normally best at the fovea. When the object of regard is imaged on the fovea, the oculomotor system ceases to initiate any eye movement. The fovea is thus the retino-motor zero point, or retino-motor centre.

Disambiguation note: the term 'zero point' is also used in relation to retinal correspondence (see section 4.5 in Chapter 4).

Note:
- In 1907 Maddox used the terms 'visual line' and 'fixation line' (Maddox, 1907).
- The visual axis must pass through the nodal point(s), and as there are two nodal points in the eye situated 7.13 and 7.41 mm behind the corneal vertex, a single visual axis cannot strictly connect the fovea with the object of regard (Rabbetts, 2007; Harris, 2010). For simplicity hereafter the terms 'visual axis' and 'primary line of sight' are used synonymously, and this is indicated in the text.
- The visual axis is not (usually) the same as the **optic axis** of the eye, which is why the anterior corneal reflection is not usually in the centre of the pupil (Fig. 1.5). The measurement of these axes is discussed by Dunne *et al.*, (2005).

The **primary line of sight** (the visual axis) is said to have the **principal visual direction**, i.e. from the fovea to the object imaged on the fovea. All non-foveal retinal receptors have **secondary visual directions**. The angular value of a secondary visual direction is calibrated by reference to the primary visual direction. The general term 'line of sight' includes both primary and secondary visual directions. Non-foveal lines of sight are referred to as 'secondary' lines of sight, or 'lines of direction' (Cline *et al.*, 1980). Hereafter,

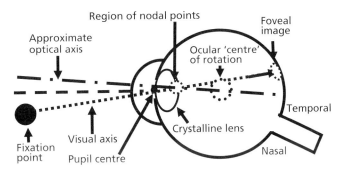

Figure 1.5 The visual, pupillary and optic axes. View of the human right eye from above, indicating the conventional directions of various axes relative to the route from the fixation point to its retinal image, via the pupil, and the assumed nodal points. The pupillary axis lies between the other two axes.

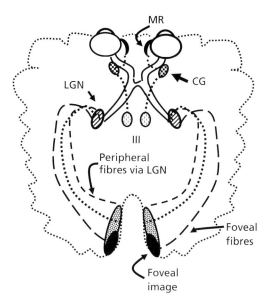

Figure 1.6 The visual system sensory and third nerve motor pathways. A schematic plan view of the visuum showing the location in the striate cortex of sensory input from the central and peripheral retina. The motor route from the third cranial nerve nuclei to the medial rectus muscles is also shown. CG, ciliary ganglion; LGN, lateral geniculate nucleus; MR, medial rectus.

'the line of sight' will refer to the primary line of sight, unless otherwise stated. **Any number of objects situated on the same (primary or secondary) line of sight will stimulate the same receptor.** This is the **law of oculocentric direction**: the direction of all these objects is the same and given by reference to the single eye involved. The law relates to the use of one eye only. So when the fovea of that eye re-fixates on an object in a different direction, the **oculocentric visual direction** moves with it.

The recognition of visual direction by retinal receptors is called **local sign**: each retinal receptor sends a neuro-visual signal and encodes the direction in vertical and horizontal coordinates, but not the distance. Each retinal receptor–cerebral sensory unit has a unique ability to detect a particular direction. These signals are conveyed through the lateral geniculate nucleus to the visual cortex (Fig. 1.6). In other words, each retinal receptor is associated with the particular direction from which it receives a stimulus. This association extends as far as the visual cortex: there is said to be **retinotopic mapping** of neurones in the visual system (Zeki and Shipp, 1988). This has been demonstrated in reverse by stimulating cortical neurones electrically. The subject sees a flash of light in the direction associated with the stimulated cortical neurone.

The local sign is the angular subtense between a retinal receptor's secondary visual direction and the primary visual direction of the fovea (Lotze, 1852). The high precision of local sign is a result of a cortical averaging process, which takes the mean of both spatial and temporal fluctuations in

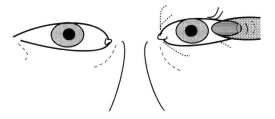

Figure 1.7 Visual local sign may be demonstrated by gently pressing on the temporal sclera. A phosphene (apparent light) is seen in the nasal visual field. The direction of the phosphene is linked with the eccentricity of the stimulated retinal area.

a stimulus (Reading, 1983). Local sign is a general attribute of sensory perception: the sensation of touch on any part of the human body surface is linked to related cortical sensory neurones. The operation of visual local sign can be demonstrated by gently (and briefly) pressing one finger on the eyelids at the outer canthus (Fig. 1.7). This is best done in a dim room. A small bright disc of light will be seen on the nasal side of the visual field. Similar mechanical stimulation of the retina occurs in retinal detachment and posterior vitreous detachment. Also by directing a small light beam onto the retina using an ophthalmoscope the impression is obtained of a small light seen in physical space. In clinical practice this subjective impression may be described as 'projection', demonstrating the inherent association of retinal points with specific visual directions. However, 'projection' is not strictly appropriate, and a term such as 'external reference', or 'apparent spatial location', may be more suitable. The ancient Greeks actually hypothesized that the eyes projected light onto the object of regard!

1.4 Binocular visual direction and retinal correspondence

The recognition of binocular visual direction is attained by averaging the simultaneous input from both eyes from the external position of an object. When objects are located by reference to the simultaneous input from both eyes, the reference position, the egocentre, is an imaginary point halfway between the two eyes. This form of localisation is **egocentric localisation**. An object fixated will be imaged on each fovea and will have an oculocentric impression of being 'straight ahead', relative to each eye. But the combined binocular percept will be as if the images were both located on the retina of a virtual shared eye in the middle of the forehead (Sheedy and Fry, 1997). A practical experiment to illustrate the difference between oculocentric and egocentric localisation consists of holding a cardboard tube between the thumb and fingers of the left hand, looking through the tube with the left eye across the room. The right hand, held before the right eye, provides the visual effect of a hole in the hand, being a stimulus upon which the left eye's restricted field is superimposed, suggested in Fig. 1.8. The egocentre is

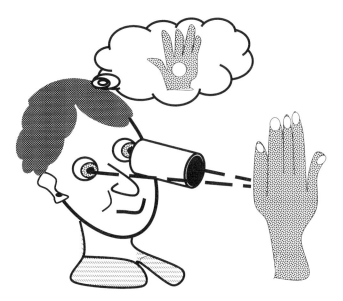

Figure 1.8 The hole in the hand. This is simultaneous perception of different images from each eye: the right and left oculocentric views are combined into a single egocentric view.

in the region of the bisector of the line connecting the two (right and left eye) entrance pupils, which are situated 3 to 4 mm anterior to the nodal points (Rabbetts, 2009). The advantage of egocentric localisation is the three-dimensional percept of the object being seen. It adds **distance** to the two-dimensional perceptions of direction produced by oculocentric localisation. Later it will be seen that even egocentric localisation can be subject to modification. For example, a dominant eye may shift the egocentre towards that eye (Ono and Barbeito, 1982). Visual illusions, lens and prism alterations may also alter the perceived localisation of an object, as will oculomotor paresis (see section 12.3 in Chapter 12). Egocentric localisation allows perception of the position of objects as seen from our egocentre. We can also localise objects in relation to each other: this is called **relative localisation** (see section 8.2 in Chapter 8).

Binocular vision needs a combination of the visual fields of the right and left eyes: the binocular visual field. The monocular visual directions have to be transformed into a binocular visual direction. This is achieved by **retinal correspondence.** The output of the fovea of one eye is linked with that of the other fovea in the visual cortex. The foveas are said to be **corresponding retinal points.** There are also non-foveal corresponding retinal points of each eye that are similarly linked to allow a binocular percept across the entire binocular visual field. So corresponding retinal points consist of a pair of retinal receptors, one in each eye, which receive stimulation from an object that is perceived to appear in the same visual direction for each eye: the law of identical visual directions. This is explained in more detail in section 4.4, Chapter 4.

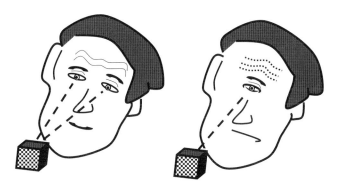

Figure 1.9 The effective human cyclopean view. The direction of the fixated object seen with both eyes open is linked with a virtual eye position midway between the right and left eyes.

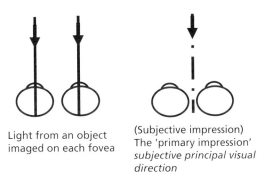

Light from an object imaged on each fovea

(Subjective impression)
The 'primary impression'
subjective principal visual direction

Figure 1.10 Primary common subjective principal visual direction. Light from an object stimulating both foveas produces a common visual direction.

The effect of egocentric localisation is to produce a **common subjective principal visual direction.** This is sometimes referred to as the **cyclopean eye effect.** Cyclops was the giant in Greek mythology with a single eye in the middle of his forehead (Fig. 1.9). Binocular visual localisation is centred on the cyclopean eye. An object imaged on each fovea is seen binocularly in the **primary** common subjective visual direction (Fig. 1.10).

Similarly, for every non-foveal point in one eye there is a related point in the other eye, which shares the same visual direction, these two non-foveal points being corresponding retinal points. The object seen by the two corresponding non-foveal points lies in a **secondary** common subjective visual direction, which is located by reference to the primary common subjective principal visual direction associated with the two foveas (Fig. 1.11). The existence of the common subjective principal visual direction can be demonstrated by masking a photographic flashlight to produce a vertical slit. One eye is covered, the centre of the vertical slit is fixated and the flash is generated. Repeat with the other eye with the slit held horizontally and the first eye occluded. The binocular after-image seen is a cross, demonstrating the common visual direction. This will work both for the foveas and the non-foveal corresponding points. In the latter case, the subject fixates a

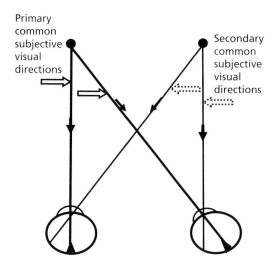

Figure 1.11 Secondary common subjective principal visual direction. Light from a non-fixated object produces a secondary common visual direction.

central target, and the flashlight is held in a fixed position away from the central area.

There are two further complications of visual localisation perception. Oculocentric visual direction gives information in two dimensions, and ego-centric visual direction extends this to three dimensions. That information would only be useful if the eyes did not move relative to the head. To measure the localisation of a new object of regard in a different binocular gaze position, or to assess the location of a moving object being followed by the eyes, information about eye movement from the extra-ocular muscle control centres is needed. This permits **headcentric localisation**: an object located on the line of sight will be seen in the same headcentric direction for any given gaze direction. The reference system is centred on the head of the subject. This facility will also allow the assessment of the relative localisation in visual space of two or more separate objects. Finally, **visuo-motor memory** will allow us into the fourth dimension, by calculating the localisation of objects in time, e.g. when and where an object rotating around us will be likely to re-appear in vision. These binocular vision faculties may appear obscure, but they are the basis for the spatial awareness skills that allow a 3-year-old child to carry a broomstick around the corners of a corridor without much difficulty, for example, and actually help the development of spatial localisation, visual prediction and – it is said – mathematics (e.g. topology).

1.5 The Vieth–Müller circle

A circle can be drawn that intersects the nodal points of each eye with the object fixated by both foveas (Fig. 1.12). Vieth and Müller predicted that any object point on the Vieth–Müller circle (VMC) would stimulate a retinal

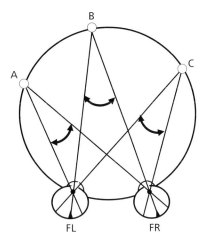

Figure 1.12 The Vieth–Müller circle (VMC; the basic form of the horopter). Three objects in space are imaged on the two retinas, each object forming images on corresponding 'points' (or areas). The geometry of the figure dictates that the angles shown are all equal to each other. The points through which the three lines pass in each eye are usually considered to represent the nodal points of the eyes, and fall on the VMC. However, opinions differ, some writers using the entrance pupils or even the assumed centres of rotation of the eyes. FL, left fovea; FR, right fovea.

point on each eye, which would have the same angular subtense relative to each fovea. Thus the VMC is a **theoretical model** of the positions of objects in space, which are imaged on corresponding retinal points. Any point on this circle would be seen binocularly as a single object.

Note: some versions of the **Vieth–Müller circle** diagram use the eyes' entrance pupils or even the centres of rotation instead of the nodal points.

The VMC is used to describe the optical **formation of images** on the retina of each eye. The VMC concept **assumes** that corresponding retinal points are placed at regular and equal horizontal distances from the fovea of each eye. However, the **measured locus** of every point in space that actually stimulates corresponding retinal points for a particular binocular fixation is called **the horopter**, and this will not be the same as the VMC (see Chapter 6).

1.6 Horizontal retinal binocular disparity

An object – let us call it object 'A' – whose image falls on corresponding retinal points of each eye will be seen as a single object. Where a second object 'B' situated on the same horizontal meridian as object 'A', is imaged on non-corresponding retinal points in each eye, the percept will be that object 'B' is seen as nearer or further from object 'A' (Fig. 1.13 and Fig. 1.14). Where the second object is situated slightly closer than the VMC, its secondary lines of sight would intersect nearer than the fixation point and

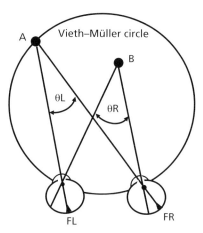

Figure 1.13 Crossed disparity. The fixated target A is situated on the Vieth–Müller circle, and the non-fixated target B is placed nearer. The right and left images of B do not fall on corresponding retinal points, but on retinal points, which are near enough for Panum's fusional area to operate. The non-fixated target B will be seen in depth, nearer than the fixation point, A. FL, left fovea; FR, right fovea.

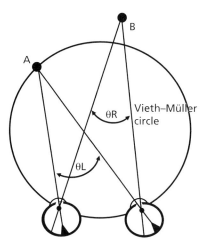

Figure 1.14 Uncrossed disparity. The fixated target A is on the Vieth–Müller circle and the non-fixated target B is placed further away. The right and left images of B do not fall on corresponding retinal points, but on retinal points, which are near enough for Panum's fusional area to operate. The non-fixated target B will be seen in depth, further away than the fixation point, A.

produce crossed disparity. Objects situated slightly beyond the VMC have secondary lines of sight intersecting beyond the fixation point and produce uncrossed disparity. A small amount of disparity is the physiological requirement for the perception of stereopsis. However, if an object is even further from the VMC, and stimulates non-corresponding retinal points sufficiently far apart, then the object will be seen in diplopia, i.e. double vision. All images of a single object falling on non-corresponding retinal points are described as **disparate.** For a particular object, the angle between the principal visual direction and the secondary visual direction in which the object is seen is called the **subtense angle.** The angular difference between the subtense angles of the right and left eyes is called the (**horizontal**) **retinal binocular disparity** (usually abbreviated to **disparity**). Although the example given above was of objects on the same horizontal meridian, the actual orientation of the retinal binocular disparity may be **horizontal, vertical** or **oblique.** The value, i.e. the quantification of the retinal binocular disparity, may be positive, negative or, for corresponding retinal points only, zero.

Horizontal retinal binocular disparity is the trigger for the perceptive faculty known as **stereopsis,** disparity sensitivity or binocular depth perception (see True binocular depth perception in Chapter 11). The disparity must be enough to produce stereopsis, but not so large as to cause diplopia. For a three-dimensional object there are different amounts of horizontal retinal binocular disparity relating to different elements of the object, some being seen nearer and some further away than the part of the object fixated by the foveas. So looking at the windscreen of an approaching car, the headlamps will be seen closer and the rear door further away. The windscreen would fall on the VMC; the headlamps would be within the VMC and the rear door beyond the VMC. The lines of sight for the headlamps would have **crossed disparity,** and those of the rear door would have **uncrossed disparity.**

Disambiguation note: all images of objects seen binocularly on the same meridian, which are situated closer or further than the VMC, will be disparate. The term 'disparity' implies stereoscopic fusion, but the term 'disparate' includes objects seen in diplopia, as well as those capable of stereoscopic fusion.

1.7 Vertical retinal binocular disparity and cyclofusion

If a vertical line in physical space is imaged on the vertical meridians of each retina of a subject, the retinal meridians are corresponding meridians, and the line will be seen without any stereoscopic effect. This is because all the horizontal elements that make up the vertical images will have zero horizontal disparity. If the line in physical space is now tilted with the top towards (or away from) the subject, the image of the line will fall on non-vertical retinal meridians. Each eye will have a different side view of the physical line. It is possible to work out the angle (D degrees) between the ocular non-vertical meridians, if the interpupillary distance ($2a$ in mm), and the distance from the eyes to the vertical line (b) are known, using the formula:

$$\tan D = 2a/b \times \tan i$$

where i is the inclination in degrees of the physical line towards the subject. The line in physical space will now be seen stereoscopically, as leaning towards (or away from) the subject. A discussion of the effect in this situation on cyclovergence and cyclofusion will be found in section 12.10, Chapter 12.

Vertical retinal disparities, together with horizontal disparities, allow cortical assessment of eye position (from the retinal data alone). However, the size of vertical disparities can be deduced from purely horizontal retinal disparity, because a vertical disparity adjusts the cortical receptive field position of corresponding points to the next higher or lower row of horizontal cortical sensors. Directions of gaze and of vergence thus can be recovered from horizontal disparity information (Read and Cumming, 2006). Where a vertical disparity occurs in near vision, any vertical diplopia is normally controlled by vertical vergence, and perceptual ambiguities because of asymmetrical convergence are resolved by the vertical disparity analysis capacity of the visual system (Brautaset and Jennings, 2005).

1.8 Cortical binocular disparity

To complicate things a little, the actual arrangement of **neural pathways** from the retina to the visual cortex determines **cortical (receptive field) binocular disparity**, with zero disparity for single, non-stereoscopic, vision. It is possible for the visual cortex to adapt, producing single vision even where zero retinal binocular disparity is not present, as where a subject has an anisometropic spectacle correction producing unequal retinal images but has adapted to see an undistorted visual percept. Here there would be zero cortical binocular disparity despite non-zero retinal binocular disparity.

Chapter 1: Revision quiz

Complete the missing words, perhaps in pencil. Only look at the answer when you have really tried. It would be useful to look back at the text and then try all these questions again.

Binocular vision has the advantage of s_____ (1) over double vision. The subtle difference between right and left viewpoints allows d_____ (2) perception, also called stereopsis. In addition, binocular vision allows visual summation, which imp_____ (3) binocular over monocular performance in a variety of ways.

Monocular visual direction allows the location of an object in t_____ (4) dimensions. Local sign is the angle between the direction of the fovea and the direction of a n_____ (5) -foveal receptor. Binocular visual direction is achieved by ret_____ (6) correspondence, the presence of which can be demonstrated by using af_____ (7) -images.

The theoretical model of the surface in physical space that locates objects that stimulate corresponding retinal points is called the V_____–M_____ c_____ (8).

Objects that are almost but not quite stimulating corresponding retinal points produce horizontal retinal binocular dis_____ (9), which is the basis for stereopsis.

Answers
(1) single; (2) depth; (3) improves; (4) two; (5) non; (6) retinal; (7) after; (8) Vieth–Müller circle; (9) disparity.

Chapter 2
THE DEVELOPMENT OF BINOCULAR VISION

2.1   Animal binocular vision

All vertebrates have two eyes. Most invertebrates have two complex eyes, often with additional simple eyes. One advantage of two eyes even without binocular overlap is that the animal can then orient itself either to face the light source or to back away, by comparing the light levels received by each eye. Marine animals can vertically orient themselves by detecting the increased light level received by the uppermost eye. For vertebrates the lateral extent of the right and left visual fields provides protection from predators, whereas for predators the overlap of the fields provides the basis for stereopsis. Stereopsis is a key attribute of even the most elementary mammals. In reduced illumination it increases the 'signal-to-noise ratio' and thereby allows the protective effect of camouflage to be negated. The tiger can be seen poised in the undergrowth despite his camouflage. Stereopsis allows depth perception to facilitate an attack on prey. Some lower animals, e.g. chameleons, can move their eyes independently over 360 degrees and see two separate objects at the same time. However, they do have the ability to switch to stereoscopic vision using both eyes to judge the distance of their prey. With an inter-eye separation of up to 90 cm, hammerhead sharks not only have 360-degree visual fields, but also have overlapping fields producing stereopsis both in front and behind the head (McComb *et al.*, 2009). For primates, the eyes are directed to the front, and all have foveas. There is binocular coordination for all eye movements. The combination of binocular overlap, stereopsis and increased motor skills gives many primates the ability to manipulate tools.

2.2   Variations in visual pathway types

Visual information from each eye, such as acuity, contrast, colour vision and the assessment of visual direction, is first combined at the optic chiasm, where some or all of the optic nerve fibres cross over, or **decussate**. Reptiles and birds have full decussation, originating from eyes that are placed on each side of the head, and a field of view that is mainly to the side. The retina of the left eye projects to the right-hand side of the brain, and the right eye retina to the left visual cortex. In this situation stereopsis is not

Normal Binocular Vision: theory, investigation and practical aspects. By David Stidwill and Robert Fletcher. © 2011 Blackwell Publishing Ltd

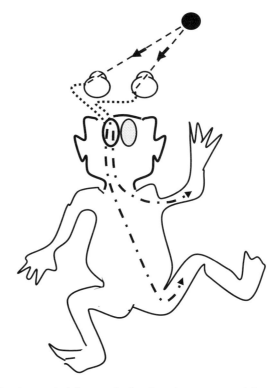

Figure 2.1 Fully decussated (crossed) visual pathways to and from the cerebral hemispheres, after Adrian (1947). Vertebrate retinal images are inverted. Here an object in the right field is naturally best investigated with the right paw or hand. With fully crossed sensory registration in the left hemisphere, the right motor response is best initiated in the left hemisphere.

possible, although panoramic vision is enhanced. Mammals have partial decussation: uncrossed fibres varying from 10% in the rabbit, 17% in cattle and horses, 25% in cats and dogs and 50% in primates, including humans. Partial (hemi-) decussation allows information from both eyes to be integrated into the same side of the visual cortex to allow processing of binocular vision. There are also advantages when sensory input from the right side of the visual field and motor control directed for right gaze both involve the same (left) side of the brain (Fig. 2.1). In addition to purely visual sensory data, there is a population of retinal ganglion cells sending information via the superior colliculus, which is used for saccadic eye movement control (Nolte, 2002).

2.3   Inborn and learned reflexes in vision

In mammals, motor control of postural reflex eye movements through the extra-ocular muscles and their cranial nerves is an inborn faculty and not learned. These include the vestibulo-ocular reflex and the optokinetic reflex (see sections 8.9 and 8.10 in Chapter 8). Similarly pupillary reflexes to light and to darkness can be elicited in a kitten on first opening its eyes. However the psycho-optical reflexes – fixation and re-fixation, version, vergence and fusion reflexes – are learned (see section 8.2 in Chapter 8). Hubel and Wiesel (1965) showed that kittens raised in total darkness for the first 3 or 4 months afterwards behaved in light as if they were totally blind. Some aspects of vision are evidently learned by exposure to a normal environment. In a human study comparing different functions associated with parvocellular (**P**) and magnocellular (**M**) visual pathways in children of different ages and in young adults, evidence was found of immaturity in the **P** (high contrast, high spatial frequency) pathway up to age 11 years, but there was no evidence of **M** (high temporal frequency, low spatial frequency) pathway development, the response being the same (mature) in this case at each age (Gordon and McCulloch, 1999).

2.4   Visual maturation and monocular occlusion

Electrophysiological study of visual striate cortical function demonstrates sensitivity to rate of movement, direction of movement and orientation of a line target stimulating the receptive field. The initial neural input to the striate cortex is directed to cells in layer 4, which therefore have a monocular stimulation (see section 10.6 in Chapter 10). From layer 4 the neural stimulation arrives at cells that can combine the input from each eye. At this level, individual striate cortex cells may respond equally to each eye, or more to one than the other.

   This distribution of cortical cell responses can be illustrated by an **ocular dominance diagram** (Fig. 2.2), derived from the activity in ocular dominance columns. These are slabs of cortical cells about one-third of a millimetre wide arranged radially (at 90 degrees) to the cortical surface and containing groups of visual striate cortex neurones. In adult mammals, the neural input comes from the right or the left eye, and each goes alternately to consecutive ocular dominance columns. In the cat, about 80% of striate cortex cells respond to stimuli from either eye. So for cats, most ocular dominance columns have an input from right and left eyes. However, 20% of ocular dominance columns do have a predominant input from one or other eye. The ocular dominance diagram profile of an adult cat is similar to that of a neonate kitten. In cats, the neural pathways for ocular dominance are present soon after birth. It is possible to modify some of these neural connections. If one eye of a kitten is kept closed from birth for 3 months and then opened and the other eye closed, the kitten behaves as if it were blind. When an ocular dominance histogram is made using data from such a kitten, it appears that hardly any cells have binocular input; the striate cortex cells respond mainly to input from the unoccluded eye. In these circumstances, the cells in the lateral geniculate nucleus receiving innervation from the occluded eye are found to be smaller than those relating to the unoccluded eye. In addition, the cortical cell columns receiving input from the deprived

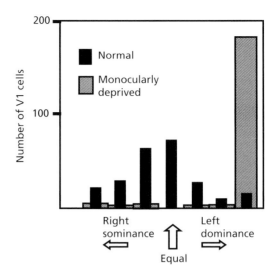

Figure 2.2 Ocular dominance distribution in visual cortex area V1 in normal cats and in monocularly occluded kittens. Modified from data after Hubel and Wiesel (1965).

eye occupy a smaller area than those stimulated by the unoccluded eye (see Chapter 10).

By replacing complete occlusion with the use of a translucent contact lens for one eye, similar results to complete occlusion are found. Thus **detailed visual stimuli** are required for normal binocular development. Deprivation of **form vision** inhibits normal **visual maturation**. The effect of producing surgical exotropia in kittens also produces an ocular dominance histogram showing striate cortex cells that respond to right or left eye stimulation but very few that respond to binocular stimulation. The same result is found in kittens subjected to alternate occlusion of each eye on successive days for an initial 10-week period. When such artificial heterotropia or alternating occlusion is induced after 3 months of age, the ocular dominance histogram is unchanged from the normal. This illustrates the existence of a critical period of development in kittens between 4 weeks and 3 months. In primates such as monkeys, although cortical ocular dominance columns begin developing prenatally, these columns still receive equal stimulation from the right and left eyes for the first 4 weeks. No integration of monocular input is possible, and therefore binocular functions such as stereopsis cannot be elaborated. The formation of independent right and left ocular dominance columns is delayed until 4–6 weeks of age, which is the time at which monkeys first appreciate stereopsis (LeVay *et al.*, 1980). A rule of thumb is that human development occurs in the same number of months since birth as weeks in monkeys. This agrees with the onset of stereopsis at 4 months in humans. During the succeeding sensitive period it is possible to reverse, to some extent, the loss of binocularity induced by visual deprivation. In the case of occlusion, the restoration of visual input to both eyes will improve the proportion of binocularly driven striate cortex cells. The degree to which binocular response is achieved depends on how soon in the sensitive period the normal visual stimulation is restored.

2.5   Children's binocular vision development

Although children are born with the ability to see and to respond to visual stimulation, the prenatal development of visual skills continues after birth. For many aspects of vision, development requires **normal visual experience**. If congenital cataract is left untreated until the child is, say, 3 years old, normal visual acuity (VA) will never be obtained in that eye. Even in a child with normal visual experience, VA reaches adult levels only at around 3–5 years of age. The period in which visual skills are developing is called the critical (or sensitive) period of development. By definition, a **critical period** will begin and end abruptly, and there is a time after which the phenomenon under consideration will no longer occur. A **sensitive period** will begin and end gradually, and have a period of maximum sensitivity. These terms are used in relation to other aspects of physiological development, including educational skills. Both terms are interchangeable to some extent in relation to visual functions, with some functions such as the development of stereopsis having abrupt start and finish points, and others such as VA that have known levels for particular steps in development but a less well-defined point at which maximum acuity can be attained.

In fact, there are different critical/sensitive periods for different visual attributes. Any interruption in visual stimulation during a sensitive period will inhibit visual development. This damaging effect is not uniform throughout the sensitive period. The visuum is most prone to damage midway through the sensitive period of development. The early instability of ocular motor control in neonates tends to limit development. Thus, although there is no obvious misalignment of the eyes in neonates, there is limited coordination of binocular fixation and of eye movements. Therefore, for most visual skills the sensitive period begins at about 4 months after birth, and follows a 'distribution curve' similar to a (tilted) normal distribution curve, with a peak at 2 years old (Nelson, 1988a). This generalised sensitive period is well under way at 4 years but then gradually declines and is largely over by 9 years of age. This is also the time frame over which anomalies of binocularity, such as amblyopia and strabismus, also appear, again with a peak at around 2 years old. For humans it is said that the sensitive period is never completely over. An old person who suffers a cerebral vascular accident and loses visual skills as a result may still regain some lost capacity afterwards. A previously visually uncorrected adult with bilateral amblyopia associated with congenital astigmatism may well regain some, although not usually all, visual acuity after a year or two of full refractive correction. Different visual skills have critical/sensitive periods starting at different times and lasting for varying periods of time (Table 2.1) (Harwerth *et al.*, 1986). Research continues to confirm the extent of these periods and to

Table 2.1 Human visual development and critical/sensitive periods

Attribute	Development
Pupil reflexes	At 30 weeks post-conception (direct and consensual)
Peiper's reflex	At 30 weeks post-conception (head jerk to bright light)
Visual attention	At birth (general motor inhibition to visual stimulus)
Blinking reflex to light	At birth (even in sleep)
Visual acuity (by VEP)	1 cpd at birth; 6–20 cpd (6/6) at 6 months
Visual acuity (by PL)	6/240 at birth, 6/6 at 3 years
Contrast sensitivity (VEP)	Between 1 and 7 months
Contrast sensitivity (PL)	Between 1 month and 14 years
Sensory fusion	Between 3.5 and 6 months
Stereopsis	Between 3 and 6 months
Motion perception	Between 2 and 3 months
Colour perception	Trichromat at 3 months
OKN	Between birth and 5 months
Accommodation	Between 1 and 7 months
Fusional vergence	Between 1 and 6 months
Accommodative vergence	Between 2 and 7 months
Saccades	Between 1 and 5 months
Smooth pursuit	Only saccadic at 1 month; full function at 6 months

cpd, cycles per degree; OKN, optokinetic nystagmus; PL, preferential looking test; VEP, visually evoked potential.

establish the variation in sensitivity related to any interruption of visual experience during development.

Visual acuity

Visual acuity in infants is most conveniently assessed by a forced-choice preferential looking (PL) test. The infant is presented with a Teller, Keeler or Cardiff PL card, and the observer determines whether the visual target is fixated or not. Using PL, at birth VA is approximately 6/300 and improves to 6/9 to 6/6 at 3 years (Fig. 2.3). Alternatively, visually evoked potential (VEP) techniques may be used, usually in a secondary care environment (Norcia and Tyler, 1985). At 3 years the normal child shows some degree of the 'crowding phenomenon', whereby a worse acuity is found using optotypes presented linearly or with adjacent distractors than for single optotypes. Single (angular) and linear (morphoscopic) acuities may take up to the age of 10 years to equalise. Even so, in the normal child the VA will be the same for each eye, whether measured with linear or single optotypes. In unilateral amblyopia there will be a greater crowding phenomenon in the eye with the worse acuity, and this is the reason why it is essential to measure VA in children using a row of letters or symbols rather than single optotype acuity tests. Binocular acuity is slightly better than monocular acuity, and this binocular summation effect is similar for other visual

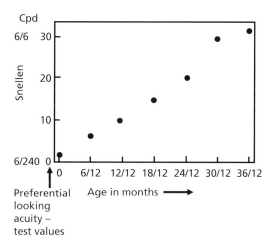

Figure 2.3 Visual acuity (VA) development in the normal child. Monocular VA from birth to 3 years old in the normal child measured using preferential looking acuity cards. The acuity is expressed in cycles per degree (cpd) and in the Snellen acuity equivalent.

attributes; see section 3.1. Visual acuity is the measurement of spatial resolution with maximal black-and-white contrast.

Contrast sensitivity

Contrast sensitivity (CS) allows the assessment of visual performance over a range of spatial frequencies, unlike VA. It is assessed by recognition of gratings; square-wave or sinusoidal, presenting varied grey on white contrasts. The bars vary in size, contrast and frequency (the number of cycles subtending one degree at the eye). Six cycles per degree involves six pairs of alternating dark and light bars, totalling one degree at the eye. For adults, best sensitivity is found at four cycles per degree, the grating being detected at 1% contrast difference between the bars. For lower and higher spatial frequencies, increased contrast is needed to detect the grating pattern. For neonates, using PL and VEP techniques, CS is undeveloped but rapidly improves by 3 months old, although with better performance in lower spatial frequencies (Atkinson *et al.*, 1977). By 7 months of age, adult-like values are found when investigated by VEP methods (Tokoro and Suzuki, 1968). Using PL psychophysical methods, adult levels are not reached until 9–14 years old (Benedek *et al.*, 2003). In adults, binocularly measured CS gives a better response than for monocular CS. This difference has not been demonstrated in normal children except at 12 months of age. Where binocular CS is definitely lower than monocular CS in children (or adults), there is likely to be significant amblyopia present. Between 3 and 5 months old a lowered CS, especially at 2.5 cycles per degree, is a risk factor for poor stereopsis.

Accommodation and convergence

The visual environment of the young child is largely situated close to the child, and binocular vision develops as accommodation and convergence become operational. **Accommodation** depends on the detection of changes in the clarity of objects. For larger targets resolvable by the poor acuity of 2- to 3-month-old infants, the accommodative performance is similar to that of adults (Braddick *et al.*, 1979). As VA rapidly develops over the first few months and the ciliary muscles become more effective, accommodative response improves even to smaller detail, and for emmetropes by 7 months it is as accurate as convergence. Hypermetropes and myopes are less accurate in accommodative response. **Vergence eye movements** are stimulated both by binocular disparity and diplopia (fusional stimuli), and by defocusing blur (accommodative stimuli). Accommodative convergence is not present at birth but develops from 1 month old (Aslin and Jackson, 1979). Between 2 and 6 months fusional convergence rapidly develops. In addition to accommodation and convergence, the child's binocular vision system has to detect **relative depth** – whether to increase or decrease convergence in order to fixate a target.

Refractive errors

Refractive errors can influence binocular vision. Ametropia at birth is +2.00 dioptres (D) (standard deviation 2 dioptres). This increases up to the age of 6 months old, and then a process of emmetropisation rapidly reduces ametropia, eventually to +0.50 DS by 6 years old. Emmetropisation is in part derived from the normal control of growth, so that as the eye enlarges the refracting surfaces become less curved and so reduce the initial hypermetropia. This is a genetically linked process. There is also evidence for a second process of emmetropisation requiring active response to visual stimuli. Here the growth of the eye is modulated to reduce refractive error (Norton and Siegwart, 1995). It is important to realise that most of the emmetropisation occurs in the first 12 months, and the higher the refractive error, the quicker the corrective process; and so the question of whether to risk reducing emmetropisation by correcting a refractive error is largely academic (Saunders *et al.*, 1995). In fact, about 75% of children show completion of emmetropisation by 12 months old. This does not happen in children with strabismus. Significant ametropia after the age of 1 year will not reduce much more, but the likelihood of amblyopia and strabismus is reduced by correcting +3.50 DS or more of hypermetropia, a more important consideration. Astigmatism is more frequently found in infants than in children over 3.5 years old. It is at that age that the earlier against-the-rule astigmatism starts to change to with-the-rule astigmatism. The mean value of 1.00 DC at birth reduces to 0.75 DC by 1 year old, and is similar to adult levels by 6 years. The average anisometropia of 0.60 DS at birth drops to 0.10 DS at 12 months old. Anisometropia of 1 D or more combined with hypermetropia of 2–3 D increases the relative risk of heterotropia compared with those individuals without anisometropia (Donahue, 2005).

Binocular oculomotor coordination

Vision is likely to be degraded by **head movements,** such as those associated with walking or other body movements. In the absence of compensatory eye movements, the retinal images would be constantly blurred. To stabilise the head there are four innate contributors: the cervico-collic reflex, which uses neck muscle proprioceptors to stabilise the head in relation to the trunk; the vestibulo-collic reflex, which stimulates neck muscles from the vestibular sense of movement; the willed control of neck muscles; and inertial forces of the head itself. The cervico-ocular reflex can initiate eye movements to reduce the effect of head movements on visual fixation but is normally secondary to the vestibular system in this regard. **Eye movements** are controlled by vestibulo-ocular reflexes, by the smooth pursuit system and by the saccadic and vergence ocular motor systems to allow central fixation of the object of regard. The fixation system then stabilises gaze. The fixation reflex, directing foveal attention to fresh peripheral stimuli, contributes to this. Thus infants are able to maintain fixation on a suitably interesting target, to follow it and to respond to peripheral stimuli. Associated eye and head movements are discussed in section 8.9, Chapter 8.

Saccadic system development

Adults changing fixation from a central to a peripheral target use a single binocular saccadic eye movement to fixate the peripheral target to within 10% of its position. This is followed, if necessary, by a smaller saccade to achieve fixation. However, infants achieve the change in fixation by using a series of small equal saccades until 5 months old, when an adult-like response is found (Atkinson, 1984). The first saccade is in the correct direction, but of inadequate amplitude, and it takes longer to initiate than for an adult. Horizontal saccades precede vertical saccades, which are not possible until about 5 or 6 weeks of age. Voluntary saccades may be initiated as a response to extra-foveal images, memory and sounds – or in adults to a scanning strategy, such as that taught to aviators and others who 'look out'.

Smooth pursuit system development

For adults the smooth pursuit system allows the fovea to maintain fixation on a moving target, e.g. the flight of a bird, which saccadic eye movements would not allow. In infants up to 4 weeks old this eye movement can, in general, only be approximated by a series of saccades (Phillips *et al.*, 1997). It has been shown that for targets subtending 12 degrees or more, and moving with slow velocity, neonates can produce smooth eye movements (Fox *et al.*, 1980). However, from 4 weeks old, smooth pursuit is possible with smaller targets but only up to 15 degrees per second. There is a rapid improvement in performance thereafter, but high levels such as 100 degrees per second arrive only in early adulthood, and then decrease by about 1%

a year until age 75 (Simons and Büttner, 1985; Kerber *et al.*, 2006). The smooth pursuit system also permits steady fixation on a non-central target towards, and past which, a subject is moving.

Note: an array of peripheral images surrounding a fixation target would still move on the retina as the subject moved towards the target. This binocular **optic flow** (synonym: visual flow) helps recognition of the subject's movement in relation to the three-dimensional environment. Optic flow actually generates the smooth pursuit movement in relation to a target moving past the subject, and suppresses other eye movements such as optokinetic response to head movements.

The development of optokinetic nystagmus

When an object triggering a smooth pursuit eye movement passes out of the binocular visual field, a rapid saccadic recovery eye movement is made to return the eyes to the primary position of gaze: the position of gaze when the fixation target is level with the eyes and on the medial plane (Erasmus Darwin, 1796; cited in Cohen, 1984). This combination of a slow smooth pursuit movement and a fast saccadic movement is called optokinetic nystagmus (OKN) and may be rapidly repeated, e.g. when watching a railway train pass an observer. Optokinetic nystagmus operates for horizontal, oblique and vertical movements of the visual target and also to allow for following-head movements (see section 8.10 in Chapter 8). Optokinetic nystagmus is seen a few hours after birth in infants. However, under monocular conditions up until 5 months old, the recovery OKN saccades occur more rapidly following a smooth pursuit movement in the temporal to nasal direction than for temporalward target movements. This is known as **naso-temporal OKN asymmetry**, or pursuit asymmetry. Up to 2 months old recovery OKN saccades for temporal target movements cannot be elicited at all. To investigate this, the targets used are vertical black-and-white stripes. By 5 months, both nasal and temporal symmetry is possible. Under binocular conditions there may be temporalward target movement for one eye and nasalward for the other, which would mask the immature monocular response.

The vestibulo-ocular reflex

The introduction of a new target into the peripheral field stimulates saccadic eye movements to allow foveal fixation. The head also moves towards the target. Generally for any change of fixation, half the movement is made by the head and half by the eyes. The head movement is detected by the semicircular canals of the vestibular system. This initiates a reflex rotation of the eyes in the opposite direction to the head movement in order to stabilise fixation on the target. The visual system coordinates the head and eye movements (see section 8.9 in Chapter 8). This vestibulo-ocular reflex is present from birth.

Vergence and fixation disparity development

The **vergence** control systems of 2- and 3-month-old infants for targets approaching from 50 to 15 cm can produce only intermittent binocular fixation. After 3 months the motor vergence reflex (fusional vergence) becomes established (Aslin, 1977). Similarly, the expected vergence response to a prism placed base-out in front of one eye is not regularly found until 4–6 months of age (Grounds, 1996). This is because Panum's areas (see section 4.12 in Chapter 4) are larger in young infants, and so a response to diplopia is less likely to occur.

Fixation disparity detection (see section 4.7 in Chapter 4) has been assessed in infants using a random dot stereogram in which a dynamic stereoscopic contour is present (Fox and Check, 1966). The random dot contour is made to move from side to side, the eyes being seen to follow the contour. As the random dot target has global stereopsis, there are no monocular clues, and therefore the (binocular) fixation disparity system must be operating. No response was obtained before 3 months, but by 3.5 months a disparity of 50–100 minutes stimulated a following-eye movement.

Fusion, binocular disparity detection and stereoscopic acuity

Fusion and stereopsis (i.e. binocular disparity detection) develop at the same time (Birch *et al.*, 1985). Fusion is the combination into one binocular image of the similar but not necessarily identical monocular images from each eye. Stereopsis is the same but with the addition of a three-dimensional percept. Binocular disparity detection development has been assessed using VEP measurement, by behavioural response to random dot stereograms, and also by eye movement analysis. These methods indicate that stereopsis develops from 2 months onwards. Stereopsis for crossed disparities appears at 12 weeks and for uncrossed disparities at 17 weeks (Held *et al.*, 1980). There is a rapid improvement in stereopsis from 2 to 6 months of age. Using VEP techniques, adult levels of stereopsis at 60 seconds of arc are then possible. However, by testing with behavioural methods, the development of stereopsis appears to take place over a longer time frame. Using clinical tests such as the Lang, modified Frisby and random-dot E stereotests, it may be as late as 3 years of age or older before values around 60 seconds of arc disparity are possible. This is the normal adult global stereopsis found on clinical testing. The size of the dots used in a random dot global stereopsis test limits measurement of small amounts of disparity to the width of one dot. Under experimental conditions, levels of about 2–6 arc seconds are possible for local stereopsis, using line stereograms. With one group of children with infantile esotropia, and one group with accommodative esotropia, Fawcett *et al.* (2005) showed that the sensitivity period for stereopsis begins at 2.4 months of age and peaks at 4.3 months for infantile esotropia. For accommodative esotropia, the sensitive period begins at 10.8 months and peaks at 20 months. By combining the two groups, it was possible to say that the end of the sensitive period for stereopsis for most children is 4.6 years. This does not mean that a later loss of binocular fixation cannot have an adverse effect. Children readily suppress the fovea when fusion is lost, with loss of fine stereopsis up to adulthood.

Dynamic stereopsis and stereo-motion perception

Dynamic stereopsis, or dynamic stereoacuity, is the ability to recognise the position in depth of a moving target, relative to another target. It develops in children naturally but can be improved by training. It is useful for participants in those sports involving rapidly moving targets. Dynamic stereopsis is less sensitive than static stereopsis. It is degraded by depth oscillations of less than one cycle per second.

Stereo-motion perception or motion-in-depth is the perception of change in depth of the position of a target (see section 10.11 in Chapter 10). It is more developed for looming movements towards the subject than for withdrawing movements (possibly for survival reasons!). The recognition of the stereoscopic depth of a laterally moving target achieves a higher threshold than for looming or withdrawing target movement.

Both static stereopsis and motion-in-depth (dynamic stereopsis) are elaborated soon after the presence of stereopsis occurs in neonate primates. There is evidence in the monkey that cells in the colliculus have a different response to retinal image displacement caused by eye movement and retinal image displacement caused by a moving target on a static eye (Robinson, 1972). Cerebral cortical neurones are also present, which identify the direction of object movement from the monocular input of each eye. They also show some binocular sensitivity for the approximate trajectory of motion of objects, and a definite indication of whether an object is moving to the right or to the left (Poggio and Talbot, 1981). This work, on rhesus monkeys, showed that about 50% of foveal-cortical cells had this property, and about 3% of the cells distinguished the fact that the retinal images were moving in the opposite direction in the two eyes. These cells therefore would have a maximum response when the monkey and its object of regard were moving directly towards or away from each other, although the cells could not detect the actual depth or stereopsis of the target. Dynamic stereopsis would also involve visual memory of successive static stereopsis evaluations.

Detection of motion

Neonates show little sensitivity to target motion. At 8 weeks old VEP testing shows a response to slow moving objects, and this rapidly improves to show responses to targets moving three to four times faster by 13 weeks.

The dominant eye

Most people have a dominant hand, foot and eye; two-thirds of the population has the right side for each of these. The clinical perception is that it is useful to know which eye is dominant. There are a variety of methods of assessing eye dominance. An objective method is to determine which eye retains fixation as the near point of convergence is reached. Subjectively the subject can use both forefingers to point to a distant target, with both eyes open. Each eye is then closed in turn, and the eye of which the line of sight/ visual axis is nearest in alignment is the dominant eye. The dominant eye is used for sighting when only one eye can be used, as in sports such as darts, archery or shooting. The cyclopean eye position is usually deviated from the midline towards the dominant eye. The dominant eye may have better visual acuity. A defocus of the dominant eye will be more apparent to the subject than in the non-dominant eye. This may be useful where it is clinically necessary to correct one eye preferentially for near vision; the prescriber usually chooses the non-dominant eye. It is possible not to have a dominant eye, and also for the eye and hand dominance to be crossed.

2.6   Hazards to binocular vision development

The development of normal binocular vision may be delayed or prevented by anatomical anomalies, sensory and neurophysiological anomalies or cortical adaptations to both of these.

- Anatomical anomalies include ametropia, and defects of the fusional system secondary to extra-ocular muscle, check ligament and pulley system defects, and neural hypoplasia, mis-direction and nerve nuclei anomalies. Congenital or acquired craniofacial problems can also affect motor aspects of binocular vision.
- Sensory and neurophysiological anomalies include congenital or acquired defects of the vestibulo-ocular reflex, retina, optic nerve, media opacities and ptosis.
- Cortical binocular vision adaptations include facultative and obligatory binocular suppression, amblyopia and loss of monocular central fixation (eccentric fixation), adaptations to heterophoria such as decompensation and foveal suppression, and adaptations to heterotropia such as more wider suppression and anomalous retinal correspondence.

The clinical spectrum of binocular vision anomalies includes: poor fusional control resulting in convergence excess or convergence insufficiency, divergence excess or divergence weakness; individual muscle under-actions resulting in diplopia in certain directions of gaze; loss of fusion causing heterotropia (strabismus) in all directions of gaze, initially with pathological diplopia and confusion; binocular rivalry; and then pathological binocular suppression, and anomalous correspondence. The incidence of individual binocular vision anomalies varies widely (Stidwill, 1997). Normal binocular vision may be compromised by a combination of factors. A common combination is the presence of congenital hypermetropic anisometropia, resulting in the development of anisometropic amblyopia and esophoria, followed in 1 or 2 years by an accommodative esotropia.

Fusion and its less attractive alternatives are discussed in Chapters 4 and 5. The investigation of motor and sensory status in binocular vision is summarised in Chapter 12. The management of obstacles to normal binocular vision is covered elsewhere: in clinical texts on binocular vision anomalies.

2.7   Summary: the development of depth perception

It has been shown that infants of 8 weeks old react to an oncoming (looming) target by blinking or attempting to avoid the target (Steinman *et al.*, 2000). It may be that this happens because of the increasing size of the retinal image rather than accommodation or convergence, and fixation disparity is not present at this age. Another technique for assessing depth perception in the first year of life is to use a visual cliff (Gibson and Walk, 1960). A table with a chequered pattern is covered with a glass or transparent plastic surface. The surface extends beyond the table over a floor, also covered with a similar pattern. The child's heart rate is measured when they are placed over the table and at the edge of the table. After 6–8 weeks of age, the heart rate increases when the child is placed at the edge of the apparent 'cliff'. So depth perception is now beginning. It is clear that normal retinal correspondence (see section 4.5 in Chapter 4) is developed before birth, but the motor control of conjugate eye movements is limited, and vergence is hardly present until about 4 months, after which binocular disparity detection and stereopsis then develop. It is at this age that the cortical pathways for binocular integration appear: ocular dominance columns and binocularly driven cortical cells. To recognise fine stereopsis, the cortical cells for binocular disparity detection gradually improve their discrimination over the succeeding months.

Chapter 2: Revision quiz

Complete the missing words, perhaps in pencil. It would be useful to look back at the text and then try all these questions again.

Most reptiles and birds have f_____ (1) decussation, whereas in primates the proportion of optic nerve fibres that decussate is about _____ (2) per cent. In primates the visual information from both eyes is received together in the s_____ (3) cortex. This information is taken to binocular cells in the o_____ d_____ (4) columns. The columns may receive predominant input from _____ (5) eye, or else equally from both. Visual skills such as acuity, contrast sensitivity, accommodation and convergence have a stage in their development called the s_____ p_____ (6). Before the sensitive period, development proceeds by genetic control rather than response to the e_____ (7).

Other physiological attributes of vision such as the vestibulo-ocular reflex are not acquired but are i_____ (8).

Answers
(1) full; (2) 50; (3) striate; (4) ocular dominance; (5) either; (6) sensitive period; (7) environment; (8) innate.

Chapter 3
BINOCULAR SUMMATION

Summation is a feature of all neuronal transmission. It is a way of enhancing the transmission of impulses (or of inhibiting them). Temporal summation occurs when a single presynaptic neurone increases the frequency of impulses so that consecutive rises in potential then algebraically combine, i.e. summate. The resulting combined potential is then large enough to reach a threshold that generates an action potential in the postsynaptic neurone. The chances of success are greater the longer the stimulus lasts. Spatial summation achieves the generation of a postsynaptic action potential by the summation of impulses from multiple sources. In the case of the eye, for retinal areas under 15 minutes of arc an action potential may be achieved spatially by either increasing the number of rods sending impulses, or by increasing the activity of a smaller number of rods. Bipolar and then ganglion cells in the retina collect (summate) the stimuli from the rods.

3.1 Binocular summation models

To understand the way in which visual information from each eye is integrated into a single percept, it is appropriate to consider the effects of a variety of visual tasks presented to each eye. These include assessment of visual acuity (VA) (spatial summation), luminance detection, the averaging of binocular brightness input and critical flicker fusion frequency (CFF). In 1904 Sherrington, following his earlier studies on spinal nerve impulse summation, first described the integration or interaction of the perceptions of the two eyes as 'visual summation' (Sherrington, 1904). This is now called binocular summation.

Adding visual information from each eye (at the threshold level, of just being detected), the combined result may be:

- **no summation** – equal to the monocular performance (Fig. 3.1)
- **complete summation** – twice the monocular performance
- **facilitation** – more than twice the monocular performance
- **partially facilitated summation** – 1.5 times the monocular performance, for example
- **inhibition** – less than the monocular performance.

Normal Binocular Vision: theory, investigation and practical aspects. By David Stidwill and Robert Fletcher. © 2011 Blackwell Publishing Ltd

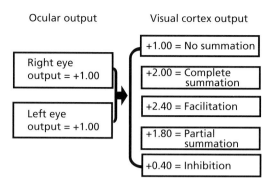

Ocular output   Visual cortex output

Figure 3.1 Binocular summation at threshold visual levels. The possible interactions of the right and left eyes' output when processed by the visual cortex are illustrated. The units are used merely to illustrate the possible additive and subtractive outcomes that could happen as a result of cortical visual processing (after Steinman *et al.*, 2000).

Visual acuity shows partially facilitated summation. Binocular acuity is slightly better than monocular acuity, e.g. right eye acuity 6/6, left eye acuity 6/6, but binocular acuity 6/5, an improvement from one minute of arc to 0.75 minutes in resolution (Horowitz, 1949). Spatial contrast sensitivity is 40% better in binocular than in monocular conditions, over a wide range of frequencies (Kintz, 1969). Thus summation enhances the perception of faint objects. It is also a characteristic of the visuum that the higher the level of stimulus intensity (luminance), the more rapid the response (perception of brightness) becomes (Le-Grand, 1968). The reaction time for a binocular stimulus is significantly briefer than for monocular stimuli (Gilliland and Hames, 1975). This confirms that binocular summation is operating during binocular vision.

The classical experiment in 1904 on summation was an investigation of CFF. Critical fusion flicker frequency is defined as the frequency when a flickering light seems to become continuous. With gradually increasing frequency, the CFF occurs at 50 Hertz (Crozier and Wolf, 1941). In 1904 Sherrington found that (square-wave) simultaneous flicker stimulating each eye produced a (slightly) greater binocular sensitivity to flicker than monocular performance (Sherrington, 1904). Sherrington's figures gave about 3% higher CFF for simultaneous (in-phase) flicker than for alternating right and left eye (out-of-phase) flicker. Summation was occurring for in-phase flicker (Fig. 3.2). If the flicker was alternated between the eyes, binocular sensitivity was less than monocular: that is, inhibition was operating. Inhibition is more likely to occur at the supra-threshold levels of luminance that Sherrington was using. More recent work has confirmed Sherrington's findings with summation, although with a greater difference between in-phase and out-of-phase stimuli; in-phase flicker typically has between 4.5% and 10% higher CFF than for out-of-phase flicker. The increased CFF is higher than calculated by probability summation and is therefore occurring because of neural summation in striate cortex binocular cells (see section 10.6).

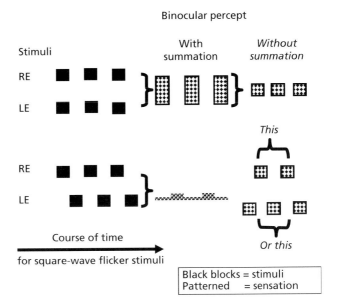

Figure 3.2 Binocular summation at threshold levels (square-wave stimuli at the critical frequency of fusion, CFF) based on Sherrington's experiment. Adapted from Steinman *et al.*, (2000). The in-phase and out-of-phase experimental results followed predictions about summation. The amounts of each stimulus or response are shown by the height of the appropriate blocks. In the upper diagram, where the right and left eyes are each presented with lights flickering at the same time, binocular summation would result in a more sensitive detection of flicker, and this is what happens. Absence of summation would produce a response equal to the monocular level as shown; this does not happen. In the lower diagram, where the stimuli for each eye are alternated, summation would produce a reduced sensitivity to flicker, and the CFF lower than the monocular level. Sir Charles Sherrington found a 3% lower CFF value, demonstrating for the first time that binocular summation does occur. LE, left eye; RE, right eye.

In 1979, Cavonius measured temporal contrast sensitivity at increasing frequencies using sine-wave flicker, i.e. gradually increasing and decreasing brightness levels (Cavonius, 1979). He showed that summation increased at low and medium temporal frequencies of stimulation (Fig. 3.3). There was less summation at high frequency (supra-threshold) levels, as in Sherrington's CFF experiment. The mechanism of binocular summation depends on three possible modalities: 'probability summation', 'neural summation' and 'signal to noise ratio'; possibly also differences between binocular and monocular status such as fixation, pupil sizes, accommodation levels or binocular rivalry for supra-threshold stimuli. **Probability binocular summation** occurs because the chance of two eyes detecting a visual stimulus is statistically greater than for one eye, even in the absence of cortical integration of the stimuli, e.g. in the case of binocular diplopia. Comparing the detection probability of seeing a low luminance stimulus under monocular and binocular conditions, it has been found that binocular conditions do give an improved (1.4 times) threshold (Pirenne, 1943). **Neural binocular summation** occurs when the

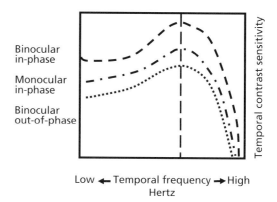

Figure 3.3 Binocular summation at threshold levels (sine-wave flicker over a range of temporal frequencies), after Cavonius (1979). Increased binocular summation effects at low and medium frequencies, typically 1.5 compared with monocular performance. High frequencies show only partial flicker summation, typically 1.1 compared with monocular performance, which is why Sherrington found only a slight difference. There is complete summation for mid-range temporal frequencies, and facilitation at low frequencies. If there were no summation, there would be no difference between in-phase and out-of-phase flicker.

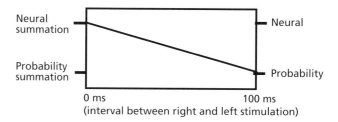

Figure 3.4 Neural and probability summation at threshold levels.

two neural pathways stimulate a single cortical binocular neurone. This was first demonstrated by comparing the absolute light detection threshold in both binocular and monocular vision (Matin, 1962). Light was presented initially to both eyes simultaneously, and then the stimulus to one eye was gradually delayed by up to 100 milliseconds (Fig. 3.4). A much greater sensitivity binocularly than monocularly was obtained with simultaneous presentation, but as the time delay was increased to 100 ms, the improved binocular performance declined to the level explained by statistical probability only.

The third possible explanation of binocular summation is the effect of background **neural 'noise'**. Neural noise from each eye would differ and fail to be summated, whereas visual signals would be similar for each eye and would result in summation (Campbell and Green, 1965). This increase in **signal-to-noise** ratio would improve the binocular threshold by the square root of 2 (roughly 1.4) compared with the monocular threshold. This means that an increase in the binocular visual threshold of up to that amount could be explained by neural summation, probability summation or the signal-to-noise ratio effect. Matin's work showing a still higher binocular threshold could realistically be explained only by neural summation. Similar stimuli location, shapes, and sizes would enhance binocular summation. These would potentiate fusion/summation rather than binocular rivalry.

To achieve neural binocular summation, it is important to equally stimulate corresponding retinal points synchronously (Westendorf and Fox, 1977). One or both of these two important requirements is lost in clinical anomalies such as unequal amounts of cataract in each eye, or in unilateral amblyopia, demyelinating disease, uncorrected anisometropia, decompensated (synonym: uncompensated) heterophoria and heterotropia. Here there may be absence of summation, or inhibition, i.e. binocular suppression (see sections 5.5 and 10.7 in chapters 5 and 10, respectively). In individuals without stereopsis (i.e. the stereoblind), binocular summation is equivalent to that expected by probability summation only: sensory binocular fusion is discussed in Chapter 4, and stereopsis in Chapter 11. In fact, the descent over time, say in a schoolchild with uncorrected anisometropic hypermetropia, from compensated to decompensated heterophoria can be plotted as a gradual reduction in stereopsis. This may then be accompanied by a reduction in VA. Such a situation would suggest investigation of accommodative convergence to accommodation ratio, the extent of fusional reserves and of ametropia, and the correction of any anomalies in these parameters. It follows that stereopsis and other assessments of binocular summation are important clinically in the routine visual assessment of preschool children. Conversely, it has been shown that closing one eye, and so preventing summation, reduces disability glare. In monocular conditions, if the area of retina stimulated is doubled, the detection threshold is lowered. There is no evidence that doubling the area by using binocular instead of monocular stimulation affects the threshold. So areal summation does not affect binocular summation (Reading, 1983).

3.2 Binocular brightness averaging, and bias towards the dominant eye

In section 3.1 the assessment of binocular visual function was related to level of detection, i.e. the threshold for perception. For stimuli of markedly higher luminance than that level, there is some degree of response saturation. Where stronger visual stimuli are used, i.e. supra-threshold stimuli, neural summation still occurs, but the binocular perception is not brighter than each monocular view; it is an average (Levelt, 1965). This averaging effect is seen in **Fechner's paradox**. Here initially one eye only views a light source. The other eye then looks through a neutral density filter, which reduces the level of light transmission. The combined visual percept is of a reduction in the light level. So an averaging has occurred, although the total amount of light must be greater with two eyes than with one eye (Levelt, 1965). This is termed **binocular brightness averaging** (Fig. 3.5). For other

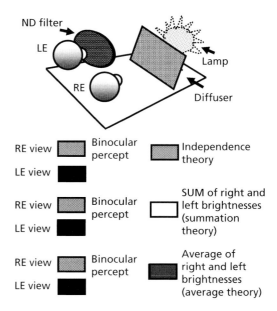

Figure 3.5 Binocular brightness averaging at supra-threshold levels (i.e. easily seen stimuli). When a neutral density filter reduces the brightness of the image reaching one eye – here the left eye – the possible effect on binocular perception is predicted in different ways by the three theories. The independence theory assumes that each eye acts on its own. The binocular percept would be the same as the brighter image in the right eye. The summation theory proposes an additive effect to produce a binocular percept brighter than in either eye separately. The **actual percept**, as the averaging theory proposes, has the binocular percept as an average of the right and left eyes. LE, left eye; ND, neutral density; RE, right eye.

visual attributes with stimulation above threshold level, there are also advantages in binocular vision; the recognition of square-wave stimuli is faster binocularly than monocularly (Harwerth *et al.*, 1980). However, Corcoran and Roth (1983) have shown that binocular brightness averaging is biased towards the brightness perception of the dominant eye. This is analogous to the shift of the position of the cyclopean eye towards the dominant eye. The same effect occurs in other visual attributes: there is evidence that more striate cortical cells are controlled by the dominant eye (Roumbouts *et al.*, 1996). In addition it has been shown that adaptation will occur in response to interocular brightness differences caused experimentally by unequally dense neutral-density filters placed before each eye. This adaptation can be predicted by Fechner's paradox (MacMillan *et al.*, 2007).

3.3 Fatigue-induced visual adaptations

There is a physiological tendency for neural responses from external stimuli to suffer **adaptation**. A finger will not feel the ring worn habitually on it, but the ring will be felt when placed on a different finger. This happens also with visual stimuli and explains why children are often better observers than adults. They observe with first impressions, rather than with a cortically edited perception. It also explains why new entoptic phenomena such as vitreous 'floaters' become less noticeable after a while. In particular, the binocular summation of **motion, spatial frequency** (= size) and **orientation** (= tilt) can be subject to fatigue-induced changes, which tend to diminish or modify the initial visual percept.

3.4 Visual masking

The perception of a visual **test stimulus** can be diminished by an interfering or **masking stimulus**. This may be presented before, with or after the test stimulus (Sengpiel and Blakemore, 1994). A monocular example is the **crowding effect**: the reduced VA associated with a row of test symbols compared with a single symbol. This is seen in preschool children. In normal children, the crowding effect is the same in each eye, but in amblyopia the crowding effect is more marked in the affected eye. For example, in amblyopia the monocular single letter acuities might be (*Snellen* visual acuity nomenclature) R 6/6 and L 6/9, but with a linear test R 6/6 L 6/18. For this reason it is essential to check the VA of children with a **crowding visual acuity test** (Fig. 3.6). Visual acuity tests are available that combine both the more scientific VA measure logMAR and the crowding effect (Elliott and Firth, 2009). Under binocular conditions, **dichoptic visual masking** occurs when the test stimulus is presented to one eye and a masking stimulus to the other eye. This can be demonstrated under experimental conditions; the participant is asked to respond to a brief test light, presented to one eye, which can be set at a range of luminance levels. The test presentation is preceded and/or followed by a longer exposure of a bright masking light source, which is presented to the other eye. The test light has then to be made brighter before it is perceived: suppression for the lower illuminance level of test light has been produced. Where the subject already has pathological binocular suppression, the masking effect can markedly increase the perception threshold, by about one logarithmic unit. An example seen under clinical conditions is the binocular sensory suppression test on the near Mallett unit, where some letters are presented binocularly and some to each eye separately. The Mallett distance and near units also have fixation disparity tests: in addition to the central binocular lock seen by both eyes, these tests depend upon delivering different images to each eye, a nonius line presented to one eye, and an unilluminated blank area to the corresponding

abcdefghijklmn   *abcdefghijklmn*

Figure 3.6 One type of visual masking. The bars above and below the text reduce the ability to identify letters. There is a 'crowding effect' due to the presence of adjacent contours.

retinal point of the other eye (as shown in Fig. 4.4 in Chapter 4). Ideally the participant reports the individual nonius line seen by each eye separately, and also the binocular lock seen by both eyes together. However, some individuals will see the blank area in preference to one of the nonius lines. This demonstrates pathological binocular suppression, but under far from normal binocular vision conditions; the fixation disparity tests are designed as tests of motor function, not as a binocular sensory test (see section 4.7). The latest near Mallett unit has a third double nonius line sensory test, which subtends a larger angle than the horizontal and vertical fixation disparity tests. This larger test is intended for binocular sensory status assessment in heterotropia.

Summation is a complex area of scientific investigation and has been discussed only briefly here. A discussion of dichoptic visual masking, binocular suppression and summation may be found in Baker and Meese (2007).

3.5 Visual advantages of binocular summation

Flicker perception is enhanced by binocular summation, providing the rate of flicker is the same for each eye. In addition to more sensitive brightness perception, a faster CFF can be detected binocularly than monocularly. If the flicker is out of phase for one eye compared with the other, the binocular CFF is slower than the monocular rate. Flicker at around 12 Hertz produces photic driving, which can produce a seizure. This effect can be diminished by closing one eye; closing both eyes would not work, because the light level although lower would still be summated.

Mesopic vision is enhanced by binocular summation. Visual acuity is usually about one VA chart row better with two eyes than with one eye. Indeed, this even happens when one eye has a slightly reduced acuity – the binocular acuity is higher than the VA of the better eye, e.g. R 6/6 L 6/9 but with both eyes together 6/5. Contrast sensitivity (CS) is also improved binocularly, and diminished by reducing the light level for one eye, or defocusing one eye significantly, say by 1.50 to 2.00 dioptres, depending on the pupil size.

3.6 Binocular summation ratio

In addition to stereopsis testing, a useful measure of binocular function (binocularity) is to compare the CS of the eye with better acuity with the binocular CS. This is the **binocular summation ratio (BSR)**. So:

$$BSR = CS \ (binocular)/CS \ (better \ eye)$$

It has been found that the BSR found in amblyopes can be simulated using a neutral density filter bar (Baker et al., 2007): horizontal sine-wave gratings were used at three or nine cycles per degree at 200 ms. Pardhan and Whittaker (2000) showed that in comparing the fovea to the retinal periphery, the BSR was similar in normal subjects, but reduced foveally in amblyopes.

Chapter 3: Revision quiz

Complete the missing words, perhaps in pencil.

Integration of visual information into a combined percept was called visual s_____ (1) by Sherrington. This would include luminance detection, averaging of binocular brightness and critical flicker fusion frequency, and v_____ a_____ (2). The results of such integration could be inhibition, full or partial facilitation, or a c_____ s_____ (3). When visual functions such as luminance detection (brightness) are integrated at the level of being just perceptible (threshold), a response like partial facilitation can occur. When the visual functions are above threshold for luminance, the binocular perception becomes an _____ (4) of the two monocular inputs. There is a further adaptation that biases the combined brightness perception towards that of the _____ (5) eye. The effect of fatigue will alter the perception of such visual attributes as motion, spatial frequency (size) and or _____ (6). This effect can be seen when a new astigmatic spectacle correction takes a few days to get used to.

Answers
(1) summation; (2) visual acuity; (3) complete summation; (4) average; (5) dominant; (6) orientation (tilt).

Chapter 4

THE BINOCULAR FUSION SYSTEM

4.1   The requirements for the binocular fusion system

The cortical combination of one image from each eye to form a combined single percept is called **binocular fusion**.

The six requirements for the binocular fusion system are as follows.

1.   The ability to move the right and left lines of sight (visual axes) onto the object of regard. This is called **motor fusion**.
2.   The visual cortex must integrate the two images. This is **sensory fusion** and depends upon retinal correspondence.
3.   The visuum must be able to maintain motor fusion by visual feedback if the lines of sight (visual axes) start to drift away from the object of regard. The **vergence** eye movement system uses **fixation disparity** (see section 4.7) to detect and correct misalignment of the lines of sight (visual axes). There must be sufficient **fusional reserves** to allow the vergence system to operate (see section 12.10 in Chapter 12).
4.   The visuum must be able to maintain fusion while fixation disparity errors are corrected, and to adapt to small rotational errors around one visual axis compared with the other, which may occur in oblique direction of gaze. This is achieved by **Panum's fusional area**, which allows sensory fusion within small limits of misalignment (see section 4.12).
5.   The sensory fusion system must be able to recognise the minor differences in the right and left eye images, which can be used to produce **stereopsis**.
6.   The fusion system must be able to **adapt** to major anomalies in both motor alignment and sensory integration with the least possible disturbance to visual perception. Such major anomalies are seen in heterotropia, which is binocular motor misalignment, and in anisometropia, which is binocular sensory incompatibility.

Sections 4.2 to 4.12 explain these requirements in detail.

4.2   Motor binocular fusion

Where motor binocular fusion (or motor fusion) merely involves a **conjugate (saccadic) eye movement**, for example for the eyes to change fixation from the current object of regard to a new object, the local sign of retinal

Normal Binocular Vision: theory, investigation and practical aspects. By David Stidwill and Robert Fletcher. © 2011 Blackwell Publishing Ltd

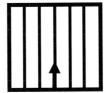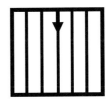

Figure 4.1 Motor fusion: to show fusion error. Try to fuse the two squares either by inhibiting convergence, or by doubling convergence effort (try holding a pen halfway between the eyes and the squares). It is possible to fuse a number of different vertical lines by adjusting the amount of convergence, demonstrated by a varying position of the two arrows.

receptors is used. For example, if a small light is presented to the side of where a baby is looking, the baby changes fixation to look at the light. The image of the light initially falls on a non-foveal retinal receptor and the direction of the new stimulus is calculated by the visuum. The primary line of sight (visual axis) of the eye then rotates through the calculated angle so that the light is now imaged on the fovea. This **fixation reflex** is a strong one, and overrules other stimuli. The same process occurs with the other eye, so that both eyes fixate the new stimulus. Although the fixation reflex is powerful, confusing stimuli may produce a **fusion error** (Fig. 4.1). The neural pathway for the change of fixation goes from the retina to the visual cortex and to the superior colliculus; also to the frontal eye movement fields of the neocortex. These both have layers of neurones, which codify the direction and amplitude of all possible saccadic movements to acquire a change in fixation, organised like a topographical map (see Bruce *et al.*, 1985; Robinson and McClurkin, 1989; Leigh and Zee, 2006). The control pathway is then thought to go via the brainstem reticular formation (in the pons) to initiate the velocity of eye movement required. This pathway also controls the holding force required to maintain the new fixation direction. The pathway then goes to the gaze-aligning centre in the nucleus prepositus hypoglossi. This structure (adjacent to the sixth and eighth nerve nuclei) has neurones that record the position of the eyes and the signals for eye velocity. Finally, the pathway goes to the brainstem nuclei of cranial nerves III, IV and VI for each eye, arranged along the medial longitudinal fasciculus. The horizontal gaze centre is the combined VI abducens nuclei. From there, nerve pathways go to the **extra-ocular muscles**. Abducens motoneurones innervate the ipsilateral lateral rectus muscles. Abducens internuclear motoneurones pass to the contralateral medial longitudinal fasciculus, which projects to the contralateral oculomotor nucleus and to the III nerve motoneurones of the medial rectus muscle. **Note**: the frontal eye fields direct **voluntary horizontal eye movements** via their connections with the contralateral paramedian pontine reticular formation (PPRF), causing movement of the eyes to the opposite side.

Where motor binocular fusion requires a **disconjugate (vergence) eye movement**, there are three elements that control these vergence movements.

1. There is a resting state of tonic vergence upon which other changes are made.
2. Any retinal blur leads to accommodative changes and accommodative vergence movements.
3. Binocular disparity produces a stimulus for vergence movement, whether the disparity is a misalignment that produces a fusible diplopia, or whether it is within the steady-state fixation disparity system, in which diplopia is not evident. Binocular disparity is especially important in a complex visual environment with multiple binocular disparities. Where the visual target is slowly moving towards or away from the subject, a smooth tracking vergence change is made. Where a sudden change is made, as in looking from a distant target to a close object, perhaps to read, a swift vergence movement is made analogous to a saccadic shift. Generally, stimuli within the central five degrees are responsible for disparity-induced vergence change, although peripheral diplopic stimuli can also initiate motor fusion. It should be noted that vergence is also affected by the subject's awareness of target proximity, and of any change in proximity: looming or withdrawal of the target of interest.

4.3   Sensory binocular fusion

Sensory binocular fusion or sensory fusion is the combination of two monocular retinal images into a single perception of visual space. It involves the neurophysiologic integration and psychological recognition of the visual input from each eye. For sensory fusion, ideally the images must be similar in sharpness, luminosity, size and colour, and fall on corresponding unit retinal areas. If the same object is imaged on retinal elements with a different local sign in right and left eyes, **retinal disparity** is produced. A small difference in local sign drives the motor fusion system. A larger difference is seen as two images: **diplopia**. If the diplopic images are close to each other, the motor fusion system attempts to fuse them. Where the difference between the images is not in the local sign, but in the sharpness, luminosity, size or colour, the right and left images may be seen in quick alternation. Alternatively, parts of each eye's image may temporarily dominate the combined perception, thus forming a changing binocular patchwork. This is seen during monocular visual field testing, when the blank view of the eye not being tested may overlap the vision of the eye under test, particularly when the non-dominant eye is being assessed. This fluctuating visual perception is called **binocular rivalry** (see section 5.7 in Chapter 5).

Sensory fusion can occur at different levels of binocular integration. Worth (1903) classified sensory fusion into the following categories.

- First grade: simultaneous macular perception and superimposition. No effort to maintain fusion: diplopia and confusion if strabismus present.

- Second grade: true fusion with some amplitude of motor fusional reserves: binocular perception without stereopsis. The term 'amplitude' was used by Worth to imply adequate fusional reserves to maintain binocular fusion (see section 12.10 in Chapter 12).
- Third grade: sense of perspective (depth perception). Blending of two slightly dissimilar visual impressions, enabling appreciation of solidity of surrounding objects and their relative distances. That is, true fusion with some amplitude of motor fusional reserves and with stereopsis.

However, this classification does not allow for the nearly 5% of the population with strabismic anomalous (retinal) correspondence allowing (anomalous) binocular single vision. To include this outcome, a tentative classification might be:

- no fusion – complete cortical suppression of one eye, or monocular vision, e.g. where there is absence of function in one eye and no need to suppress
- simultaneous vision – both eyes operating but no fusion (diplopia and confusion)
- simultaneous normal binocular single vision – fusion but with no stereopsis present; this could happen in an individual with amblyopia in one eye
- simultaneous anomalous binocular single vision – fusion of images from the right and left eyes, but in the presence of heterotropia (there may be gross stereopsis (3000 seconds of arc) – anomalous retinal correspondence is present to fuse the image from the non-aligned eye)
- normal stereopsis with fusional reserves – the highest level of binocular vision.

It should be realized that classifications are for the purpose of understanding concepts. In reality, most biological attributes are on a continuous spectrum of function, rather than in steps. Also these attributes may fluctuate from time to time. For the following, see Chapter 5: binocular diplopia, binocular confusion, binocular suppression, binocular rivalry and binocular lustre.

4.4   Sensory binocular correspondence

When light enters the eye and stimulates an area of the retina, there is a perception in visual space of a stimulus of a certain colour, shape ('form') and brightness, and with an apparent direction. The stimulus is **localised** in visual space in this apparent direction. The rather inappropriate term 'projection' is sometimes used. The retinal photoreceptors that are stimulated transmit a neural impulse to neurones in the lateral geniculate body, thence to the visual cortex and then to further neurones in the cerebral cortex. The retinal receptors and subsequent local retinal neurones responding to the visual stimulus are known (collectively) as a **retinal element**. Where retinal elements of each eye have the same local sign they share the same **common subjective visual direction**. For most of each retina, every retinal element or 'retinal point' shares a common relative subjective visual direction with an associated retinal point in the other eye. The **law of identical visual directions** states that **a single target that is imaged on right and left eye corresponding retinal points will be localised for each eye in the same apparent monocular direction**. There are some peripheral retinal elements that never actually share a common visual direction because they receive images from objects in the monocular visual field of each eye. Retinal elements of each eye that do have the same common subjective visual directions are called **corresponding retinal points**. For a given retinal element in one eye, all retinal elements in the other eye except the corresponding retinal point are **non-corresponding points**. The objects stimulating corresponding retinal points may themselves be separated in physical space (Plate 4.1). For a discussion on the properties of corresponding retinal points, see Hillis and Banks (2001).

The fact that **corresponding retinal points have common relative subjective visual directions** is called the **law of sensory binocular correspondence**. The orientation of objects relative to each other in visual space is determined by reference to the principal common visual direction of the two foveas. That is, the visual directions of non-foveal corresponding points are at fixed angles relative to the **foveal common visual direction** (see Fig. 1.9 in Chapter 1).

4.5   The development of normal and anomalous retinal correspondence

Where the monocular images for each eye are substantially similar, and fall on corresponding retinal points, they are processed by the visuum simultaneously and integrated into a binocular percept: this is the sensory binocular fusion described above. Together with sensory binocular correspondence, this produces **normal retinal correspondence** (NRC). The fusion process is not itself purely retinal but retino-cortical. As the child's interpupillary distance enlarges with head growth, so the retinal correspondence must adapt to maintain normal depth perception. The fundamental clinical indication that normal retinal correspondence is operating is the presence of good stereopsis. The small differences in binocular disparity that produce stereopsis are still part of normal correspondence.

If there are larger differences between the images for each eye, however, the visual processing swaps from fusion to **pathological binocular diplopia** and **confusion** (see sections 5.2 and 5.3 in Chapter 5). The visual input from each eye to the visual cortex is then said to be rivalrous, and this results in **binocular rivalry** (see section 5.7 in Chapter 5). These differences between the left and right images may arise from anisometropia, or from strabismus, or from both. Strabismic children under the age of 7 (exceptionally up to 15 years old; Stidwill, 1998) can adapt to pathological diplopia and binocular confusion and the accompanying binocular rivalry. This adaptation consists of a series of binocular sensory and motor changes. Initially the central binocular visual field of the deviated eye is totally suppressed. The remaining peripheral binocular rivalry then produces a physiological adaptation called **anomalous retinal correspondence** (**ARC**). The visuum learns to **fuse** the straight-ahead visual scene received by the peripheral retina of the non-deviating eye, with the same scene, imaged on non-corresponding areas of the deviated eye. This is a triumph of cortical adaptation. It may be related to the larger size of Panum's fusional areas in the periphery of the binocular visual field. The ARC appears to develop from the cortical representation of the retinal peripheral binocular field towards the cortical representation of the two foveas. A central binocular suppression area remains, the size of which depends upon the size, and variability, of the heterotropia angle, and the level of visual acuity in each eye. A large angle heterotropia, unsteady angle of deviation or poor visual acuity results in a larger central suppression area. Where those factors are less intrusive, there may remain only:

- a one-degree suppression area at (the cortical representation of) the fovea of the deviated eye
- a one-degree suppression area at (the cortical representation of) the point in the deviated retina, now receiving the image intended for the fovea (Mallett, 1988).

Note: the suppression (area) relates to the visual information from one eye, but it is technically called binocular suppression, as there is no longer a normal binocular cortical percept in this situation.

ARC allows a low grade of (anomalous) simultaneous binocular vision, although without significant global stereopsis. For a small and constant angle strabismus with deep ARC there may be significant local stereopsis. In the child, the newly developed ARC (and the central suppression area/s) gradually becomes almost impossible to reverse, because the sensitive period applies to adaptations as it does to normal visual development. After the sensitive period it is increasingly difficult to change things. The possible mechanisms operating in ARC are discussed in Evans (2007). The motor adaptation consists of a change in the zero motor fusional response, which coordinates the binocular eye movements to maintain binocular fixation on the object of interest. This is, in effect, a modified form of fusional reserves (see section 6.7 in Chapter 6). Version and vergence movements still have to be coordinated, but now with the eyes at a constant misalignment in order to allow the ARC to operate efficiently.

Disambiguation note: the retinal point on a deviated strabismic eye, which receives the straight-ahead image also found on the fovea of the fixating, non-strabismic eye, used to be called the false fovea, and is now sometimes called the zero point. In other words, it is the point that has the same visual direction as the fovea of the non-deviated eye. However, the term 'retino-motor zero point' is best used only in relation to motor aspects of vision – specifically the retinal point in a normal eye that does not induce a fixation reflex eye movement when an image falls upon it (see section 1.3 in Chapter 1). As the 'zero point' of a strabismic eye normally has a central suppression area, it can hardly be involved in fixation. However, the central five degrees of the binocular visual field is sensitive to the anomalous binocular disparity even in ARC, and this anomalous disparity is the signal for the oculomotor saccadic and vergence systems to maintain (anomalous) binocular fusion at the strabismic deviation angle.

Retinal correspondence types

- Following the initial appearance of heterotropia, children can develop ARC, which is strictly termed **harmonious anomalous retinal correspondence** (HARC). HARC develops readily up to the age of 6 years, and occasionally as late as 10 or 15 years. Using a sensitive sensory test for binocular sensory status, such as the Bagolini striated lens test, about 80 to 90% of concomitant heterotropia shows HARC. As discussed above, there is also evidence of a central suppression area or areas.
- Children can also develop total **pathological binocular suppression** up to 10 years, and occasionally later still. This affects the entire binocular field of the affected eye. About 10 to 20% of concomitant heterotropia shows total pathological binocular suppression. It is generally seen in large angle exotropia, or where there is deep amblyopia in the deviated eye. In this case there is said to be **absence of retinal correspondence**.
- Advanced as the adaptation of HARC is, it is confounded when an individual with heterotropia and HARC has surgery to straighten the angle of deviation. Following surgery, the eyes are then straight or approximately so, but the ARC now produces diplopia. The ARC is no longer harmoniously fulfilling the function for which it developed and is now unharmonious: **unharmonious anomalous retinal correspondence** (UARC). This is because the fovea and the surrounding retinal area of the originally fixating eye are not associated with the new area on the deviated eye that is now receiving the straight-ahead image. It is still associated with an area on the deviated eye that was receiving the straight-ahead image until the surgery, but that eye is now rotated. In practice, this problem of post-operative pathological diplopia and confusion is resolved by the rapid replacement of UARC with total suppression of the binocular field of the deviated eye – provided the strabismus surgery is completed by about 6 years of age. The diplopia produced by UARC is suppressed, generally within 24 hours.
- There is evidence for **covariation**, in which a lightly ingrained form of HARC is maintained even when the heterotropia angle varies from day to day (Nelson, 1988b). This could happen with an under-corrected

hypermetropia, in which the amount of accommodation, and therefore the heterotropia angle, could vary with the amount of clarity needed to identify visual targets. The usual situation in heterotropia, however, is for the deviation angle to be constant, with a deeply ingrained anomalous correspondence.

- It is worth noting that the innate NRC, and the adaptations of pathological binocular suppression and of HARC once made are retained in the memory of the visuum. Under exceptional circumstances, such as illness or stress, it is possible for the post-operative pathological binocular suppression to be suspended, and for the innate NRC and the acquired ARC adaptation simultaneously to operate again. If there remains a small heterotropia (it is usual to under-correct the deviation during surgery) then the individual is likely to see double, i.e. binocular diplopia, or possibly even binocular triplopia. The object of regard is imaged on the fovea of the fixating eye, and also on a non-foveal area in the other eye, which has both innate NRC and acquired ARC connections. Luckily, the multiple vision usually resolves within a few hours or days, being replaced by pathological binocular suppression again. That is extremely rare; however, slightly more frequently in adulthood, often with fatigue, a different situation occurs in which the post-operative residual angle of heterotropia may increase, and here the central suppression area is not large enough to remove diplopia at the increased angle of strabismus deviation. Usually the deviation can be restored to its previous angle, often with botulinum toxin therapy.

Motor aspects of retinal correspondence

The difference (under binocular conditions) between the sensory foveal visual direction of the deviated eye in strabismus and the motor angle of deviation is called the angle of anomaly. This sensory angle equals the motor angle of heterotropia in harmonious ARC: the angle of the anomaly is then zero. For strabismus with NRC, the angle of the anomaly is non-zero and is the difference between the objective (motor) angle, as measured by cover test for example, and the subjective (sensory) angle. In this situation, diplopia and confusion would be expected, but may then be avoided by pathological binocular suppression. Where there is a large suppression area the motor angle may vary, with accommodative effort or tiredness, for example. Where HARC is present there is anomalous motor correspondence to maintain a constant deviation angle, in all directions of gaze, and in convergence. The motor adaptation consists of a change in the zero motor fusional response, which coordinates the binocular eye movements to maintain binocular fixation on the object of interest. This is, in effect, a modified form of fusional reserves (see section 6.7 in Chapter 6). Version and vergence movements still have to be coordinated, but now with the eyes at a constant misalignment in order to allow the HARC to operate efficiently.

Retinal correspondence and interocular transfer evidence

Studies of interocular transfer and other electrophysiology techniques show that the **sensitive period for retinal disparity detection** starts at about 4 months of age, reaches a peak of integration at 2 years and gradually declines up to the age of 9 years. So this is the period when the innate NRC is being most actively refined. It is also the time span when HARC can develop in a strabismic individual. Furthermore, it is the treatment period when any attempt to switch back from HARC to NRC is most likely to be effective, ideally as soon as possible after heterotropia has become manifest.

Note: interocular transfer is a research technique that may be illustrated by the common experience: where after stopping a vehicle, the road still appears to be moving – a motion after-effect. If this is repeated with one eye closed, and then that eye is opened and the original eye closed, the motion after-effect is still seen. This indicates that the brain cells registering the after-effect must receive stimulation from binocular cortical cells. This interocular transfer is less effective when the non-dominant eye is stimulated compared with the dominant eye. For different after-effects, varying amounts of interocular transfer occur. The transfer is also affected by the pooling of activity from different types of monocular cortical cells (before binocular fusion), and by some binocular cells that act like computer 'OR' and 'AND' gates. After-effects have been shown for **motion, size** (spatial frequency) and **tilt** (orientation) (see Paradiso *et al.*, 1989). A tilted image is presented to one eye: say of a black-and-white grid tilted to the left of vertical. The effect is transferred (via binocular cortical cells) to the perception of the other eye. If this eye then looks monocularly at a vertically orientated black-and-white grid, the percept is that it appears tilted to the right of vertical. There has been a binocular adaptation to the tilt, to try to 'correct' it. There is a very strong adaptive impulse to see the environment as having horizontal and vertical contours, rather than oblique. On the Hong Kong Peak Tramway, which travels on a steep incline, the tram appears to be travelling horizontally, and all the skyscrapers outside appear to have been built at an angle of 45 degrees! So when a non-tilted grid is presented, the adaptation makes it appear to be tilted, in this case to the right. This is one method of investigating the sensitive period for retinal disparity detection.

The transferred tilt effect would hardly occur in a child whose strabismus occurred at the peak of the sensitive period, at about 18 months of age, as then the cortical binocular cells would not be receiving stimuli that can be fused: their right and left eye inputs would be completely different, because in strabismus corresponding points do not receive similar images. Strabismus onset either side of that age would show some but less than normal transfer of the tilt after-effect. Movshon *et al.* (1972) showed that about 70% of subjects with no strabismus and normal stereopsis demonstrated interocular transfer of the tilt after-effect. Interocular transfer was shown for 49% of non-strabismic subjects without stereopsis and only 12% of strabismic subjects. Later work by Mitchell and Ware (1974) confirmed a transfer rate of 70% for stereo-normal subjects, but in four stereo-blind subjects, three of whom had strabismus, no interocular tilt transfer was seen. In similar work a year later, Mitchell *et al.* (1975) found no transfer in early-onset strabismics for central retinal stimuli, but transfer was present for these early-onset strabismics in which the stimuli were large enough to include the peripheral retina. Q: It might be asked why HARC does not take over the transfer? A: Possibly because the immediate effect of heterotropia is to produce pathological diplopia, and then a large binocular suppression area followed by the gradual development of HARC from the periphery of the binocular visual field, and there is always a central binocular suppression area of some size. There is therefore no fusible binocular input to cortical cells until the HARC has become well established and the retina-cortex topography has been redrawn. The peripheral HARC likely to be present in early-onset strabismics would possibly account for the tilt transfer for targets from the retinal periphery.

4.6 Fusional reflexes

Heterophoria exists where the two eyes have a tendency to deviate from the object of regard. This tendency is controlled by the **fusional reflexes**, which initiate a **fusional movement**. A fusional movement occurs when a person with heterophoria changes fixation using saccadic (sideways) or vergence (in depth) eye movements. Because a new object is replacing the previous object, fusion does not operate until the new object is fixated. The trigger for fusional movements is a disparity in the retinal images. The fusional reflexes are a group of reflexes, some innate, and some initially acquired as conditioned reflexes that are controlled and reinforced by cerebral systems and then become unconditioned reflexes.

- The vestibulo-ocular system contributes the innate **gravitational reflex** (or compensatory fixation reflex) using the vestibular saccules to activate the oblique extra-ocular muscles, and the utricles to activate the vertical rectus muscles.
- The **following reflex** uses the slow pursuit system to follow horizontally moving targets.
- The **vergence fixation reflex**, the **motor fusional vergence reflex** and the **accommodation reflex** together form the accommodation convergence reflex.
- The **fixation reflex** moves the eyes to a new target, and to any subsequent target. In babies it is involuntary and can be used to assess ocular motility and gross visual field extent. Most adults can inhibit this reflex (except when performing visual field tests!).

Some authorities also recognise **disjunctive fusional reflexes** during convergence and divergence. Also **conjugate fusional reflexes** when changing lateral and vertical gaze without loss of binocular fixation (Straube and Büttner, 2007).

4.7 Fixation disparity

The horizontal fusional reflexes provide fairly precise bilateral ocular retinal correspondence. There is often, however, a small inaccuracy in alignment of the vergence angle: the angle between the two lines of sight. This small misalignment, in which one axis misses the object of regard by an angle of a few minutes of arc, is called a **fixation disparity**, previously known as 'retinal slip' (Ames and Gliddon, 1928). An under-convergence produces an exo-disparity and over-convergence produces an eso-disparity. This is considered 'normal' if no symptoms exist, and normal binocular vision is possible. Indeed the vergence 'error' (the fixation disparity) is needed to maintain vergence control. The larger the fixation disparity, the greater the fusional vergence response that will be required. An even larger misalignment incapable of stimulating fusion would result in diplopia. Under experimental conditions using small foveal targets, fixation disparity cannot generally exceed about 12 minutes of arc, as the disparity must lie within Panum's fusional area, and 10 to 12 minutes of arc is the horizontal dimension of Panum's area at the fixation point on the horopter in these conditions. In more normal viewing conditions, fixation disparities up to 2 degrees can be accommodated (see section 4.13).

Note: 12 minutes of arc is about one-fifth of a prism dioptre. A prism dioptre is the unit of light deviation (strictly of 587.6 nm wavelength, on a surface normal to the light ray) that forms the angle subtended by 1 cm at 1 metre, and has the Greek symbol delta (Δ); 1Δ approximately equals 0.57 degrees, and 1 degree equals 1.75Δ.

- Thus fixation disparity has a **dual nature**. Lesser amounts are part of a normal feedback mechanism that maintains binocular fixation. Larger amounts are associated with a defective control of fusion: a horizontal fixation disparity between 0.5 and 10 minutes of arc may be associated with symptoms of **decompensated heterophoria** (synonym: 'uncompensated heterophoria'), or with **foveal suppression** (Ogle, 1954; Parks and Eustis, 1961; Mallett, 1964).
- The **aligning prism** (previously known as the 'associated heterophoria') needed to eliminate fixation disparity symptoms and signs in decompensated heterophoria is larger than the fixation disparity itself; and the heterophoria is larger still. The fixation disparity cannot be larger than the size of Panum's area under the prevailing conditions (Charnwood, 1951). The correcting response system has two components for horizontal disparities: a fast disparity vergence system (Rashbass and Westheimer, 1961) and a slow disparity vergence system.
- The **fast disparity vergence system** uses retinal image disparity and responds to changes in horizontal vergence demand at the rate of one prism dioptre or less per second (Ciuffreda and Tannen, 1995), with a latency of 180 to 200 ms. When a horizontal prism is placed before

one eye of an orthophoric subject, the fast system changes the oculomotor control to avoid diplopia. The fast system uses a neural leaky integrator with a time constant of about 12 seconds (Leigh and Zee, 2006).

- The **slow disparity vergence system** or **vergence adaptation system** uses the motor output of the fast mechanism as its error signal (Schor, 1979). The slow system also has a neural leaky integrator, but with a time constant of 4 to 5 minutes. The slow system provides prism adaptation, which allows an orthophoric subject to adapt to the prism, so that a cover/uncover test would now show no heterophoria present, even though the introduced prism is still in front of one eye. Effectively the slow system resets the level of tonic vergence. This then allows the fast system to use fusional reserves to keep the eyes aligned. The fixation disparity system provides that when a cover/uncover test is used to assess heterophoria, the speed of the recovery from dissociated to bifoveal vision may be used to determine whether the heterophoria is compensated – a rapid recovery – or decompensated – a slower recovery. The cover/uncover test is described in section 12.1 (Chapter 12). The reader should consult a textbook on abnormal binocular vision for details of situations in which the cover/uncover test may be ineffective.
- The **vertical vergence system** has a slow mechanism only and is generally limited to heterophoria of up to 2Δ in either vertical direction, up or down. A step change in vertical (and cyclofusional) disparity requires 8 to 10 seconds for completion of the response (Perlmutter and Kertesz, 1978). Larger amounts of vertical heterophoria fusion occur exceptionally in individuals who have adapted to the effects of vertical ocular muscle paresis.
- The **cyclofusional system** also has a slow mechanism only, with about 12 degrees of cyclodisparity control available. It also requires about 10 seconds for the full response to occur (see section 12.10 in Chapter 12).

Fixation disparity measurement is described in section 12.8 (Chapter 12).

4.8 Prism adaptation: the (slow) vergence adaptation system

The fusional reflex system has the function of correcting misalignment of the lines of sight/visual axes. An example has already been given in which an anisometropic spectacle correction produces increasing and asymmetric amounts of induced prismatic effect as the subject looks further from the optical centres of the spectacle lenses. Similarly, where a prism is introduced before one eye, the fusional reflex corrects the resulting misalignment of the visual axis, often before diplopia is noticed. Any minimal fixation disparity still remaining is also corrected. This correction will only happen if the prism is not too strong for the visuum to overcome. The slow vergence adaptation system is slower than the fast disparity vergence system, and may take 4 or 5 minutes to stabilise. After this time, a fixation disparity test shows alignment of the visual axes. However, in symptomatic subjects with decompensated heterophoria, this process of prism adaptation is less effective, particularly with increasing age, where there is linear reduction in adaptive ability. Here the prescription of prisms maintains asymptomatic fusion (North and Henson, 1992).

Disambiguation note: the term 'prism adaptation' is used:

- to describe what happens when the vergence adaptation system operates as described above
- as a clinical test to establish the efficacy of prescribed prisms – the pre-prescribing prism adaptation test
- as a test of the likely effectiveness of planned eye surgery – the prism adaptation test (PAT)
- as a test used by psychologists to evaluate cerebral adaptation to new visual experience, using prisms deflecting both eyes in the same direction
- with the same prism arrangement in the treatment of stroke patients.

4.9   The vergence position integrator

At the end of a vergence adaptation eye movement, there has to be a cortical mechanism for maintaining steady eye positions at a given amount of convergence or divergence: the **vergence position integrator**. It would appear that the vergence position integrator is not driven by visual information, as tonic muscle activity keeps a constant eye position even in darkness (useful for driving at night). It is likely to be derived from the velocity instruction that brought the eyes to their current position. There is some evidence that this function is largely found within the anatomical structure known as the nucleus reticularis tegmenti pontis. Incidentally, there is likely to be a separate, similar system for a **conjugate position integrator** for post-saccadic stabilisation, although its location and pathways may be shared with the vergence integrator (Leigh and Zee, 2006).

4.10   Accommodative input to vergence adaptation

In the same way that there is a fast and a slow fusional system, there is an analogous accommodative arrangement. The fast accommodative feedback mechanism uses retinal defocus as an error signal. It can react in a few hundred milliseconds. The slow accommodative feedback system uses for its error signal the output of the fast mechanism. This takes some seconds to operate. There are also neural cross-linked pathways that provide a connection between accommodation and vergence. One pathway provides accommodation-induced convergence (AC), and another provides convergence-induced accommodation (CA) (see section 9.4 in Chapter 9). It is possible that defects in these cross-linkages may be the source of convergence and divergence excess and insufficiency.

4.11   Motor and sensory fusion synergy

The zone in which fixation disparity initiates a correcting vergence movement is called the **motor fusion field**, the approximate dimensions of which are shown in Fig. 4.2. Disparate images within this zone trigger a motor fusional response. The minimum disparity necessary is of the order of 0.05 prism dioptres (about 2 minutes of arc). The motor fusional reflex is initiated and monitored by the extra-foveal retina (Fig. 4.3). The operation of the fusional system can be demonstrated by putting prisms in front of one or both eyes within the limits set by the motor fusion field. However, if too large a strength of prism is placed in front of one eye, the motor fusional reflex is not triggered; the eyes remain stationary and the subject experiences diplopia. The perimeter of the motor fusion field is therefore the threshold for diplopia. Objects imaged outside Panum's area but within the motor fusion field may not necessarily produce diplopia of which the subject is conscious. If you look from 3 m away, to a pen held just further away than the near point of convergence, you will notice a brief period of diplopia until the pen is fixated by both foveas. The motor fusional reflex generally reduces the fixation disparity, but not to zero disparity within Panum's area; the remaining disparity is managed by **sensory fusion**. Binocular sensory fusion is a function primarily of the foveal area.

The fusional system, motor and sensory, has to cope with complex heterophoria problems. For example, where an individual needs a correcting

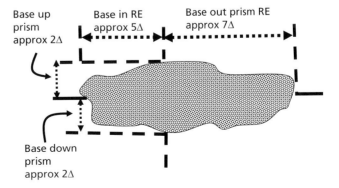

Figure 4.2   The motor fusion field. An illustration of the approximate binocular visual area in an individual subject, over which the binocular motor system is able to make corrective eye movements in order to maintain binocular fusion. The limits of fusional movements in different directions are given in prism dioptres. RE, right eye.

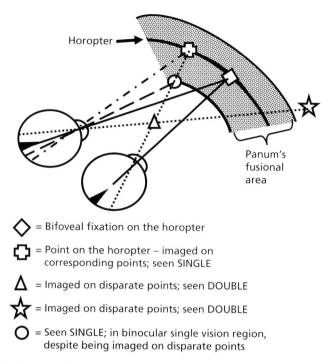

= Bifoveal fixation on the horopter

= Point on the horopter – imaged on corresponding points; seen SINGLE

= Imaged on disparate points; seen DOUBLE

= Imaged on disparate points; seen DOUBLE

= Seen SINGLE; in binocular single vision region, despite being imaged on disparate points

Figure 4.3 Panum's fusional area. The grey area indicates the depth in the horizontal plane in which an object may be placed and retain fusion as a single percept. Objects beyond or closer than Panum's area are seen double.

spectacle lens for one eye only, any eye movement away from the optical centre of the correcting lens produces a prismatic effect for the corrected eye only. This effect gradually increases as the primary line of sight (visual axis) moves from the optical centre. In effect, the person has a heterophoria of constantly varying amount. Gradually the vergence system takes this in its stride, even if astigmatic and progressive lenses produce even more complex prismatic variations. The measurement of fusional reserves is described in section 12.10 in Chapter 12.

4.12   Panum's fusional area

Corresponding retinal points consist of a pair of retinal receptors, one in each eye, that receive stimulation from an object that appears in the same visual direction for each eye. This allows the object to be seen as single. Panum (1858) demonstrated that single vision could also be obtained by stimulating a point on one retina and a small **area** around the corresponding point of the other eye (Fig. 4.3). In other words, there is a **point-to-area correspondence**. If two similar stimuli are presented, one for each eye (so that each is in a different visual direction but still within Panum's fusional area), then a single impression of the two stimuli is seen. This is an

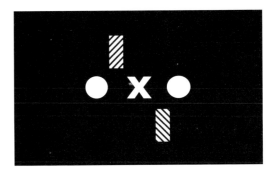

Figure 4.4 Panum's fusional area: binocular and dichoptic stimuli. For a subject with decompensated heterophoria, a fixation disparity test apparatus presents potentially disparate binocular stimuli that lie within Panum's fusional area and are fused, seen here as 'O X O'. The apparatus also has potentially disparate dichoptic stimuli, which are presented to each eye simultaneously, but separately, seen here as the nonius bars above and below the 'O X O'. The nonius bars are cross polarised, as indicated, so that each eye sees only one bar when viewed through cross-polarised viewing spectacles. The oculocentric directions of the bars are correctly perceived in different directions, because in decompensated heterophoria the eyes are not aligned. This figure is based on the Mallett unit arrangement as seen through polarised lenses in decompensated heterophoria.

example of binocular disparity. However, if a marker line (**nonius line**) is added to each stimulus so that it is seen by that eye only, the resulting perception is that the binocular stimuli are seen as one image, but the two nonius lines are displaced away from each other. Their oculocentric directions are correctly perceived (Fig. 4.4). The stimuli identically presented to each eye are **binocular stimuli**. However, the nonius lines are **dichoptic stimuli**, being seen by each eye but in different directions from each other. The fused binocular stimuli are perceived at a different distance away from the subject from a pair of targets falling on precisely corresponding points.

Note: it is this binocular disparity that creates the stereoscopic effect.

In a fixation disparity test, the different visual direction related to each fovea is shown by oculocentric separation of the test unit nonius lines in visual space. At the same time, point-to-area correspondence is demonstrated by the single egocentric perception of the test unit 'binocular lock', which is the element of the test seen by both eyes. To summarise, Panum's fusional area is the locus of all objects on a surface, whose retinal images either fall on corresponding points in each eye, or are derived from objects close enough in depth from this surfaces to allow fusion and the perception of stereopsis. Panum's fusional area permits single perception of the object of regard, even while the motor vergence adaptation system is responding to, and controlling, any fixation disparity. This allows for minor imprecision in ocular alignment during fusion, or caused by the gaze stabilisation system (see section 8.3 in Chapter 8), and also allows for objects to be seen in stereopsis.

4.13 Measurement of Panum's area

The actual size of Panum's fusional area depends on several visual factors. These include:

- the effect of fusional eye movements
- the retinal eccentricity of the point-to-area being measured
- the size of the targets being used to determine the area being investigated
- the sharpness, and speed of attempted separation of the images falling on each eye (the size of the fusional areas varies but can be as much as 15 times wider for rapidly moving out-of-focus images compared with slowly moving, focused images
- anomalous enlargement of Panum's fusional area in heterotropia accompanied by anomalous retinal correspondence (note: this factor is not part of 'normal binocular vision').

The usual method of measuring Panum's fusional area uses the concept of the **Wheatstone–Panum limiting case**. An object is presented to each eye and is imaged on each fovea. A second (similar) object is presented to one eye only so that its image is close to the fovea of that eye (Fig. 4.5). The effect is to produce the impression of a single object seen in stereopsis (depth). If the second object is moved so that its retinal image moves further from the fovea, there will come a point at which stereopsis is lost and two objects are seen instead of one (Fig. 4.6). The limiting case is the position in which the second object is seen as diplopic 50% of the time. This retinal extent, i.e. Panum's fusional area, is recorded for movement of the object both to the right and to the left of the fovea. It can also be measured for

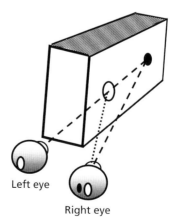

Left eye

Right eye

Figure 4.5 The Wheatstone–Panum limiting case, in which two discs are fixed to a wall, the black disc B hidden from the left eye by the white disc A. The left eye has a single retinal image of the two discs. The right eye sees both discs, with retinal images of A and B; the right-eye and left-eye images of A are fused. All three retinal images are needed for stereopsis, three being the lower limit – hence the classical description of 'limiting case'.

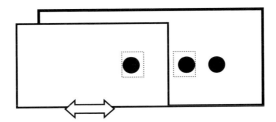

Figure 4.6 Panum's limiting case stereogram. This printed stereogram consists of two cards. The single disc, as seen by the left eye, is to be fused with the left-hand disc of the pair seen on the larger card by the right eye. The smaller card slides laterally to change the disparities of the binocular retinal images. Thus the stereoscopic percept is lost when diplopia supervenes, presumably when the left retinal image moves away from Panum's area. The reader should use a simple stereoscope and make such a stereogram for personal experiments.

vertical movement using polarising filters. It is called 'limiting' because it is the limit between single vision and diplopia.

Historically it was found that Panum's area took the shape of a horizontally elongated oval. There is evidence that the horizontal lengthening is caused by a larger horizontal motor fusion capacity than for vertical movement, and if the target objects are briefly exposed, Panum's area becomes more circular (Mitchell, 1966). The area, however, becomes larger further away from the fovea, by about 2 minutes of arc for each degree further from the fovea, starting at 10 minutes of arc centrally (**under experimental conditions**) and increasing to 40 minutes at 15 degrees from the fovea (Ogle, 1950). This peripheral enlargement of Panum's fusional area:

- matches the increasing receptive fields of the peripheral retina
- accommodates up to 7% magnification difference between the eyes peripherally (anisoeikonia), so making pathological binocular suppression less likely in the retinal periphery
- allows for torsion (rotation of the eye around the line of sight) in oblique eye movements (the effect of torsional misalignment is greater the further the receptive fields are from the fovea – this is because the retinal periphery moves more than the centre of the retina during a rotational movement; see section 8.13 in Chapter 8).

It should be borne in mind that if there is no detailed foveal image, and fusion is dependent on relatively large retinal images, then Panum's fusional area may be as large laterally as the 10 to 40 minutes of arc visual axis misalignment, as discussed above. Panum's areas extend in depth about 500 seconds of arc beyond and closer than the horopter, near the fixation point. However, for objects within this depth of Panum's area but very close to the horopter, there may not be sufficient disparity to produce stereopsis. These measurements were obtained with fairly stabilised eye positions. Collewijn *et al.* (1991) found that when subjects were allowed to view stereograms that were moving to stimulate convergence changes, normal stereopsis – and therefore sensory fusion – was possible with up to 2 degrees line of sight (visual axis) misalignment. So in **normal viewing conditions, Panum's fusional areas** may be fairly flexible.

Chapter 4: Revision quiz

Complete the missing words, perhaps in pencil.

Binocular fusion may be divided into motor and s_____ (1) fusion. When the eyes move from an old to a new object of regard, the f_____ (2) reflex is said to operate. When the eyes are almost aligned, then sensory fusion can operate. The highest level of fusion is normal stereopsis with f_____ (3) reserves. Retinal elements ('retinal points') that share the same common subjective visual directions are called c_____ (4) retinal points. The fusional reflexes maintain fusion. A small motor misalignment of the visual axes is called a _____ (5) disparity. The area over which a small motor misalignment can be controlled is called a _____ (6) fusion field. The area over which a small misalignment of right and left images can be sensorily fused into a single stereoscopic percept is called P_____ f_____ (7) area.

Answers
(1) sensory; (2) fixation; (3) fusional; (4) corresponding; (5) fixation; (6) motor; (7) Panum's fusional.

Chapter 5

DIPLOPIA AND CONFUSION, SUPPRESSION AND RIVALRY

5.1 Physiological diplopia

Where an object is fixated binocularly and the images fall on each fovea the object is seen singly. Similarly, other objects in the binocular visual field that are imaged on non-foveal corresponding retinal points are also fused into a single percept for each object. When the same object is imaged on well-separated non-corresponding points of each retina, the visual percept will be of two identical objects located in different visual directions. This is double vision, technically **diplopia**. As it is not possible for all objects in the binocular visual field to be imaged on corresponding retinal points, it might be thought that the normal visual percept is of most objects being seen in diplopia. This would be inconvenient! In fact we concentrate on the object on which we are fixating and generally ignore the diplopic images formed by objects closer or further than the fixation point. The lower acuity of non-foveal retinal areas and the active process of **physiological binocular suppression** achieve this (see section 5.4).

In some circumstances of normal binocular vision, the subject may notice diplopia. This is **physiological diplopia**. Hold two pencils directly in front of you, one closer than the other. Whichever pencil you fixate, the other will be seen in horizontal diplopia. It may be necessary to move the non-fixated pencil a little in order to appreciate the diplopic images. Failing that, if you close each eye in turn, the non-fixated pencil will appear to jump from side to side (Fig. 5.1). You are now well on the way to understanding the theory of retinal correspondence!

When looking at the further pencil, the images of the nearer (non-fixated) pencil is formed on the temporal retinas either side of the foveas. This is called **crossed diplopia** (Fig. 5.2) because the non-foveal image on the left retina is seen in the right side of the binocular visual field, and the non-foveal image falling on the right retina is seen in the left side of the binocular visual field. Conversely, if the closer pencil is fixated, the further pencil is seen in **uncrossed diplopia**. It is uncrossed because the right eye percept is of an object to the right. The left eye percept is of an object to the left of fixation (Fig. 5.3).

Disambiguation note: crossed and uncrossed diplopia differ from crossed and uncrossed binocular disparities only in that the disparities are derived

Normal Binocular Vision: theory, investigation and practical aspects. By David Stidwill and Robert Fletcher. © 2011 Blackwell Publishing Ltd

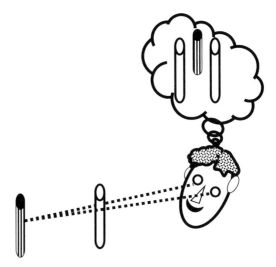

Figure 5.1 Physiological diplopia. On fixating the further bar (or pencil), the nearer one appears double, and vice versa.

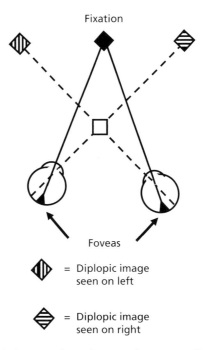

Figure 5.2 Crossed diplopia. When the two foveas are fixated upon a distant object, the images of a nearer object are found on the temporal retina of each eye. The nearer object is seen in physiological diplopia, and because the diplopic images are on the opposite side to the eye receiving them, the condition of 'crossed diplopia' is said to exist.

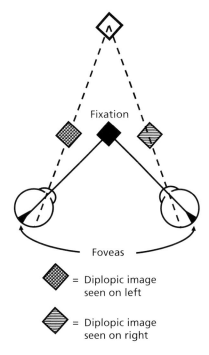

Figure 5.3 Uncrossed diplopia. When the two foveas are fixated upon a near object, the images of a distant object are found on the nasal retina of each eye. The further object is seen in physiological diplopia, and because the diplopic images are on the same side as the eye receiving them, the condition of 'uncrossed diplopia' is said to exist.

from retinal images that are close enough (within Panum's fusional area) to fuse and produce stereopsis. Diplopic images are outside Panum's area, and cannot be fused, and so are seen as two separate images.

5.2 Pathological binocular diplopia

There can be an abnormal situation in which only one eye is fixing the object of regard. Here the other eye is fixating in some other direction of gaze (visual direction). This can occur in a normal individual, at the extremes of ocular motility, when one eye may be able to move slightly further than the other eye. More commonly during motility testing – checking the function of the extra-ocular muscles – the fixation target may be placed beyond the view of one eye. Perhaps the nose occludes one eye only: bilateral fixation is lost. On moving the fixation target back into the binocular field of vision, there may be momentarily misalignment of the lines of sight (visual axes): the target is seen double. In this case, **pathological binocular diplopia** is briefly present, although no clinical anomaly is present: a single object is being seen in two visual directions. A more serious condition producing pathological binocular diplopia is **strabismus** (heterotropia). This is a permanent or intermittent deviation of the line of sight (visual axis) of the

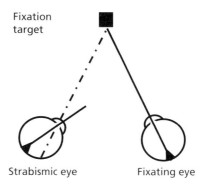

Fixation target

Strabismic eye   Fixating eye

Figure 5.4 Pathological diplopia. Because the visual axis of the strabismic eye is not aligned with the object seen by the fixating eye, that object is imaged on a non-foveal point on the retina of the strabismic eye. The object of regard is processed by two different cortical areas and so is seen as two separate objects.

strabismic eye, so that it is not aligned with the object of regard as fixated by the other eye (Fig. 5.4). It is possible for pathological binocular diplopia to be **suppressed** or **ignored**, particularly if one image is well separated from the other, or if one image is less defined, or deliberately degraded. Where pathological binocular diplopia is intractable and can neither be suppressed nor ignored, some form of occlusion may be needed, as for example with a high power fogging (blurring) contact lens.

5.3   Binocular confusion

Pathological binocular diplopia is often accompanied by **binocular confusion**. Here, two objects are seen in the same visual direction. This is because a different image is falling on the fovea (or other corresponding points) of each eye. For example, a subject with strabismus may fixate a fir tree with one eye, but the deviated eye may be fixating an oak tree to the side of the fir tree (Fig. 5.5). As each tree is fixated by one fovea, both trees appear to lie in the same visual direction. The oak tree appears to be superimposed on the fir tree. This effect is called **binocular confusion**. This is a clinical term for which a more scientific term would be 'interocular confusion'. The real confusion is that the whole visual field is seen twice, in different visual directions, not merely the object fixated. The accompanying pathological diplopia, incidentally, will mean that a non-foveal point in each eye also sees the non-fixated tree. (You may need to read this explanation again!)

5.4   Physiological binocular suppression

When both eyes fixate the same object, the foveas of each eye receive identical images. Another object sufficiently closer to or further from the fixation object as to be outside Panum's fusional area would normally be seen double. In normal visual circumstances we are not aware of this: the physiological

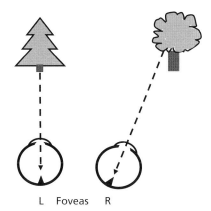

L   Foveas   R

Figure 5.5 Binocular confusion in strabismus. The fovea of the fixing left eye receives the image of the fixation target (a fir tree). The fovea of the right, non-fixating eye (with exotropia) receives the image of another object (an oak tree). Two different objects are perceived to lie in the same egocentric direction; this is binocular confusion.

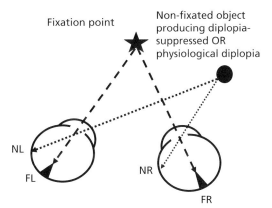

Figure 5.6 Physiological suppression. The fixated object is imaged on each fovea and fused. The non-fixated object is located outside Panum's fusional area, and is imaged on the right nasal retina in the right eye, and the left nasal retina in the left eye. These are non-corresponding areas, and so the double images of the non-fixated target may either be seen double as physiological diplopia, or may be suppressed, which is physiological binocular suppression. The diplopia of such a non-fixated object is normally suppressed, i.e. ignored. However, the object itself does not disappear, just the diplopic perception. If the non-fixated object is then moved, or has its luminance varied, suppression will be difficult, and physiological diplopia will appear. FL, left fovea; FR, right fovea; NL, left nasal retina; NR, right nasal retina.

diplopia is suppressed. This is one example of **physiological binocular suppression** (Fig. 5.6). Again, in scientific papers the term 'interocular suppression' is preferred. The (physiological) suppression of physiological diplopia can be reversed, often with some difficulty, for purposes of orthoptic exercises. Where binocular confusion is minimal it may be possible for the visuum to initiate **local suppression**. This may involve a delay of 70 to 150 ms (Schor

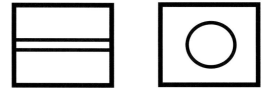

Figure 5.7   Local suppression. In this stereogram, two horizontal bars are seen by the left eye, and a circle by the right eye. The square frame is seen by both eyes and fused. Local suppression occurs at the intersections of the circle by the two bars. There are therefore four small areas of local suppression in this figure.

et al., 1976). An example is where a circle is seen by one eye, and two horizontal lines by the other eye (Fig. 5.7). Local suppression occurs at each intersection of the circle, so that it is now seen as two semicircles separated by the horizontal lines. Thus only the overlapping parts of each eyes' images are subject to local suppression. Local suppression is transient and disappears when the conflict of images is removed. Where binocular confusion is more marked, the process of **binocular rivalry** appears (see section 5.7).

Disambiguation note 1: 'suspension' was previously used as a synonym of 'suppression'. The term 'suspension' is better used to describe a monocular event, as in the note below. The term 'suppression' is more appropriate for inhibition of binocular summation, as in pathological binocular suppression.

Disambiguation note 2: there is **monocular physiological suspension** of visual awareness of blind areas in vision. For example, the normal blind spot is not apparent to the individual. It appears that the cortex 'fills in' the missing visual area with similar information to that surrounding the blind spot. It is also impossible to visualise or be aware of the limits of the normal visual field. Although nothing can be seen outside the visual field, any edge, or area of blackness, is not perceived. Although suspension is a monocular event, it can occur in both eyes at the same time: both physiological blind spots would produce a failure of stereopsis over the areas that they cover, for example. Another monocular suspension event is called the **Troxler effect**. This occurs during extended steady fixation (Plate 5.1). Here the micro-instability of normal fixation (see section 8.3 in Chapter 8) is thought to be insufficient to stimulate the larger peripheral receptive fields, so the retinal images are relatively stabilised, and a stabilised retinal image can induce transient monocular suspension/suppression.

5.5   Pathological binocular suppression

A more serious and persistent **pathological binocular suppression** (synonyms: 'pathological suppression', or 'suppression') may occur in the visual cortex, when the image received from one eye is entirely different from that imaged on the other eye, as in strabismus; or differs in being blurred, distorted, magnified or of low contrast, as in anisometropia (Sengpiel and Blakemore, 1994). The term 'pathological binocular suppression' is used, because it occurs only in binocular vision. However, it is the image of only one eye at a time that is suppressed. 'Pathological interocular suppression' would be more descriptive. The visual effect of different images for each eye may be to produce **foveal suppression**, or more widespread **general suppression**, both of which may lead to **amblyopia**. Foveal suppression is more likely in anisometropia, and general or total suppression in the minority of individuals with strabismus who do not have anomalous retinal correspondence.

Where there is recent strabismic (pathological) diplopia, the development of foveal suppression (of the deviated eye) would remove binocular confusion. Diplopia would be removed by the development of extra-foveal suppression. The extra-foveal point in the deviated eye receiving the image intended for the fovea would particularly need to be suppressed. In fact, in strabismus two small suppression areas can develop in the deviated eye (Mallet, 1988). A single large suppression area may cover both these areas. These developments are almost universal in strabismic children but rare in an adult who suddenly acquires strabismus.

The mechanisms available for producing both foveal and general suppression are thought to include:

- a multitude of inter-cortical potential pathways, between both adjacent cortical cells and between cortical visual areas, including the corpus callosum function (see section 10.19 in Chapter 10)
- inhibitory effects at the lateral geniculate nucleus (LGN) laminas from right and left eye input (see section 10.3 in Chapter 10)
- centripetal pathways from the cortex to the LGN.

Binocular suppression is primarily a cortical activity, conducted along the same pathways as binocular rivalry, and subsequent to the monocular level of cortical activity (Sengpiel and Blakemore, 1994). Suppression is the clinical description of inhibition (see section 10.7 in Chapter 10). It is possible that over time interocular inhibition develops permanent changes both at the LGN and in the visual cortex. The process of amblyopia genesis is then underway.

In alternating heterotropia, **alternating binocular suppression** can occur in two ways.

1. A stimulus is derived from inhibitory pathways from the cortex to the LGN. Inhibition of one lamina of the LGN by an adjacent layer from the other eye would still occur. Alternating pathological binocular suppression causes no anatomical changes in the LGN laminas or in the cortical ocular dominance columns.
2. The conclusions of Wolfe and Blake (1985) in binocular rivalry as described in section 5.7 are likely also to apply to binocular suppression: in addition to a visual cortex binocular layer 4 channel, there are layer 4 channels for right and left eye input, which would alternately inhibit

each other. The binocular channel would not operate in alternating pathological suppression, except where there was an intermittent alternating heterotropia. In this case when the heterotropia was absent, the binocular pathway would operate.

Clinically, pathological binocular suppression is classified as **facultative** where it is transient and does not have any effect on monocular vision, and **obligatory** where the suppression is so ingrained and prolonged that it is associated with a drop in monocular visual acuity – that is, amblyopia. The discussion of amblyopia is not included here, as it is abnormal, and generally a monocular condition. It is worth noting, however, that there is some evidence in amblyopia of binocular complications, in that the acuity of the better eye may be slightly compromised, and also binocular accommodation may be reduced. For details of the clinical aspects of pathological binocular suppression, amblyopia and eccentric fixation, a textbook on abnormal binocular vision should be consulted.

5.6 The characteristics of a suppression area

In pathological binocular suppression, the term **suppression area** (or 'suppression zone') is used because part of the cortical input from one retina is suppressed. Some degree of dissimilarity between right and left eye images can be tolerated in the retinal periphery. This is because of the large Panum's fusional areas there, and also because of the much lower visual (form) acuity in the peripheral vision. A suppression area is therefore more likely to occur for central vision. It will be triggered by the detailed (spatial frequency) difference between each eye's stimuli. The eye receiving a low spatial frequency image is more likely to be suppressed, as shown in Fig. 5.8 (O'Shea *et al.*, 1997). Diminished colour, brightness (luminance), sharpness, movement or contrast of the stimulus received by one eye compared with the other are also factors for pathological binocular suppression. As suggested in section 4.5, in strabismus a suppression area occurs related to the fovea of the deviated eye, and another suppression area occurs related to the peripheral retinal point in the deviated eye receiving the image intended for the fovea. ('Related to' because the suppression is cortical rather than retinal.) These two functional scotomas (suppression areas) swap to the

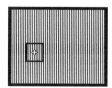 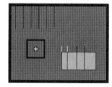

Figure 5.8 Suppression zone: high- and low-frequency suppression differences. The reader should fuse the two stereogram images. Concentrate on fusing the two small cross marks. Note the tendency to suppress the six dark low-frequency lines at the top, rather than the dark low frequency lines at the lower right.

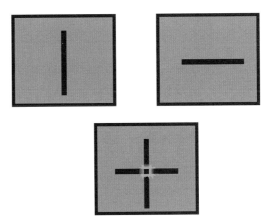

Figure 5.9 Suppression zone: mutual suppression. The reader should fuse the two stereogram images, showing a vertical and a horizontal bar, respectively. The 'halo (of suppression) effect' around the strong image of each bar produces a mutual suppression zone at the intersection.

other eye in alternating strabismus. The dimensions of the peripheral scotoma increase in larger angles of strabismic deviation. In some cases, the two areas coalesce. In large angle constant exotropia there may be a complete suppression area covering the whole binocular field of that retina, rather than the more usual regional suppression area.

Under experimental conditions (in eyes with normal binocular vision) in which a bold image is presented to one eye and at the same location for local sign in the other eye, a uniform background is presented to the other eye; the bold image induces physiological binocular suppression of the featureless background. Binocularly a 'halo effect' is seen around the strong image – a suppression zone, where even the featureless background is absent. This may be illustrated by presenting a vertical black bar on a white background to one eye, and a horizontal black bar to the other eye (Fig. 5.9). The intersection of the two bars shows an additive effect of increased contrast to the background, except where the bars cross. At the crossing point the percept of each bar is faded because of mutual interocular suppression.

Disambiguation note: the term 'suppression zone' is generally used to describe what happens under experimental conditions with normal binocular vision. The term 'suppression area' generally relates to the effects on binocular vision of suppression as a clinical anomaly; however, both terms may be used.

5.7 Binocular rivalry

Where markedly dissimilar images for each eye are both of moderate to high contrast, an alternating type of physiological binocular suppression can occur. This is known as **binocular rivalry** (previously known as 'retinal rivalry'). It is most pronounced with images containing very different contours (shapes). Marked differences of colour or illuminance of the right and left images will also produce binocular rivalry. It has been proposed that there are parastriate layer 4 channels for right and left eye input, using the layer 4 monocular cortical cells. If these right and left monocular channels receive visual stimuli too dissimilar to fuse, they alternately inhibit each other for input of equal intensity (Wolfe and Blake, 1985). If the right and left monocular input is of unequal intensity, only the more stimulating data proceeds to consciousness. However, if the two monocular channels have similar, fusible input, it proceeds to the layer 4 binocular cells.

A classic experiment arranges that the images for each eye consist of a series of lines (i.e. 'gratings') oriented at 90 degrees difference between the right and left eye (Blake and Fox, 1974). The two images are not seen as an overlapping series of lines. The dissimilar input arrives in consciousness as a constantly varying mosaic of samples of left and right eye images across the visual field: **spatial zones of binocular rivalry** (Plate 5.2) (Blake et al., 1992). This is particularly the case for large areas and is known as **mosaic dominance**. Where the gratings are at low contrast it is possible for summation to produce a stable tartan-like effect. To experiment with binocular rivalry, the equipment described in Appendix 1 (section A6) may be used.

In the retinal periphery, a 'spatial suppression zone' will appear, where rivalrous stimuli are presented to each eye. The size of the zone is related to the cortical representation of the peripheral visual field; the cortical magnification factor allows about one-third of the visual cortex to represent the macula, but smaller areas of the visual cortex represent the peripheral retina. The zone, where rivalrous stimuli are alternately seen (rather than mosaic dominance), therefore enlarges towards the retinal periphery. By contrast, for dissimilar images with low contrast, some degree of binocular integration – simultaneous vision – may occur. The combined images are seen together, especially when accompanied with a high-contrast fused image, as with the spotlight in the Bagolini striated lens test (Bagolini, 1967) (Fig. 5.10). For smaller areas, the images seen by each eye may be suppressed alternately, described as **exclusive dominance**. Binocular rivalry is most evident when deliberately presented under experimental conditions.

Note: somewhat similar effects may occur in the course of an optometric examination. One example is the (unfortunate!) need to close one eye when using a monocular ophthalmoscope to avoid binocular rivalry. Similarly, visual field examination can be problematic when the dominant eye is occluded and the non-dominant eye is under test.

A beneficial effect of binocular rivalry has been described (Nakayama and Shimojo, 1990). A monocular cue to depth perception is the overlapping of a distant object by a nearer one. Where the overlapping totally occludes the view of the object of regard by one eye, and only partially occludes the view of the other eye, a rivalrous situation occurs, aiding depth perception: this is called **da Vinci stereopsis** (Fig. 5.11).

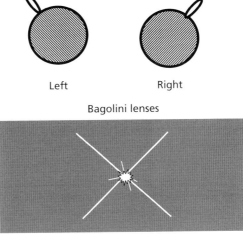

Left　　　　　Right

Bagolini lenses

Percept

Figure 5.10　Simultaneous vision. By placing Bagolini lenses in front of each eye, with striations at 90 degrees to each other, the percept is of a cross, composed of two streaks (one seen by each eye). Rather than rivalry, there is simultaneous vision.

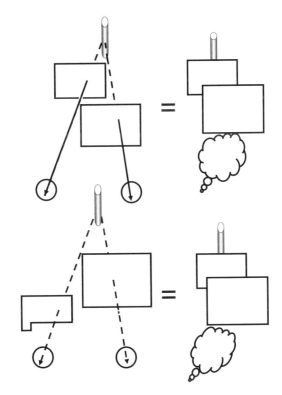

Figure 5.11　Overlap (Da Vinci) stereopsis. In the upper figure, the closer rectangle partially occludes the further rectangle, which in turn partially occludes the rod, so correctly indicating the relative proximity of each object. In the lower figure, the relative proximity of objects is misinterpreted by the visuum, because the objects have been chosen to simulate overlap stereopsis.

5.8 Visual stimulus threshold in physiological and pathological binocular suppression and in binocular rivalry

The **visual stimulus threshold** is the strength of stimulus required to allow a change in binocular percept (Levelt, 1965). The stimulus may be a change in contrast, luminance or motion. Any of these stimuli can be presented to each eye, in the conditions of:

1. physiological binocular suppression
2. binocular rivalry
3. pathological binocular suppression as in strabismus or anisometropia (this suppression is a binocular function, and **not** the monocular condition of amblyopia, although that may also be present).

Comparing these three alternatives with normal binocular fusion (Table 5.1):

• Typically any of the three types of visual stimulus (contrast, luminance and motion) suffer the same elevation of threshold in the suppressed part of the visual field for (1) and (2).

Table 5.1 A comparison of visual processes in physiological binocular suppression, pathological binocular suppression and binocular rivalry

Characteristic	Physiological suppression	Pathological suppression	Binocular rivalry
Speed of onset	75–150 ms	1 to 2 min	About 5 ms
Is there wavelength-specific sensitivity loss?	Yes	No	Yes
Must right and left images differ?	No	No	Yes
Does the binocular percept fluctuate?	No	No	Yes
Does a change in suppressed image affect binocular percept?	No	No	Yes
Are similar parts of the visual field removed from binocular percept?	Yes	Yes	Yes
How much is the visual stimulus threshold raised in the suppressed eye?	0.5 log units	≪0.5 log units	0.5 log units
Does the strength of the dominant stimulus affect suppression of the non-dominant stimulus?	Yes	Yes	No
Does the strength of the dominant stimulus determine the length of suppression of the non-dominant stimulus?	No	No	Yes
Likely site of neural control	Cortex + pre-cortex	Cortex + pre-cortex	Cortex

- About a threefold increase in stimulus strength is required for the stimulus to be perceived by the suppressed eye compared with the non-suppressed eye, i.e. 0.3 to 0.5 log units, for (1) and (2).
- Pathological binocular suppression is more readily interrupted by a visual stimulus in the region of 0.1 log units. The reason is that the active functioning of the non-suppressed eye triggers the suppression of the other eye's image from the binocular percept. This suppression initiation is equally strong in physiological binocular suppression and binocular rivalry, but needs to be less strong where the eye requiring suppression is already strabismic (Holopigian *et al.*, 1988). For binocular rivalry to occur, the images from each eye must differ. Both physiological binocular suppression, and particularly pathological binocular suppression, can operate with identical images from each eye. But pathological binocular suppression may take up to two minutes to occur (e.g. when changing from monocular to binocular vision), whereas physiological binocular suppression has an onset time of around 180 ms.
- Both physiological binocular suppression and binocular rivalry share some similar characteristics – for example, that a stronger local stimulus for one eye will cause suppression of the image received by the other eye at that position.
- Physiological binocular suppression and binocular rivalry differ in that physiological binocular suppression will maintain a fixed degree of suppression at any particular point of the combined image. In binocular rivalry there is a continual alternation in suppression between the two eyes, even if one eye averages a longer percept caused by a stronger stimulus (Blake *et al.*, 1971; Kalarickal and Marshall, 2000). In addition, any change in the suppressed image with binocular rivalry (but not with physiological binocular suppression), such as a change in contrast, orientation or spatial frequency, will bring the image back into perception (Walker and Powell, 1979). The suppressed image is still being monitored by the visuum during rivalry. See Appendix 1 (section A6) for experiments with suppression of vision.
- In binocular rivalry, equally strong visual stimuli are likely to be seen for equally long alternations of vision. Where a stimulus is of lower contrast, it is suppressed for a greater proportion of the time than the other stimulus (Levelt, 1965). Suppression in binocular rivalry appears equally affected by the luminance, movement or contrast of the stimulus. However, achromatic stimuli are suppressed less readily than chromatic stimuli (Ooi and Loop, 1994).

5.9   The cortical control of binocular rivalry

To assess the factors that control binocular rivalry, an alteration in the contrast, luminance and duration of each eye's input can be arranged. This permits us to determine the stimulus that is perceived as the **dominant**

stimulus. The stimulus that is suspended from perception is called the **suppressed stimulus**. The depth of suppression can be affected by factors other than luminance or contrast (Blake and Camisa, 1979).

Binocular rivalry is not an instantaneous response; very short presentation of rival images produces a combined, rather than alternating, perception. Wolfe and Blake (1985) proposed the presence of a binocular channel for similar images and separate right and left channels that inhibit each other alternately as they fatigue in turn. This process is thought to occur in (the visual cortex layer 4) monocular cells before they feed into binocular cells (in adjacent layers). The evidence that recognition of rivalry occurs at a high cortical level is that a suppressed stimulus can cause adaptation, even though the stimulus itself is not perceived (Lehmkuhle and Fox, 1975). The ability to produce adaptation lies in the visual cortex. For the suppressed stimulus to cause adaptation, the process of rivalry perception must be at a higher level than the level of adaptation itself. Similarly, rivalry processing has been shown to occur at a higher level than the processing of orientation and spatial frequency.

5.10   Binocular lustre

A special type of binocular rivalry occurs when the right and left images differ mainly in luminance. The image is perceived not as an average of the two luminances but as an imperceptible alternation of the two images. The shimmering effect is described as **binocular lustre** and is commonly associated with faceted jewels such as diamonds, but also with shiny black objects such as anthracite coal. Where the two images differ in hue, the effect is similar and called **binocular colour mixing** (Walls, 1942). It has been used to aid **hue discrimination** in colour vision anomalies. Wearing a red tinted contact lens in one eye only, red objects are seen without lustre but green objects are lustrous because of the different luminance arriving at each eye. In this situation, the lustrous appearance indicates the presence of a green stimulus (see Fletcher and Voke, 1985). Unexpectedly, it is possible to design stereograms that combine both lustre (caused by opposite contrasts) and stereopsis (caused by disparity differences) (see Julesz and Tyler, 1976). This indicates that the two processes of binocular rivalry and stereopsis are not mutually exclusive, but must be processed by separate systems working for the same location in visual space.

5.11   Summary

In summary, **binocular fusion** is encouraged by the similarity of binocular stimuli. **Pathological binocular suppression** is stimulated by the long-term dissimilarity of stimuli, particularly where one eye consistently has a degraded stimulus.

Binocular rivalry is produced by stimuli that are dissimilar but equally stimulating to each eye, and occur generally for short-term presentations of dissimilarity.

Chapter 5: Revision quiz

Complete the missing words, perhaps in pencil.

When the eyes fixate an object and another object substantially nearer or further away is seen double, this is called _____ (1) diplopia. If the diplopia is not apparent to the subject, then _____ (2) suppression is operating. When the eyes do not both align on the object of regard because of a failure of the visual system, the consequent double vision is called _____ (3) diplopia. This will usually be accompanied by totally different images being received on each fovea, producing binocular _____ (4). Where the difference in the right and left images is minimal, only the intersection of the two images may disappear, which is called _____ (5) suppression. Where the difference between the right and left images is because of gross misalignment of the eyes, or to unequally clear images, then an anomalous and permanent adaptation may occur called _____ (6) suppression, which may lead to amblyopia.

Answers
(1) physiological; (2) physiological; (3) pathological; (4) confusion; (5) local; (6) pathological.

Chapter 6

THE NORMAL HOROPTER

As Franciscus Agulonius said, '*Horopter recta est linea per axium opticorum congressionem ei, quae centra visuum conectit, paralleluus incedens*' (cited in Meissner, 1854).

6.1 The development of the concept of the horopter

There is (unfortunately and surprisingly) a difference between the actual position of an object in physical space and its apparent position in visual space. The distance between train rails is fixed in physical space, but to human eyes the rails appear to approach each other (in visual space) as they recede into the distance. Even at relatively short distances, differences can appear. If a subject is asked to place drawing pins on a horizontal board (looking along the board from one end) to form parallel lines, the actual result is that the lines curve away from each other. These effects can be explored using the methods described in Appendix 1 (section A10).

Lines of sight from the physical object stimulate a retinal area. The subjective equivalent to the line of sight for the fovea is the principal visual direction, and this locates the physical object in visual space (and secondary visual directions locate stimulation on non-foveal retinal elements). If the foveas fixate on an object point in physical space, the retinal images are subjectively associated with an external single point in visual space. Where object points lying on a relatively simple surface (in physical space) stimulate corresponding foveal and corresponding non-foveal images for each eye, their visual directions indicate the subjective **boundary** of that surface (in visual space). This boundary is the locus at which the points are seen as single rather than in diplopia. The terms 'singleness horopter' or 'identical visual direction horopter' have been applied. From the Greek terms *horos* (a boundary or limit, hence 'horizon') and *horao* (to 'look at' or 'see'), the description **horopter** developed in the seventeenth century. This term is chiefly used for a horizontal locus of points.

In the nineteenth century, Vieth (1818) and Müller (1826) suggested, for near objects, that the horopter takes the form of a circle running through the nodal points of the eyes, usually lying between the two outer canthi

---

Normal Binocular Vision: theory, investigation and practical aspects. By David Stidwill and Robert Fletcher. © 2011 Blackwell Publishing Ltd

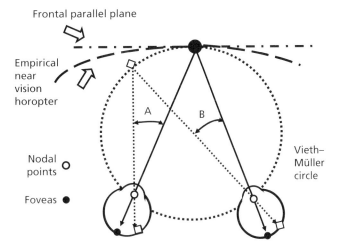

Figure 6.1 The Vieth–Müller circle (VMC) and the empirical horopter. In the theoretical geometric model of visual space, angles A and B would be of the same size wherever the peripheral object (a square) is displaced from the fixation point on the VMC circular locus. When the horopter is measured empirically, it is found in fact to be less curved than the VMC, for distances less than about 2 metres from the subject. The frontal parallel plane is a plane parallel to the frontal plane of the subject (see Fig. 6.2).

(Fig. 6.1). Ocular movement prompts the idea of 'mean nodal points'; such ocular movement will disturb the shape of the horopter.

As a simple introduction to the horopter, imagine horizontal ocular version movements over a small world map placed on a wall at arms' length. Consider the vertical 'longitudinal' strips of the map, imaged on small vertical narrow sections of the retinas. Then maintain fixation steadily in the centre of the map, apart from small fixation-maintaining eye movements. The two-dimensional map lies in a (physical space) frontal parallel plane – that is, a plane parallel with the face plane, technically known as the 'fronto-parallel plane'. The visual space representation of the map can be plotted: the horopter. Tschermak-Seysenegg (usually called Tschermak) used a term, *langshoropter*, for the longitudinal (horizontal) horopter (Boeder, 1952). Experimentally, Hering used vertical rods to plot the frontal plane horopter, known as the apparent fronto-parallel plane horopter, shown in Fig. 6.2 for the concept (and later in Fig. 6.5 for detail) (Hering, 1868). With steady central fixation at about two metres, rods are moved to appear to be all at the same distance from the eyes, and to lie in a plane parallel to the subject's frontal plane. Although the rods visually are in a plane, for most fixation distances they are actually on a physically curved surface. Subsequent treatment of the form of the horopter, by Helmholtz and more recently by Ogle, used mathematical descriptions applied to the complex three-dimensional surfaces, which result from varying the binocular fixation direction (Fig. 6.3) (Ogle, 1932, 1963). Non-uniformity of the

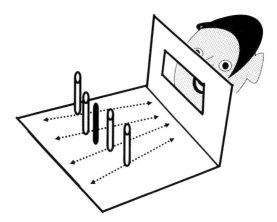

Figure 6.2 Hering's rod experiment. A fixed central rod is used for binocular fixation. Four other rods are moved so that they all appear to be at the same distance away from the subject's eyes as the fixed rod, and in a plane parallel to the frontal plane of the subject's face. The surface on which the rods now lie is the apparent frontal plane horopter. Although apparently flat, usually this horopter is actually a curved surface.

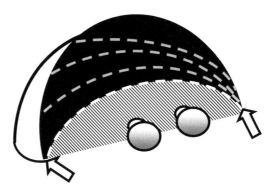

Figure 6.3 The VMC for different fixation positions. This illustration shows the upper half of the imaginary semi-spherical area of visual space in front of the two eyes and is based upon work by Ogle, and also by Luneberg, in the middle of the twentieth century. Here, half a Vieth–Müller locus lies horizontally in front of the eyes, which are converged and elevated. The object is thought to lie upon another locus tilted upwards, as from the ends of the diameter shown.

spacing of retinal elements and their visual directions, as well as the differences in retinal images in anisoeikonia, and changes in contrast, ocular torsion and other factors, conspire to distort the horopter (see section 6.12). So the apparently straight line or apparent fronto-parallel plane horopter (the experimental longitudinal horopter) is different from the theoretical Vieth–Müller circle (VMC). The difference is known as the **Hering–Hillebrand deviation**; the amount of this deviation varies with the fixation distance. These concepts are now explained in more detail.

6.2 The different forms of the horopter

A stimulus in physical space, imaged on the fovea of each eye, is seen as a single percept in visual space. Other stimuli in physical space that are imaged on non-foveal corresponding retinal points of the right and left eyes are also be seen as single percepts in visual space. A stimulus not imaged on corresponding retinal points should produce a double image in visual space. For discussion purposes, the simplified horopter proposed by Vieth and Müller comprises a circle in physical space connecting the fixation point with the nodal points of each eye. This surface in visual space perceived by stimulation of corresponding points in each eye is called the **geometric horopter**, or theoretical point horopter. All points on this horopter appear to be at the same distance from the subject (Fig. 6.1). This theoretical concept of a horopter is useful for investigating and explaining how physical space is converted into visual space. It is used to assess visual attributes such as judgment of depth and the effects of fixation disparity.

The *experimentally plotted horopter* can be thought of as a single entity, which may be measured in different ways, or alternatively as different types of horopter resulting from the different methods of measurement. Thus the actual form of the measured or **empirical horopter** varies for different **horopter measurement criteria**, as follows:

- the **apparent fronto-parallel plane** – the positions in visual space where any target presented in physical space appears at the same distance from the subject as the fixation point **identical visual directions** – the law of identical visual directions states that a target that is imaged on corresponding retinal points of each eye is monocularly localised with the same local sign; the horopter criterion is the locus of all the target points that have the same visual directions for each eye
- **single perception** – the arc and depth of visual space at which Panum's fusional area allows single perception
- **zero motor fusional response** – the locations in visual space that do not initiate a (motor) vergence response
- **stereoscopic threshold**: the points in visual space providing maximal stereopsis.

The experimental methods for measuring the above horopter measurement criteria on an individual are described in sections 6.3 to 6.8. For one fixation distance only, the physical and visual spaces are similar – a flat surface – variously located between 1 and 6 m, according to circumstances, from the subject (known as the **abathic distance**). Beyond that, the **horizontal (or longitudinal) horopter** is a convex surface curved away from the fixation point (i.e. convexity towards the subject). Within the abathic distance, the horopter is a concave surface curved around the subject. Most investigation of the horopter has been carried in the horizontal plane through the fixation point. The **vertical horopter** is a nearly vertical line through the fixation point, which is tilted away from the subject above the horizontal, and towards the subject below the horizontal (Siderov, 1999). The vertical horopter has little bearing on the study of binocular space perception, and will be ignored in the following discussion.

6.3 The geometric horopter

The geometric horopter (the VMC) comprises the theoretical locus of points in visual space associated with corresponding points in each retina. It assumes that there is complete ocular symmetry of each eye and so successive corresponding points have equal angular displacement:

- from the fovea towards the retinal periphery
- in both temporal and nasal directions
- and the eyes rotate about their nodal points and not their centres of rotation.

If these theoretical conditions were true, all the pairs of corresponding points in the horizontal meridian would lie on a circle intersecting the nodal point of each eye and the fixation point at whichever distance it was located. This is the **geometric horopter**, or the VMC (Fig. 6.1). The closer the fixation point, the smaller the circle becomes. Suppose the right retinal image is made larger than the left one. A 'size lens', described later, would do this. Alternatively, an anisometropic spectacle correction could be involved, provided there was no compensatory cortical adaptation. A new horopter would be formed (Fig. 6.4). The horopter would be tilted towards the right eye, but the impression of visual space (the fronto-parallel plane) would be rotated towards the left eye, considering just the horizontal horopter. If the anisometropia was a recent development, the new horopter might cause disorientation at first.

Objects that are not on the horopter are seen double. An object nearer to the eyes than the fixation point will be seen in crossed physiological diplopia (see Fig. 5.2 in Chapter 5). An object further from the eyes than the fixation point will be seen in uncrossed physiological diplopia. Diplopia results from the retinal images of the two eyes having retinal disparity greater than the small amount of retinal disparity that produces stereopsis. Remember, points on the horopter activate corresponding retinal points in the eyes with zero **retinal image disparity** relative to each other (see section 1.6 in Chapter 1). **Receptive field disparities** are a later product of the coordination of right and left images by the neural pathway, lateral geniculate body and the visual cortex. Receptive fields for each eye are corresponding only if they activate a binocularly driven single cortical neuron. Non-corresponding cortical receptive fields are said to be **disparate**. The visual cortex recognises small changes (from corresponding receptive fields to disparate receptive fields) as a **change in depth**. Larger changes produce diplopia. As disparities change from uncrossed to crossed, objects

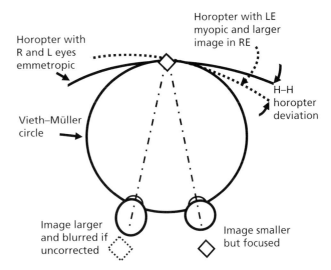

Figure 6.4 The geometric horopter in binocular emmetropia, and also with spectacle-corrected myopia in the left eye only, are shown. The effect of the left eye myopia is to make the right eye retinal image relatively larger (anisoeikonia), and to produce a new location of the geometric horopter. In this case the horopter is tilted towards the right eye, but the impression of visual space (the fronto-parallel plane, not shown) will be tilted towards the left eye. LE, left eye; RE; right eye.

appear to alter from being further from the fixation point to closer than this point.

6.4 Measurement of the apparent fronto-parallel plane horopter

The theory of stereopsis holds that stimulation of disparate points is necessary for the perception of relative depth by stereopsis. If there is no depth difference between any object point and the fixation point, the two points must stimulate non-disparate, corresponding retinal points. The subject is asked to arrange a series of vertical rods so that they appear to be on an **objective fronto-parallel plane** in physical space: that is, with no depth difference between them. However, the rods are actually placed by the subject on the **apparent fronto-parallel plane** (also known as the equal-distance horopter or the stereoscopic depth-matching horopter) in visual space. The objective fronto-parallel plane is defined as the true plane in physical space passing through whichever fixation point is chosen, and is parallel to the face plane, which is the plane formed by the forehead and the eyebrow superciliary notches. The objective fronto-parallel plane is where the subject is attempting to place the road, and the apparent fronto-parallel plane is where it is actually placed. This is the apparent fronto-parallel plane horopter method.

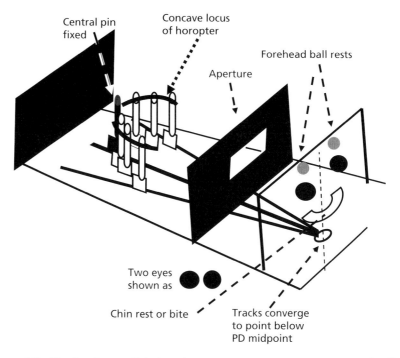

Central pin fixed

Concave locus of horopter

Aperture

Forehead ball rests

Two eyes shown as

Chin rest or bite

Tracks converge to point below PD midpoint

Figure 6.5 The fronto-parallel plane horopter measurement apparatus. The fixation rod (or 'pin') is shown as solid black. Only two of the lateral tracks are shown, to avoid confusion, although each pin would move on its own track. PD, interpupillary distance.

Apparatus to measure the apparent fronto-parallel plane horopter is shown in Fig. 6.5 and also in Appendix 1 (section A11). The subject fixates the central rod, with the head still, moving the side rods until they appear to lie in the same plane through the fixation point, parallel to the plane of the subject's face. The horopter may be measured at a variety of fixation distances, and at eccentricities to the right and left up to about 10 degrees. For each different fixation distance the subject always views a fixation rod placed in the median plane. Thus the lines of sight (visual axes) are converged symmetrically on to the fixation rod – the horopter has a different form where **asymmetric convergence** is present. The apparent fronto-parallel plane and the true/objective fronto-parallel plane do coincide at one fixation distance, the abathic distance, which depends upon the individual. Rods nearer than this are placed by the subject on a concave surface (Fig. 6.6) and rods further away are placed on a convex surface (Fig. 6.7), very likely because corresponding points are compressed in the nasal retinas relative to those in the temporal retinas (see section 6.10). The practical result for fixation distances less than the abathic distance is that the rods form a shallow curve (Fig. 6.8), perceived by the subject as in a flat plane but actually arranged in an arc. In this situation, the true (actually flat in physical space) objective fronto-parallel plane is perceived

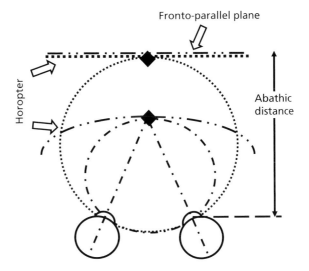

Figure 6.6 The horopter found at the abathic distance compared with the concave horopter for closer fixation points.

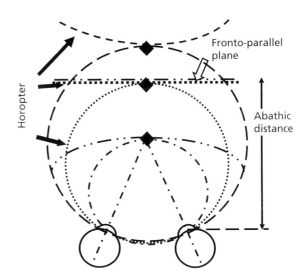

Figure 6.7 The horopter found at the abathic distance compared with the convex horopter for further fixation points.

as the mirror image of the rod-setting curve. If the vertical rods were correctly placed on the objective plane, in this example, they would appear to be curved away from the subject. So the shape of the apparent fronto-parallel plane horopter varies with different fixation distances (see later in Fig. 6.17).

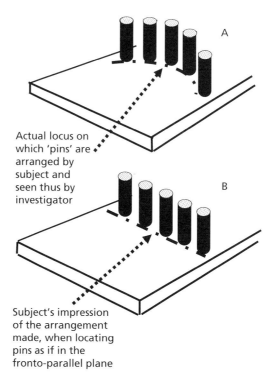

Actual locus on which 'pins' are arranged by subject and seen thus by investigator

Subject's impression of the arrangement made, when locating pins as if in the fronto-parallel plane

Figure 6.8 The fronto-parallel plane. The subject's impression of the vertical pins compared with their actual locus on the fronto-parallel plane horopter apparatus, for fixation distances less than the abathic distance.

6.5 Measurement of the identical visual directions

As corresponding points give rise to identical visual directions, the position of an object that stimulates a pair of corresponding points can be located if each eye sees a different part of the object, say the top and bottom of a vertical rod. If the two parts are seen in the same direction, the object is in the position at which it stimulates corresponding points. This is the **grid nonius method** of horopter measurement (Plate 6.1 and Fig. 6.9).

This type of horopter is assessed when both eyes view a fixation object, such as a stationary vertical rod in the primary direction of gaze. A second, moveable, rod is placed to the side of the fixation rod. Using Polaroid filters or a mechanical septum, one eye is permitted to see the upper half of this rod. The other eye sees its lower half (Fig. 6.10). In most experiments, such rods must be relatively thin. The subject moves the adjustable rod towards and away from him/her until the upper and lower halves appear to be in an identical visual direction. A single unbroken rod is then seen. This task is repeated at increasing lateral separations from the stationary fixation rod. As the eyes are aligning each of two halves of a target, this is also known as the **vernier method** of horopter measurement. Because of the use of vernier measurement, the nonius horopter is the most precise form of crite-

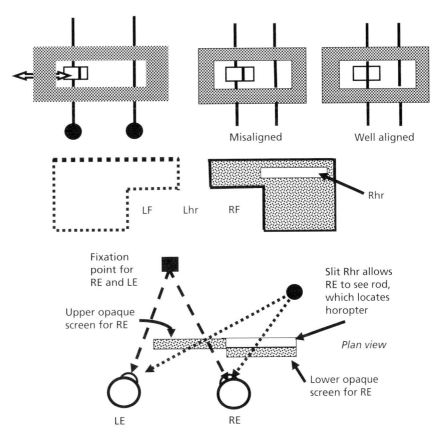

Figure 6.9 The Tschermak and the Ames vernier (nonius) horopter methods. The upper figure shows an empirical vernier (nonius) horopter location method based upon Tschermak's method with two plumb lines, aligned to locate the empirical horopter. The central figure shows the modified binocular screen system used by Ames *et al.* (1932), a method ascribed to Van der Meuklen (1873). LF and RF are the retinal areas used by the subject to see a central fixation point. **Lhr** is the area for the left eye (LE) view of a horopter rod on the right of fixation. **Rhr** represents one of three slits allowing the right eye (RE) to see part of the horopter rod. The left screen is merely outlined. The lower figure shows the plan view of this system.

rion measurement, and may be plotted to eccentricities each side of fixation up to 14 to 16 degrees from the central fixation point. Objects closer than the horopter are seen in crossed diplopia. Objects further away than the horopter are seen in uncrossed diplopia.

It is worth considering why the objects on this horopter appear single. The original method used a series of grids next to the subject's eyes to allow the upper and lower half of the test rod to be seen by only one eye (Tschermak, 1900). The vernier method was originally used by the Portuguese mathematician Nunez (in Latin, *Nonius*) for calibrating astronomical instruments. The measuring stimuli for right and left eyes are called nonius lines (or bars). So the identical visual directions horopter is sometimes called the **Nonius horopter**.

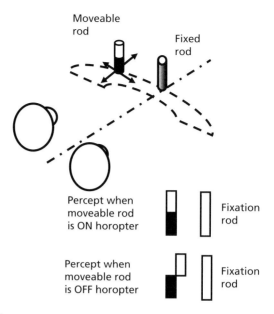

Figure 6.10 The principle of the vernier (nonius) or identical visual directions measurement of the horopter. The subject fixates a fixed rod and a moveable vertical rod is seen half by one eye and half by the other eye. When the two halves are vertically aligned, they appear to be in an identical visual direction. The arrangement for each half to be seen by a different eye is achieved by having slits in a screen as in Fig. 6.9, or by cross-polarisation, or by having different targets on transparent sheets as in Plate 6.1.

6.6   The haplopia (singleness) horopter

The haplopic method (method of the region of single binocular vision) is based on the primary definition of corresponding points: that is, retinal points that give rise to identical visual directions and, as a consequence, single vision. If diplopia is observed, disparate points are being stimulated. Therefore the haplopic method involves determining the boundaries of single binocular vision. The haplopia horopter measures the area of single vision, rather than identical visual directions. Fig. 6.11 shows the experimental arrangement, and Fig. 6.12 shows the subjective impression of single or double images. Like the identical visual directions horopter, the area of single vision plots Panum's area. This area increases in depth peripherally because of the reduced acuity there, i.e. the elevated spatial localisation threshold. The haplopia horopter is taken to lie in the centre of the zone of single vision. If the technique is repeated above and below the longitudinal (i.e. horizontal) horopter, the area of single vision vertically is limited to a vertical cylinder, going through the fixation point. The haplopia horopter is more difficult to plot than the Nonius horopter.

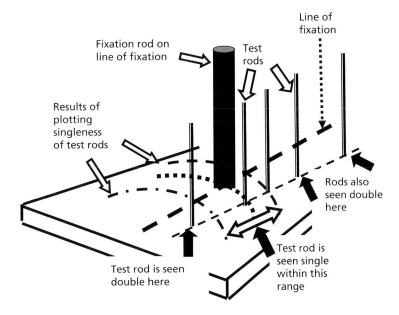

Figure 6.11 The haplopia (singleness) horopter, showing the experimental arrangement. The horopter is taken to lie in the centre of the zone of single vision.

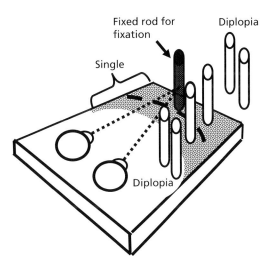

Figure 6.12 The haplopia (singleness) horopter showing the subjective impression. Both eyes fixate a central rod. A peripheral vertical rod, also seen binocularly in its entirety, is moved to and from the subject, plotting points at which single perception is lost, and the rod is seen in diplopia. Measurement is repeated at increasingly peripheral locations to right and left of fixation. Rods seen as single are within Panum's fusional area, and those seen double are outside it.

Note: for both the identical visual directions horopter and the haplopia horopter, the horopter location may be shifted towards or away from the subject by the presence of fixation disparity in the subject's visual system.

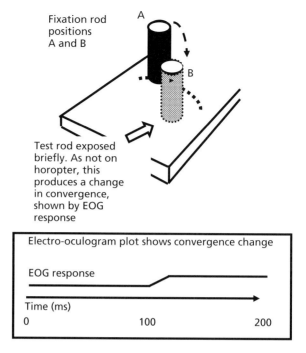

Figure 6.13 The zero motor fusional response horopter ('zero vergence horopter'). The subject fixates a fixed vertical rod. A test rod briefly appears. If it appears within or beyond the horopter, there is a change in the subject's vergence, and an electro-oculograph (EOG) apparatus identifies this. A version change alone would not indicate a shift from the horopter.

6.7　The horopter of zero vergence

The horopter of zero vergence (also known as the zero fusional response horopter) records the locus of points on a horizontal line going through the binocular fixation point that do not trigger a motor fusional movement. The subject binocularly fixates a central target such as a vertical rod. A test target seen by each eye is then presented briefly. Fig. 6.13 illustrates the principle of this technique and Fig. 6.14 shows the subjective impression. Suppose the test target was imaged in each eye on slightly non-corresponding retinal points. In this case a motor fusional movement would be triggered to allow sensory fusion of the disparate test target images, and the disparity then induced in the central target would be corrected by sensory fusion. This horopter is rather theoretical because it has yet to be successfully measured experimentally. In harmonious anomalous retinal correspondence, the horopter is adapted to utilise anomalously corresponding retinal points.

6.8　Maximum stereopsis sensitivity horopter

Stereopsis becomes more sensitive the closer a stereoscopic target is brought to the horopter. Differences in stereoscopic disparity, i.e. from no disparity

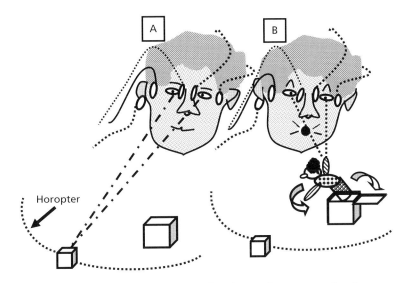

Figure 6.14 The subjective impression of a change in vergence for the zero vergence horopter measurement. This figure is purely to illustrate the principle, not the actual apparatus! The electro-oculograph (EOG) equipment, used to monitor the change in fixation, is outlined.

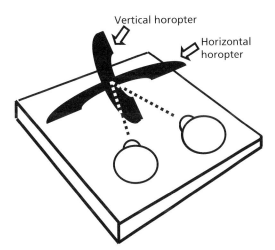

Figure 6.15 The maximum stereopsis sensitivity horopter. The subject fixates a central target. Maximal stereopsis is found on the horopter, and reduced stereopsis closer or further from the horopter.

to a slight disparity, are more acutely perceived as the horopter is approached (Blakemore, 1970). This may be assessed by fixating on a central rod and judging the movement in depth of a second, test rod set either nearer or further than the central rod. The subject is asked to say when the test rod has moved in depth. The amount of depth will be least as the horopter is approached. That is, the disparity thresholds are lowest, and the stereoacuity is highest, at the horopter (Fig. 6.15).

6.9 The shape of the horizontal horopter in normal binocular vision

The VMC (Fig. 6.16), the theoretical proposition of the shape of the horopter, passes through the fixation point and the nodal points (or entrance pupils) of each eye. However, when the horopter is actually measured on experimental apparatus, the shape is generally less concave and also more elliptical than the VMC at distances less than 6 m. It forms a plane surface at a distance from the subject of around 1–6 m, depending upon the subject and the experimental conditions: the abathic distance. The horopter is convex beyond 6 m (Fig. 6.17, after Ames *et al.*, 1932). The abathic distance is given by the formula:

$$H = 2a/b$$

where *2a* is the interpupillary distance and *b* is the fixation distance, measured in the same units.

The VMC is based on the assumption that there is a uniform distribution of light receptor cells in each retina. In fact, the temporal retinal receptors and therefore their 'local signs' are spaced further apart than those of the nasal retina. So the temporal corresponding points of one eye and the nasal corresponding points of the other eye are located at different angular subtenses from the common subjective principal visual direction. This produces a mismatch between the actual location of an object and its perceived

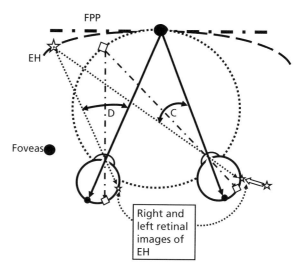

Figure 6.16 The Hering–Hillebrand deviation of the empirical measured horopter compared with the theoretical Vieth–Müller circle. The figure illustrates that the retinal images are separated by different amounts for each eye, yet the images actually fall on corresponding areas of the two retinas, which share a visual direction. Clearly angle D is more than angle C. The Vieth–Müller circle does not allow for the 'nasal packing' of retinal receptors and other physiological asymmetries. EH, a point on the experimentally measured horopter; FPP, front-parallel plane.

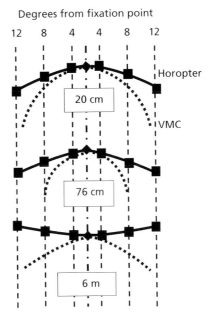

Figure 6.17 The apparent fronto-parallel plane horopter measured at three distances, and compared with the Vieth–Müller circle (VMC). Adapted from Ogle (1950).

location: our perception of space is **warped**. Thus beyond 6 m (depending upon the individual subject) a series of vertical rods placed on a plane surface are perceived as being horizontally convex to the subject.

Note: It is helpful to recall the relative extents of the nasal and temporal visual fields.

6.10 The Hering–Hillebrand horopter deviation

The difference between the VMC and the empirical (measured) shape of the horopter is called the **Hering–Hillebrand deviation coefficient** and has been given the **value *H***. This usually has a value between +0.10 and +0.20, indicating a horopter flatter than the VMC (Fig. 6.16) (Ogle, 1963). Positive values of *H* indicate less curvature; and negative values, more curvature, than the VMC. The value *H* is a measure of the **varying relative magnification** over the two-dimensional horizontal visual field. If the eyes are fixating in the primary position of gaze, *H* could be caused by the non-uniform arrangement of retinal elements, and therefore local signs. The closer arrangement of nasal retinal elements is referred to as **nasal packing**.

However, if instead of considering the horopter in two dimensions, using point objects to plot *H*, they are replaced by vertical line objects (nonius lines), then a three-dimensional **space horopter** can be obtained. The **rectilinear horopter** is the name of the complex surface in space accommodating those lines, which are imaged as corresponding retinal lines. The difference (in three dimensions) between the theoretical VMC and the plotted space horopter is not because of retinal asymmetry, but depends upon how converged the eyes are, and also the amount of eye rotation (torsion) associated with that amount of convergence (see section 8.13 in Chapter 8). To summarise, the Hering–Hillebrand horopter deviation may be affected by the optical imperfections of the eye, by nasal packing of the retina, by other forms of neural magnification along the visual pathways and visual cortex, and by convergence and torsion.

Note: although it is completely unrelated to binocular vision, normal or otherwise, the gradually increasing horizontal magnification associated with nasal packing is also produced along the base-apex meridian of an ophthalmic prism. In fact, a telescope can be produced by stacking four prisms with each base at 90 degrees to the next! Equally, looking through ophthalmic prisms distorts the horopter, both by this magnification effect, and by ocular torsion associated with the resulting change in convergence or divergence.

Difference of magnification

Where there is a difference of magnification of the images of each eye, the empirical horopter curve rotates about a vertical axis through the fixation point (see section 6.15). Although the shape of the horopter alters at different fixation differences, the differences (**H**) in curvature between the horopter and the VMC remain constant. This indicates that the arrangement of corresponding points in each retina is not affected by changes in vergence. When the eyes fixate to the right or left of the median plane, an additional distortion of the horopter occurs. This is caused by torsional (rotational) movement of the eyes in non-primary directions of gaze. The result is to tilt the horopter at an angle to the horizontal, depending upon the amount of torsion (rotational eye movement).

Note: the empirical (i.e. measured) horopter, in addition to showing the Hering–Hillebrand horopter deviation may also show localised deformation associated with retinal distortion, e.g. in macular oedema, or associated with spatial distortion changes in anomalous correspondence in heterotropia.

6.11 Adaptations of the horopter

In clinical anomalies there will be changes in the horopter. These are summarised in Table 6.1, but reference should be made to texts on binocular anomalies for details.

6.12 The horopter and anisoeikonia

The retinal image gives rise to a percept apparently located in visual space. This percept and its dimensions are affected by the retinal image, the anatomic characteristics of the retinal elements, and by cerebral processing

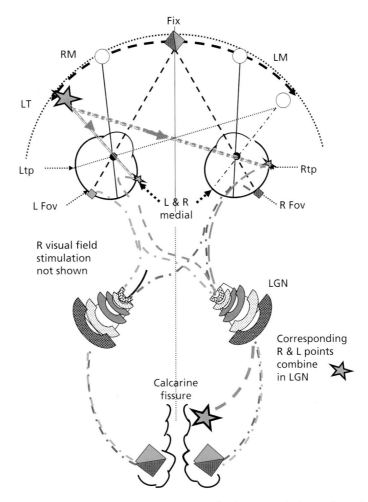

Plate 4.1 Corresponding retinal points. The star, which is on the horopter, is imaged on the nasal retina of the left eye, and the temporal retina of the right eye. These retinal points have the same angular sub-tense from each fovea (the same local sign), and so are corresponding retinal points. Their images are therefore brought to the identical cortical location and fused there. Similarly, the bi-coloured diamond, also on the horopter, is imaged on each fovea and fused at the same foveo-cortical point, also shown as a bi-coloured diamond. There is, however, dual representation of the foveas, one in each hemisphere, and these two representations are linked through the corpus callosum. Fix, bi-foveal fixation point; L fov, left fovea; LGN, lateral geniculate nucleus, showing the six layers; LM, left medial visual field; LT, left temporal visual field; Ltp, left temporal point on the retina receiving the star image; R fov, right fovea; RM, right medial visual field; RT, right temporal visual field; Rtp, right temporal point on the retina receiving the star image.

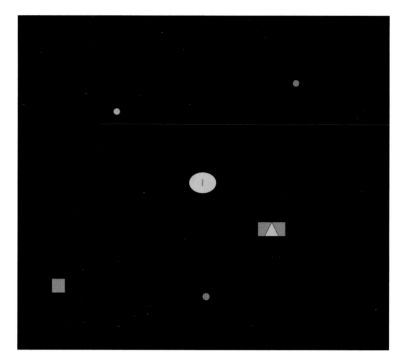

Plate 5.1 The Troxler effect or phenomenon. With steady central fixation, a type of 'fatigue' occurs and visual discrimination in the periphery becomes less reliable. At a reading distance, the reader should binocularly fixate the small central red vertical line, previously having noted the features of the more peripheral stimuli. Slight changes of appearance in the lighter area around the red line give clues to the inevitable unsteadiness of fixation over more than a few seconds. When fixation is most steady the percept of the peripheral stimuli alters.

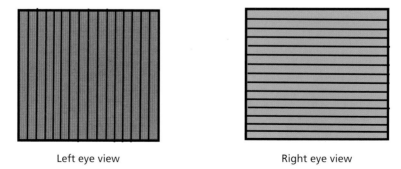

Left eye view   Right eye view

Plate 5.2 Binocular rivalry. The reader should fuse the two stereogram images. A constantly changing mosaic of binocular rivalry patterns is seen. Although smaller details (contours) that are at different orientations to each other may be suppressed, larger contours alternate in perception – that is, their perception is rivalrous.

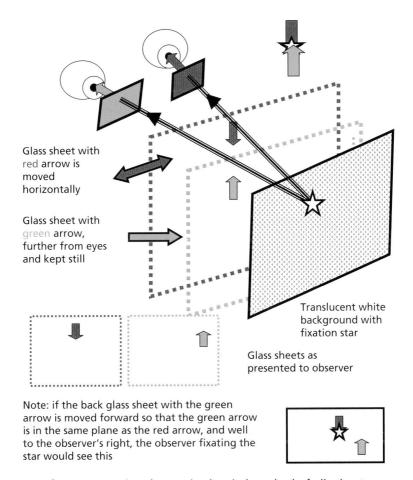

Glass sheet with red arrow is moved horizontally

Glass sheet with green arrow, further from eyes and kept still

Translucent white background with fixation star

Glass sheets as presented to observer

Note: if the back glass sheet with the green arrow is moved forward so that the green arrow is in the same plane as the red arrow, and well to the observer's right, the observer fixating the star would see this

Plate 6.1 One type of apparatus using the vernier (nonius) method of aligning two arrows at different distances from each other and from a fixation object. The red arrow is moved horizontally until it and the green arrow appear to touch. The subject's combined binocular percept would then be as shown. This method, derived from Hering's 'plate haploscopy' involves the parafoveal areas as corresponding parts of the retinas.

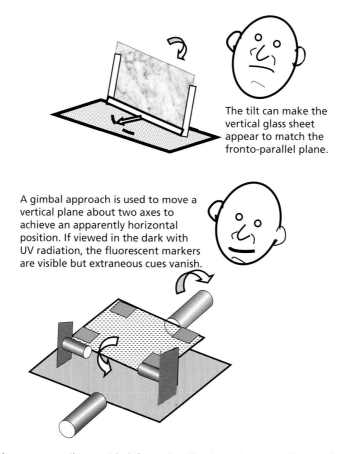

The tilt can make the vertical glass sheet appear to match the fronto-parallel plane.

A gimbal approach is used to move a vertical plane about two axes to achieve an apparently horizontal position. If viewed in the dark with UV radiation, the fluorescent markers are visible but extraneous cues vanish.

Plate 6.2 Tilting planes are easily provided for anisoeikonic estimation. The vertical glass sheet can be tilted to make it appear to match the fronto-parallel plane. A gimbal approach is used to move the vertical plane about two axes to achieve an apparently horizontal position. An improved effect is obtained if the board is covered with fluorescent paper and an ultraviolet (UV) light source is used. If viewed in the dark with UV radiation, the fluorescent markers are visible but extraneous cues vanish.

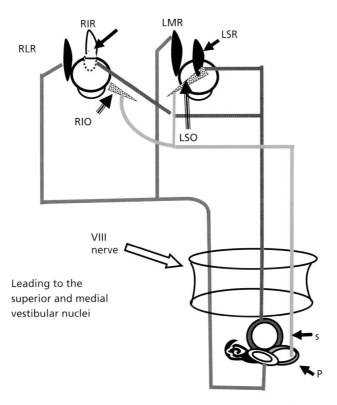

Plate 8.1 The stato-kinetic reflex pathway. Varied vestibular connections influencing ocular stato-kinetic reflex movements. On account of the complexities, this diagram omits synapses and neurones connecting via the oculomotor nerve nuclei. The vestibular superior (S) and posterior (P) canals only are indicated. LMR, left medial rectus; LSO, left superior oblique; LSR, left superior rectus; RIO, right inferior oblique; RIR, right inferior rectus; RLR, right lateral rectus.

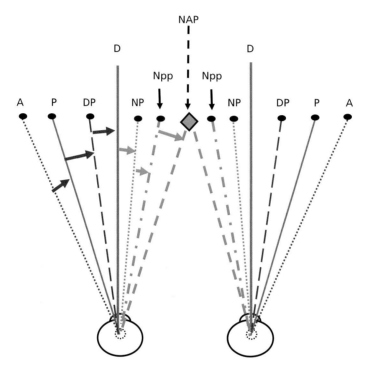

Plate 9.1 The subdivisions of convergence eye movement. A to P = tonic convergence; P to DP = initial convergence; DP to D = distance fusional convergence; D to NP = near accommodative convergence; NP to Npp = near proximal convergence; Npp to NAP = near fusional convergence. A, anatomical rest position; D, distance active position; DP, distance passive position (fusion free); NAP, near active position; NP, near passive position (fusion free); Npp, near proximal position; P, physiological rest position.

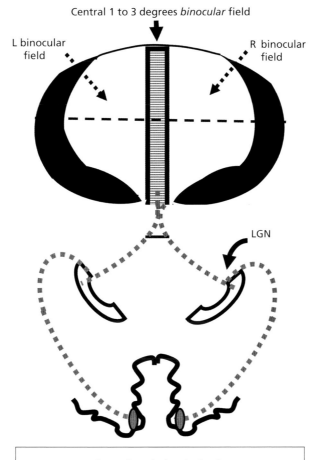

Central 1 to 3 degrees *binocular* field

L binocular field

R binocular field

LGN

Central vertical retinal strip
in each field imaged in both R and L cortical
regions on account of overlapping
representation, possibly via corpus callosum
bridging

Plate 10.1 The fine stereopsis pathway from the central 1–3 degree macular receptor strip for each eye, to a duplicate representation in the macular area of the visual cortex of each hemisphere. LGN, lateral geniculate nucleus.

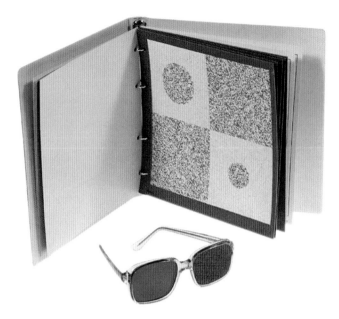

Plate 11.1 The TNO stereotest. This measures global stereopsis between 2000 and 15 arc seconds, using red and green anaglyph spectacles. Reproduced with kind permission of Haag-Streit UK Ltd.

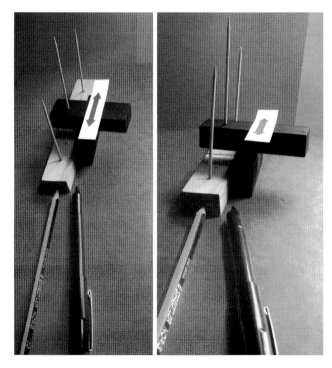

Plate A1 The pen and pencil represent the visual axis of each eye.

Table 6.1 Horopter variations

Anomaly	Visual effect
Anisometropia	Produces anisoeikonia (see section 6.12)
Astigmatism	Magnification in one meridian causes apparent shape changes
Asymmetric convergence	Produces anisoeikonia (see section 6.12)
Constant esotropia	Anomalous retinal correspondence with spatial distortion
Cyclovergence, e.g. convergence in down-gaze	Floor appears tilted (but see section 1.7 in Chapter 1)
Intermittent exotropia	The horopter is within the VMC
Prescribed prisms base-in	Distort the horopter to be horizontally convex; and the visual percept looks relatively concave, and tilted
Prescribed prisms base-out	Distort the horopter to be horizontally concave; and the visual percept looks relatively convex, and tilted

of the final perception. If the two ocular images are identical in dimensions, the two eyes are said to be **isoeikonic**. **Anisoeikonia** is a visual anomaly associated with size (and sometimes shape) differences between the right and left halves of the visual system produced either where the two ocular images differ in their dimensions, or by neural magnification effects further along the visual pathways. It is also spelled 'aniseikonia'.

Disambiguation note: if magnifying effects are applied equally to both eyes, the term 'anisoeikonia' does not apply.

Optical and neural anisoeikonia

A common cause of **anisoeikonia** is a difference in the refraction of each eye, called anisometropia. This may be **refractive** or **axial** anisoeikonia (or a combination of both), producing **refractive** or **axial anisometropia** (or both). Where the **retinal images** are identical in size, it is still possible to have **neural anisoeikonia**: for example, if there is retinal distortion from macular degeneration or other disease processes. However, physiological neural anisoeikonia of 0.5% to 1% occurs in about half of all emmetropes without producing adverse effects. Over 2% difference between the two eyes may produce visual disturbances, to which the individual may be able to adapt. Over 6% will reduce global stereopsis. For differences beyond 10%, diplopia or pathological binocular suppression will occur.

6.13   Measurement of anisoeikonia

A readily available clinical method of measuring anisoeikonia is to use **anisoeikonia stereograms** in a Holmes stereoscope, such as Charnwood's designs (Charnwood, 1952). The anisoeikonia stereograms are graduated in amounts of image difference, and by finding one that apparently gives a normal

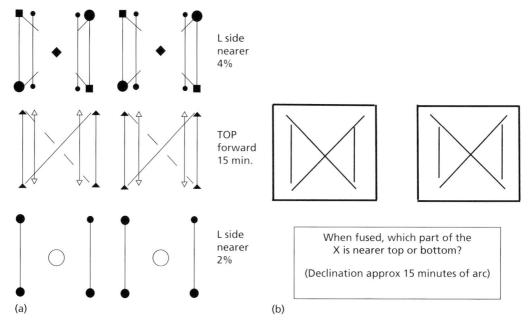

Figure 6.18 (a) Anisoeikonia stereograms, based on stereograms by Charnwood and used in the American Optical space eikonometer to estimate horizontal magnification. This series of stereograms may be viewed in a stereoscope, or fused by free fusion, by over-converging or under-converging. Under-converging fusion may only be possible if this figure is photocopied and enlarged to increase the separation between the right and left images. A horizontal prism may help. The stereograms show the effect of different amounts of magnification in one eye compared with the other. By inverting the stereograms, the opposite effect may be produced. Hence they may be used to estimate the presence and amount of anisoeikonia in a subject. (b) Anisoeikonia stereograms, based on stereograms by Charnwood and used in the American Optical space eikonometer to estimate vertical magnification.

percept, the degree of anisoeikonia may be estimated, subject to any error introduced by the stereoscope itself (Fig. 6.18a and b). Another method is to use two spotlights at 6m, horizontally separated, and viewed through a Maddox rod with one eye: the Brecher Maddox rod anisoeikonia test (Brecher, 1951). That eye sees two Maddox rod vertical streaks and the other eye sees two horizontally separated spotlights. If the subject is isoeikonic, the streaks run through each spotlight. If the subject is anisoeikonic, only one spotlight has a streak running through it. The second spotlight and vertical streak are horizontally separated from each other (Fig. 6.19). The Maddox rod (and spotlights) can be rotated to measure anisoeikonia in any meridian. To assess the amount of anisoeikonia it is necessary either to measure the apparent separation of the images, or to use a special correcting lens called a **size lens**. This can be used to magnify the smaller image received, and so to neutralise the anisoeikonia. Any thick spectacle or trial lens produces a change in the apparent size of an object. For near objects even a thin plate of glass or plastic such as the Frisby stereotest produces a magnification of the object viewed. (Indeed, the Frisby test has been calibrated to allow for this magnification effect upon the original stereopsis value.) The magnification caused by the **refractive power** of a size lens is given by the **power factor**, *Mp*:

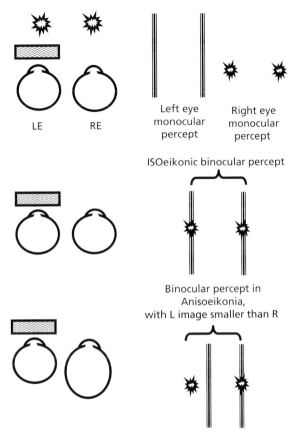

Figure 6.19 The Brecher Maddox rod anisoeikonia test. The subject looks at two spotlights separated horizontally (or at any other angle for which anisoeikonia is to be investigated). A Maddox rod with the axis horizontal in front of one eye (here, the left eye) would produce the binocular percept (if there were no image size difference between the eyes) of two spotlights, each with a vertical line through it. If there is anisoeikonia, as illustrated in the lower diagram (enlarging the right eye retinal image size), the subject will see two spotlights, one with a vertical streak through it, and the other streak located between the two spotlights. A horizontal prism may be placed in front of the Maddox rod to shift the mis-aligned streak onto the spotlight. (The other streak can be ignored.) If the spotlights are positioned 100 cm apart at a fixation distance of 600 cm, and a one-prism dioptre prism aligns the streak with the spot, there would be a 1% image size difference. Over 3–5% image size difference creates difficulties in adaptation for normal subjects. LE, left eye; RE, right eye.

$$Mp = 1/(1 - af_v)$$

where a is the vertex distance from lens to eye, and f_v is the back vertex power of the lens.

The magnification given by the **back surface power and thickness** of the lens is called the **shape factor**, Ms:

$$Ms = 1/(1 - (t/n')f_1)$$

where f_1 is the front surface power, t is the lens thickness, and n' is the refractive index. The **total magnification** of the size lens is the sum of Mp and Ms.

An illustration of overall and meridional magnifying size lenses is given in Fig. 6.20. Fig. 6.21 shows the experimental arrangement of a large space eikonometer as used by Ogle to investigate anisoeikonia, and to demonstrate anisoeikonia using size lenses on a normal subject. There is a computer program called Aniseikonia Inspector (Optical Diagnostics), which allows

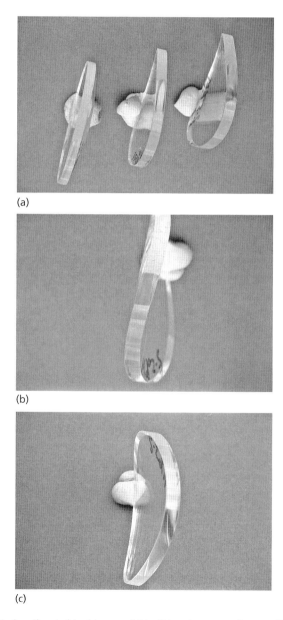

(a)

(b)

(c)

Figure 6.20 Anisoeikonic (size) lenses. (a) Left lens has overall magnification 1.25%. Centre lens has meridional 1.25% magnification. Right lens has 2.5% meridional magnification. (b) and (c) give improved view of the bi-toric meridional lenses.

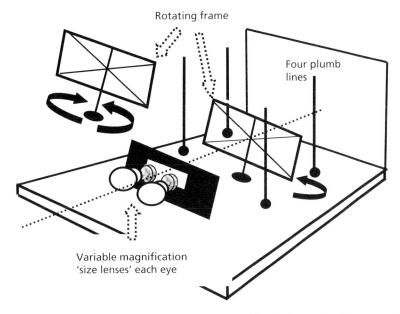

Figure 6.21 The large space eikonometer as used by Ogle *et al.*, with cross wires rotating on a vertical axis.

measurement of anisoeikonia and calculation of correcting spectacle lenses (de Wit, 2008). Apparatus to investigate the effect of a size lens is described in Appendix 1 (section A12), and the Hawkswell eikonometer is shown in Fig. 12.3 in Chapter 12.

Summary of sources of magnification effects

1. Optical magnification
    i. external, e.g. owing to spectacle lenses
    ii. internal, e.g. owing to ametropia
2. Uniform magnification – retinal crowding, neural – cortical representation anomaly
3. Asymmetric magnification – astigmatism
4. Irregular and localised magnification – retinal lesions

6.14 The anisoeikonic ellipse

Consider, for simplicity, purely optical image size differences between the two eyes. If one eye has a magnification of the retinal image in only one meridian, that eye will see an ellipse where the other eye sees a circle. If the same meridional magnification occurs in both eyes, both eyes will see the same ellipse, and the magnification effect can be found from the difference in the longer and shorter dimensions of the ellipse, i.e. the major and minor axes. A more complicated situation arises when meridional magnification is found along a different meridian for one eye compared with the other. Remole (1981) describes an algebraic and graphical analysis in which an anisoeikonic ellipse is considered to represent a single magnifier in front of one eye, combining the magnifying effects of both eyes. This treatment allows measurement of the magnification, and of the resulting tilt of the fronto-parallel plane. The method also allows calculation of the effect of non-uniform magnification produced by ophthalmic prisms, and prediction of the effect of anisometropic ophthalmic lenses, including pincushion and barrel distortions.

6.15   Overall and meridional magnification effects

Overall magnification will be produced by a spectacle lens at the rate of 1.4% per dioptre difference between the left and right eyes. You can experience a similar effect by holding a pencil directly in front of one eye so that it is closer to that eye than the other. There will be a marked difference in image size. Fig. 6.20 illustrates the appearance of an anisoeikonic (size) lens with overall magnification, and of two strengths of lens with meridional magnification. **Meridional magnification** causes more complex distortions than overall magnification. If a meridional size lens is set in front of one eye with its axis vertical and magnification therefore horizontal, the apparent fronto-parallel plane is **rotated** about a vertical axis (Fig. 6.22). The horopter is rotated towards the eye with the size lens. The percept (of whatever is being regarded) is rotated away from the eye. So the magnification stretches the binocular disparities from their previous size, and creates an artificial stereoscopic effect rotating the horopter towards, and the objects perceived, away from that eye. This rotation does not accord with tactile space, or with any monocular depth perception clues. It is called the **geometric effect**, because the degree of rotation can be calculated. The formula is:

$$\tan a = (m-1)/(m+1)\,d/a$$

If a meridional size lens is set in front of one eye with its axis horizontal, it produces a vertical magnification. This does not produce horizontal disparities between the eyes and so would not be expected to affect the

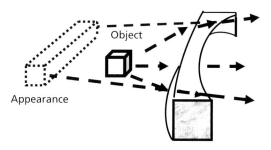

Figure 6.22   Meridional magnification in the horizontal meridian only. The lens is afocal in both principal meridians, which do not affect vergence of light from a distant object.

fronto-parallel plane. In fact, the effect of such a lens is the same as a horizontally magnifying lens placed before the other eye. Because this effect cannot be calculated (although it can be measured) it is called the **induced effect** (Ogle, 1938). More than a small vertical magnification would produce vertical diplopia. **Oblique magnification** at 45 degrees, or at 135 degrees, produces a **tilt** away from the vertical plane, of the fronto-parallel plane about a horizontal axis (Fig. 6.23). Magnification along the meridian 45 degrees in the right eye, and along 135 degrees in the left eye, produces a

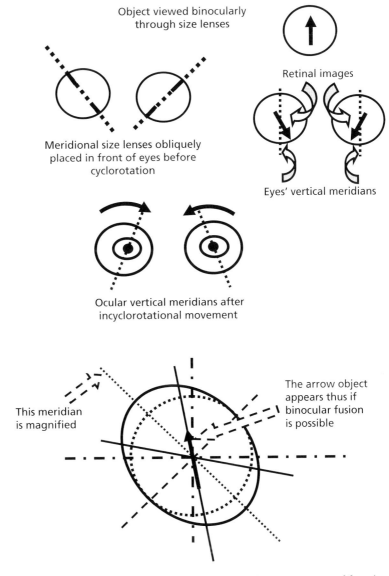

Figure 6.23 Oblique magnification. The perceptual consequences of fused retinal images, which have been modified by oblique orientation of binocular meridional size lenses. There is a tilt, away from the vertical, of the fronto-parallel plane.

tilt or **inclination** of the upper part of the fronto-parallel plane towards the subject. The opposite effect is **declination.** Magnification at **other oblique axes** produces a combination of tilt and rotation. All these asymmetrical magnification effects result in either the centres of the right and left images being fused and the periphery of one image suppressed, or one eye being entirely suppressed. Alternatively, the individual learns to ignore the conflicting binocular evidence and rely upon the monocular clues to depth perception. When horizontal and vertical magnification of up to 2–3% is present (**overall magnification**), the geometric and induced effects cancel out, and no rotation of the fronto-parallel plane is seen.

Distortion of the perception of physical space

Binocular perception of tables or floors is sometimes anomalous in normal subjects. Existing or changed conditions – for example when adjusting to newly prescribed spectacles or contact lenses – can be responsible. The novel retinal images often make floor or wall surfaces appear to slope. Moveable plane surfaces allow the extent of such appearances to be demonstrated and measured. Tilting planes like those shown in Plate 6.2 are easily provided, and measurements can be made using an eikonometer such as that described by Hawkswell (see Fig. 12.3 in Chapter 12). A rule of thumb in clinical practice is that changes of over 0.75 dioptre, or astigmatism axis changes over 10 degrees are likely to cause initial spatial awareness changes.

Magnification investigation using a leaf room

Magnification effects caused by anisoeikonia, where one eye's retinal image is a different size to the other, are produced by horizontal binocular disparities. But different information about the depth of the objects viewed may be available from **monocular depth perception clues** (see section 11.1). These monocular clues include linear perspective, retinal image size and overlap of a further object by a nearer object, increased surface detail for closer objects and accommodation and motion parallax. Where binocular and monocular clues conflict, perceptive confusion can occur and the monocular clues may diminish the effect of anisoeikonia. For experimental investigation of uniocular magnification under binocular conditions, monocular clues can be removed in a **leaf room** (Fig. 6.24). In a leaf room even small amounts of meridional magnification produce a noticeable distortion in perception, and this environment is particularly suitable for investigating the subjective effects of size lenses.

6.16 Calculating curvature and tilt of the theoretical point horopter

The theoretical locus in physical space of the points imaged on corresponding points of each retina is the VMC. For the right eye, consider the angle

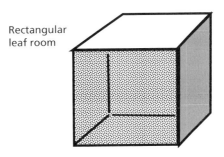

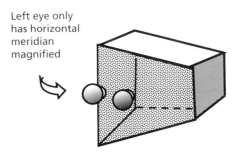

Rectangular leaf room

Left eye only has horizontal meridian magnified

Figure 6.24 The leaf room. The actual (cube) dimensions of the leaf room are apparently distorted by placing a size lens, in this case with horizontal magnification only, in front of the subject's left eye.

between the line connecting the nodal point of that eye and the fixation point, and the line connecting the nodal point and a second point away from the fixation point but still on the VMC: call this angle A_1. For the left eye consider a similar angle, A_2 (Fig. 6.25). These angles are called **external longitudinal angles**, as they are measured externally to the eye. They represent the visual directions relating to stimulated retinal elements, although the internal optics of the eye may have some unknown effect on the actual ray paths within the eyes. The subtended angle between two points in space, **angle A_1**, will be equal to **angle A_2** provided both the fixation point and the other point are both on the VMC. Next consider the situation when the fixation point remains on the VMC but the second point (**C**) is not on the VMC but either in front or behind it. A new angle, **angle A_3**, is formed. Because **C** is not on the VMC, **angle A_3** does not equal angle A_1 and angle A_2. This situation would occur using the grid nonius method of determining the apparent fronto-parallel plane where one eye's image was magnified compared with the other eye. Both eyes view a fixation point, a thin vertical rod, binocularly. The second point, also a vertical rod, is viewed by one eye seeing its upper half and the other eye seeing its lower half. Where the retinal image of one eye is **magnified** compared with the other eye, the two halves of the second rod are perceived as being in the same direction, but are displaced in physical space. The **relative magnification (R)** of the right and left eye images is given by the formula:

$$R = \tan A_1 / \tan A_2$$

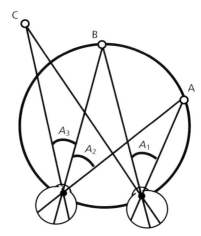

Figure 6.25 External longitudinal angles and the VMC. Any object point on the VMC stimulates corresponding retinal points, and the perception is that the object points are on the fronto-parallel plane. Any object point not on the VMC is not imaged on corresponding retinal points, and the perception is that the objects are not in the fronto-parallel plane (see also Fig. 6.1). Here both eyes fixate object B, and the external angles A_1 and A_2 are equal. This is because both objects A and B are on the VMC. Object C is not on the VMC, and the external longitudinal angle A_3 does not equal A_1 and A_2.

where there is no relative magnification then $R = 1$, and the angle of an object relative to the fixation point is the same in **physical space** as in **visual space**. For example, if the angles A_1 and A_2 were both 10 degrees, then:

$$R = \tan 10°/\tan 10° = 1.00$$

where there **is** a relative magnification between the two eyes, the objects will be perceived to lie in the same direction in visual space, but will no longer be at the same place in physical space, and R will not equal **1**. For example, the left eye's image will be magnified relative to the right eye when $A_1 > A_2$ and then $R < 1$. Say $A_1 = 10$ degrees and $A_2 = 8$ degrees, then:

$$R = \tan 10°/\tan 8° = 0.176/0.141 = 1.248$$

Similarly, if changes in angle A_2 are plotted against R, both the relative magnification and the subjective tilt of the horopter can be found. This is done by plotting the graph of:

$$R = H (\tan A_2) + R_0$$

where H is the slope of the plot and R_0 is the y-axis intercept.

For a full and well-illustrated discussion of the possible shape of the horopter with different amounts of convergence, elevation and torsional (rotational) effects associated with fixation in tertiary positions of gaze, see Schreiber *et al.* (2006).

Chapter 6: Revision quiz

Complete the missing words, perhaps in pencil.

The surface in physical space where objects may be placed, and each object is seen as single, is called the _____ (1). The circle connecting the fixation point and the nodal points of each eye has been suggested as such a surface and is called the _____ (2) circle. It is also known as the theoretical _____ (3). Measurement of the apparent fronto-parallel horopter is achieved by asking a subject to fixate a central rod and move adjacent rods so that they appear in the _____ (4) plane. The identical visual directions horopter is measured by observing the stationary fixation rod, and also a non-fixated moveable rod, the top of which is seen by one eye and the bottom by the other. This rod is moved until the two halves appear to be in the _____ (5) direction. Where the same object is imaged on each retina but with different image sizes for each eye, the condition of _____ (6) is present.

Answers
(1) horopter; (2) Vieth–Müller; (3) horopter; (4) same; (5) same; (6) anisoeikonia.

Chapter 7

THE EXTRINSIC, OR EXTRA-OCULAR, MUSCLES

A study of binocular vision must involve knowledge of extra-ocular muscle (EOM) actions, and anatomical arrangement. While greatest detail is provided by Bron *et al.* (1997) and not essential here, much simpler information is found in the English translation of Saude (1993). The present selection and emphasis draws on many sources helpful for most undergraduate and professional purposes. Some matters of recent interest and suggestions for further study are included.

Relatively simple mechanical views of ocular kinematics have been popular for many years, but recently challenges have arisen, based on new histology, magnetic resonance imaging (MRI) scans and other techniques. There is now attention to the layers of the muscles and their effective origins, involving pulley sleeves with attachments to the orbit, which change the effective direction of the muscle actions when the gaze alters. There is some evidence that sympathetic, as well as parasympathetic, neural involvement takes place. The vexed matter of possible proprioception persists.

7.1 Eye movements and the EOM

Horizontal eye movements, around a vertical (z) axis, are chiefly produced by the medial rectus (MR) for adduction and convergence and the lateral rectus (LR) for abduction and divergence of the lines of sight (visual axes). Vertical eye movements around the horizontal x-axis (normal to the z- and y-axes) are mostly caused by contractions of the superior and inferior recti (SR and IR). The former is anatomically associated with movement of the upper eyelid by the levator muscle.

The superior and inferior oblique (SO and IO) muscles have prominent cyclorotational actions around the y-axis (the line of sight), causing extorsion or intorsion of the top of the eyeball. These muscles have secondary actions, to be described later, depending on their insertions into the eye, their origins and where the eye is looking. The superior oblique has an effective origin at the **trochlea**, acting as a pulley, through which its superior oblique tendon passes, determining the direction of its pull. Muscle sleeve effects on other muscle actions are considered below. The IO, the shortest of these muscles, has its origin on the orbital floor, some 37 mm on the anterior nasal side; it

---

Normal Binocular Vision: theory, investigation and practical aspects. By David Stidwill and Robert Fletcher. © 2011 Blackwell Publishing Ltd

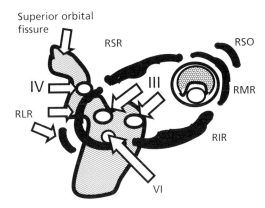

Figure 7.1 The annulus of Zinn. The origins of the extra-ocular muscle, other than the inferior oblique muscle. The levator palpebris superioris originates just above the central annulus. After Whitnall (1932). RIR, right inferior rectus; RLR, right lateral rectus; RMR, right medial rectus; RSO, right superior oblique; RSR, right superior rectus.

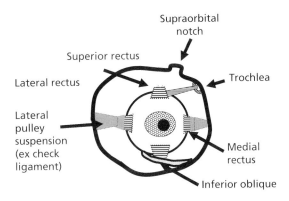

Distance from muscle insertion to limbus

Muscle	Average (mm)	Likely range
medial rectus	6	5.5 to 7.00
lateral rectus	7	6.7 to 7.10
superior rectus	8	6.5 to 11
inferior rectus	6.5	5.5 to 8.00

Figure 7.2 The spiral of Tillaux, right orbit, front view. The superior oblique tendon from the trochlea lies under the superior rectus, and the inferior oblique under the inferior rectus.

passes back to its insertion in the posterior lateral quadrant of the globe. The other EOM originate at the back of the orbit in the **annulus of Zinn,** which is approximately circular (Fig. 7.1). The recti are inserted around, and just behind, the limbus in the **spiral of Tillaux,** shown in Fig. 7.2.

The globe is supported by orbital fat and by the fascia bulbi, Tenon's capsule (a somewhat spherical sheath of fibrous tissue), which extends back from the conjunctiva to the optic nerve's dural covering; this capsule has loose attachments to the EOM and orbital sides and rim, forming hammock-like septa. Inferiorly, a structure historically called the ligament of Lockwood merges with inframedial smooth muscle. Formerly the name 'check ligaments' was used for various supports chiefly associated with the EOM, now regarded as pulley suspensions, or double insertions, giving support from attachments to the orbital walls. The extent to which ocular rotations are restricted by these elastin, collagen and smooth muscle bands is debatable; formerly fascial intervention was considered to graduate and to smooth saccades. The sheath of the SR attaches anteriorly to the levator muscle, both muscles sharing the same branch of the third cranial nerve, so elevation of the globe occurs with that of the upper eyelid. Figs 7.3 and 7.4 indicate the positions.

Ocular rotation takes place around a locus at the centre of the eye – a small volume rather than a 'centre' of rotation – known as the centrode.

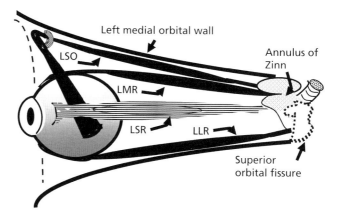

Figure 7.3 Left orbit from above. LLR, left lateral rectus; LMR, left medial rectus; LSO, left superior oblique; LSR, left superior rectus.

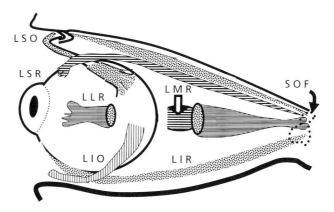

Figure 7.4 Left orbit, side view. LIO, left inferior oblique; LIR, left inferior rectus; LLR, left lateral rectus; LMR, left medial rectus; LSO, left superior oblique; LSR, left superior rectus; SOF, superior orbital fissure.

The directions of eye movements depend upon the positions of the EOM, according to the starting position of the primary line of sight (visual axis), as indicated in Figs 7.5 and 7.6. The position of the centrode has been located at various distances behind the corneal apex, some 12 to 16 mm.

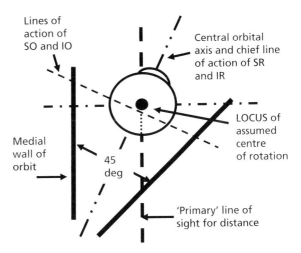

Figure 7.5 Lines of action of the vertically acting extra-ocular muscles. deg, degrees; IO, inferior oblique; IR, inferior rectus; SO, superior oblique; SR, superior rectus.

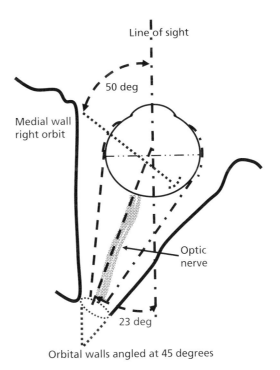

Figure 7.6 The approximate angles of the extra-ocular muscles relative to the orbital walls and optic nerve with the eye in the primary position, looking ahead.

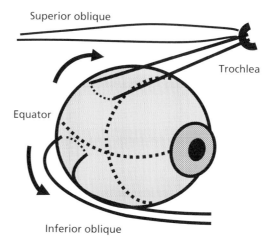

Figure 7.7 The insertions of the oblique muscles on the posterior half of the globe, with their directions of rotations of the eye.

Perkins *et al.* (1976) found a range between 11.35 and 15.33 mm on 80 subjects. Park and Park (1933) made measurements within that range with the 'centre' of rotation moving nasally during fixation changes of some 50 degrees from nasal to temporal sides. Appendix 1 (section A20) describes a simple way to locate this region. All these muscles have secondary actions, depending on their insertions into the globe, their origins and where the eye is looking. The rotational effect of the superior and inferior oblique muscles is shown in Fig. 7.7. The superior oblique has an effective origin at the trochlea, which determines the direction of its pull. Fig. 7.8 and Table 7.1 indicate the complexity of the co-operative muscle actions.

7.2 Origins and insertions

The recti muscles contact the eyeball tangentially, then move close to the globe of the eye to insertions at tendons. The insertions of the oblique muscles are shown in Figs 7.9 and 7.10, while Figs 7.11 and 7.12 reveal the vertical and torsional actions involved. The directions of the primary line of sight (visual axis) and the angles at which the tendons reach the eye determine the primary and secondary actions of each EOM; in practice, the effects of the muscle sleeves (pulleys) influence such actions, as they act as effective origins. Some elementary insight is provided by personal construction of an ophthalmotrope, described in Appendix 1 (section A14).

Well-established opinions identify the influences of orbital periosteum and two distinct layers of each EOM. The global layer is distinctly adherent to the eyeball. A more orbital layer is associated with the orbital fascia, and some efferent nerve supply is present, so there are distinctive differences in muscular and neural composition between these layers. As long ago as 1932, Whitnall described Fisher's 1904 consideration of some 'pulley' actions

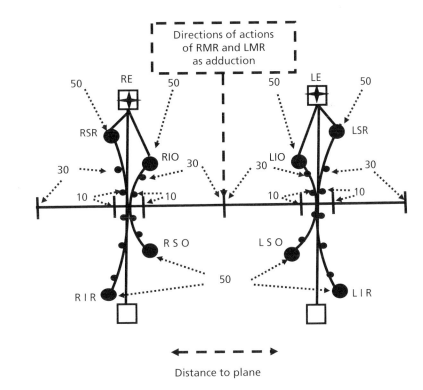

Figure 7.8 Actions of muscles shown by lines traced by the line of sight on a sheet of glass viewed at the distance indicated, through which the observer views the traces from the other side. Hering's representation, modified by Tschermak, and further modified. The superior rectus elevates, with incycloduction and adduction actions. The combined actions of the superior rectus and inferior oblique result in vertical elevation, shown as a star within a box. Note: both superior rectus and superior oblique produce incycloduction when the eye is in the primary position of gaze. All these muscles have secondary actions, depending upon their insertions into the globe, their origins and where the eye is looking. The rotational effects of the superior and inferior oblique muscles are shown in Fig. 7.7. The superior oblique has an effective origin at the trochlea, which determines the direction of its pull (see Table 7.1). LE, left eye; LIO, left inferior oblique; LIR, left inferior rectus; LMR, left medial rectus; LSO, left superior oblique; LSR, left superior rectus; RE, right eye; RIO, right inferior oblique; RIR, right inferior rectus; RMR, right medial rectus; RSO, right superior oblique; RSR, right superior rectus.

involving the areas where the sheathes of the EOM pierce the fascia (Whitnall, 1932). Developments of this idea are described later in section 7.4.

7.3   The innervation of the extra-ocular muscles

The cerebral cortex sends commands for eye movements along the **medial longitudinal fasciculus,** which serves the coordination of normal impulses to the EOM. These commands reach the appropriate cranial nerve nuclei in the midbrain.

The **oculomotor (III) nerve** has nuclei to the right and left of the midline. Most of the oculomotor nerve fibres travel directly to the ipsilateral EOM,

Table 7.1 Extra-ocular muscle actions in primary and other gaze positions

Muscle (Nerve supply) (Origin and course)	Gaze	Main action	Secondary action	Tertiary action
Medial rectus (III nerve) (Annulus of Zinn then follows orbital axis)	Primary	Adducts	None	None
	Upgaze	Adducts	Elevates	None
	Downgaze	Adducts	Depresses	None
Lateral rectus (VI nerve) (Annulus of Zinn and lateral orbit wall)	Primary	Abducts	None	None
	Upgaze	Abducts	Elevates	None
	Downgaze	Abducts	Depresses	None
Superior rectus (III nerve) (Annulus of Zinn and above orbit axis and optic nerve)	Primary	Elevates	Incycloduction	Adducts
	23 abduct	Elevates	None	None
	54 adduct	Incycloduction	Elevates	None
Inferior rectus (III nerve)	Primary	Depresses	Excycloduction	Adducts
	23 abduct	Depresses	None	None
	54 adduct	Excycloduction	Depresses	None
Superior oblique (IV nerve)	Primary	Incycloduction	Depresses	Abducts
	36 abduct	Incycloduction	None	None
	54 adduct	Depresses	None	None
Inferior oblique (III nerve)	Primary	Excycloduction	Elevates	Abducts
	39 abduct	Excycloduction	None	None
	51 adduct	Elevates	None	None

The terms 'upgaze' and 'downgaze' refer to the muscle actions in the specified direction of gaze. The numbers 23, 54 and so on refer to the primary, secondary and tertiary effects of the specified muscle when the line of sight/visual axis is moved horizontally by the specified number of degrees in the direction stated. Thus 'Superior rectus III 23 Abduct' means the primary, secondary and tertiary effects of the superior rectus muscle, when the eye is abducted by 23 degrees.

the LR, MR and IR, while those destined for the SR cross over and pass within the third nerve branches to the opposite orbit. Fig. 7.13 indicates the locations of the different parts of the nucleus. Emerging at the front of the brain stem, the oculomotor nerves pass forward through the cranium, via the cavernous plexus, to divide into two main branches before entering the orbit through the superior orbital fissure, inside the annulus of Zinn. The appropriate nerves separate to enter the muscles towards the rear of each one.

The trochlear (IV) nerve nuclei lie next to the oculomotor nuclei, but the IV nerve fibres cross over to innervate the SO of the opposite eye. Each of these nerves is thin and relatively long, leaving the midbrain on the dorsal aspect, then running round the peduncle forwards and almost joining the third nerve before penetrating the belly of the SO as several small branches; it does not reach the trochlea.

Each **abducens (VI) nerve** leaves its nucleus via the lower part of the pons in several initial branches, and fibres proceed to the ipsilateral eye, upwards through the cavernous plexus and the superior orbital fissure to the medial region of the lateral rectus (Fig. 7.14). Before reaching the cavernous plexus,

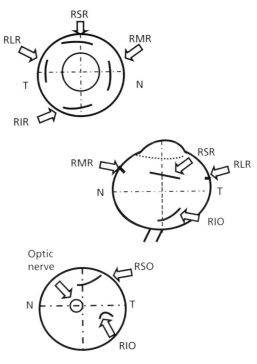

Figure 7.9 The insertions of the extra-ocular muscles in the right eye. After Salzmann (1912). N, nasal; RIO, right inferior oblique; RIR, right inferior rectus; RLR, right lateral rectus; RMR, right medial rectus; RSO, right superior oblique; RSR, right superior rectus; T, temporal.

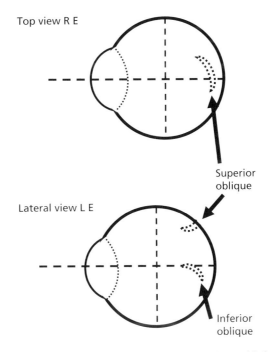

Figure 7.10 Schema of oblique muscle insertions of right and left eyes from two aspects (after Merkel and Kallius (1901) and other sources). LE, left eye; RE, right eye.

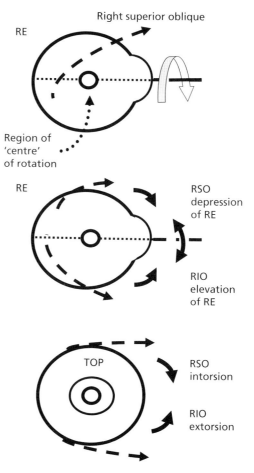

Figure 7.11 The oblique muscles, right eye, after Spooner (1957). The ocular rotations of these muscles, in concert with the rectus muscles, are shown. RE, right eye; RIO, right inferior oblique; RSO, right superior oblique.

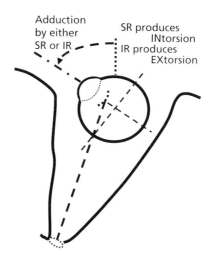

Figure 7.12 Adduction of the right eye. When the right eye is adducted, the superior rectus (SR) produces intorsion, and the inferior rectus (IR) produces extorsion. Both produce adduction in this position.

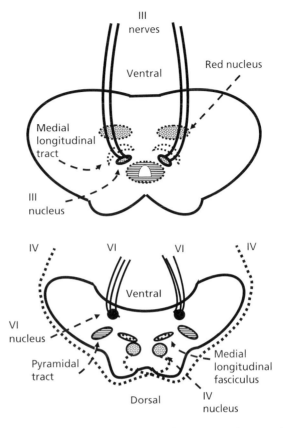

Figure 7.13 Cranial nerve nuclei related to the extra-ocular muscles. The third nerve nucleus is shown at a higher level of section, the fourth nerve and the sixth nerve lower down. Note the decussation of the fourth nerve and its movement around the peduncular mass.

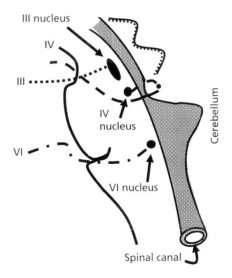

Figure 7.14 Lateral view of extra-ocular muscles' cranial nerve nuclei and initial origins.

the nerve bends over the petrosal section of the frontal bone, a somewhat dangerous manoeuvre.

7.4 Pulley sleeves

Some 16 mm behind the insertions of the recti on the globe, Demer (2007) has described pulley sleeves in an extensive review of orbital mechanics (Fig. 7.15). The muscles move through these sleeves, which have been termed double insertions of EOM by Ruskell *et al.* (2005) in an extensive research report, considering implications of the 'active pulley hypothesis' and the influences of the presence of smooth muscle fibres. Just as the trochlea acts as an oblique region from which a muscle running along from the back of the orbit passes, so the sleeves form secondary origins for the EOM. New movements of the eye probably influence the positions and tractions of the pulleys, suggested in Fig. 7.16. Side slipping during globe rotation is more restricted than was formerly thought, and significant movements of the sleeves as indicated in Fig. 7.17 should somewhat vary the muscle actions. Listing's law (see section 8.13) may well be simplified by these structures, which contain collagen, elastin and varied amounts of smooth muscle in their suspensions. There is evidence of the involvement of the superior cervical ganglion, nitrous oxide from the pterygio-palatine ganglion and neurotransmitters such as acetylcholine. Very complex commutative mechanical activity is probably involved, rather than just neural controls of the mechanics of the EOM. Some of the recent discoveries have been based on MRI and fresh histological studies.

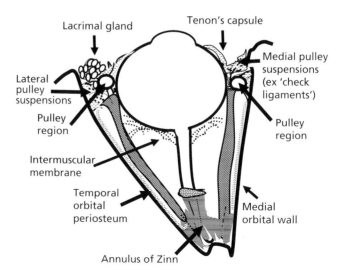

Figure 7.15 View of the left orbit from above. The medial and lateral pulley suspensions, previously described as 'check ligaments', are shown.

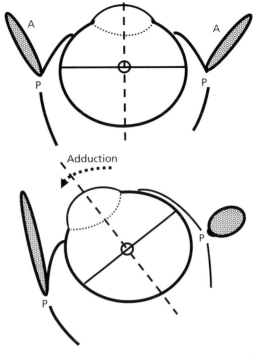

Adduction

Figure 7.16 Possible movements of pulleys (P) and fascial attachments (A) as the right eye moves from the primary position into adduction. Modified after Demer (2007).

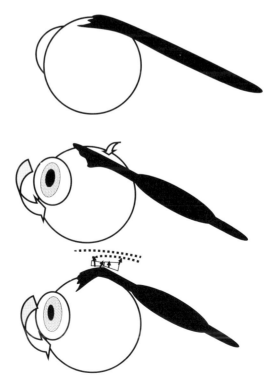

Figure 7.17 Possible extra-ocular muscle slippage over the globe on rotation. The lowest sketch follows recent proposals that a 'double insertion' sleeve of pulley attachment to the orbital wall prevents the slip.

7.5 Muscle structure and function

The term 'motor unit' introduced by Sherrington is used to describe neurones stimulating muscle fibres. As age progresses, fewer muscle fibres appear in the EOM, while variations in the number of neural elements seem to be smaller. Muscle fibres mostly terminate in the middle regions of the muscles, the slower *felderstruktur* fibres being in a minority compared with those of *fibrillenstruktur* type. The distinction is emphasised in Fig. 7.18. Three varieties of nerve termination are present on the tendons of the EOM. Muscle spindles are present, although some appear to be inoperative in the usual manner, while 'false spindles' have been described. The schematic view of a muscle spindle in Fig. 7.19 indicates the afferent and efferent supplies, with a transverse sectional representation in Fig. 7.20.

The EOM differ from skeletal muscles: for instance, myosin in the EOM fibres somewhat resembles relatively undeveloped skeletal muscles. Kjellevold-Haugen (2001) presented clear indications of different morphologies among a range of animals. Muscle fibres are built from filaments of

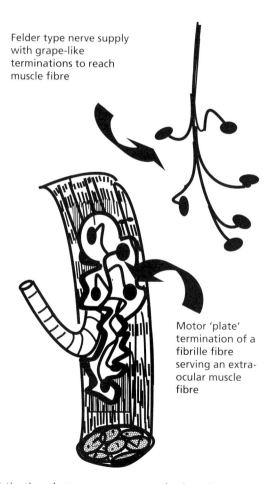

Felder type nerve supply with grape-like terminations to reach muscle fibre

Motor 'plate' termination of a fibrille fibre serving an extra-ocular muscle fibre

Figure 7.18 Distinctions between neuromuscular junctions on muscle fibres.

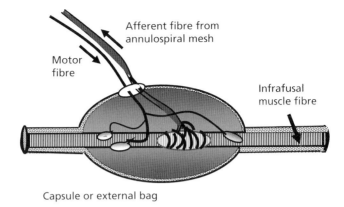

Figure 7.19 Stylised view of muscle spindle or stretch receptor.

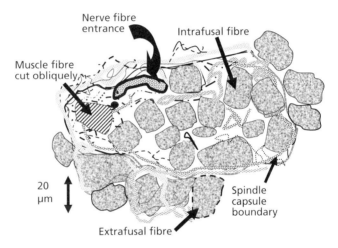

Figure 7.20 Transverse section of muscle spindle at nerve entry, some muscle fibres outside the capsule. Scheme based on preparations by Ruskell (1989) and Bruenech and Ruskell (2001).

protein, which combine to form long microfibrils. These filaments are rearranged during muscle contraction, sliding in relationship to each other, and there are some elastic elements within muscles, contributing to movements of the main body. The characteristic striations are produced by variations in proteinous content, and the two main types of fibres, *felderstruktur* and *fibrillenstruktur*, show several anatomical and functional differences. Fibrille fibres are innervated through a motor 'plate' termination (*en plaque*), where an action potential is produced, rapidly resulting in uniform contraction by depolarisation as a twitch reaction. It amounts to an all-or-nothing event. These fibres are found as several subtypes, reaching the EOM at about its mid region. Büttner-Ennever (2007) has labelled the twitch muscle fibres with a single end-plate zone 'SIF'. Also the label 'MIF' was applied to non-twitching muscle fibres having multiple end-plate zones, which mammalian

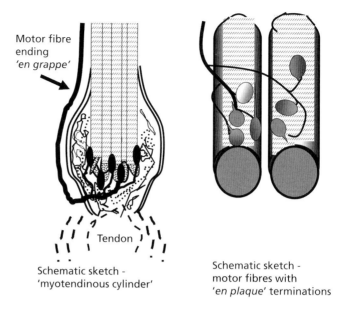

Motor fibre
ending
'en grappe'

Tendon

Schematic sketch -
'myotendinous cylinder'

Schematic sketch -
motor fibres with
'en plaque' terminations

Figure 7.21 Types of neuromuscular junctions found for extra-ocular muscle. The *'palisade en grappe'* junction between muscle and junction was described by Ruskell (1978).

muscles do not usually have. Only in mammals, 'palisade-ending' nerve terminations are found in the MIF zones of the global layer of the EOM. These neural 'cuffs', or fences, at myotendinous junctions are possibly sensory, even combining motor functions for a few muscle fibres. Figs 7.21 and 7.22 further illustrate some features of varieties of innervation, spindles and Golgi structures with motor and sensory aspects related to alterations in muscles and tendons.

Neuromuscular junctions

The felder fibres are supplied with nerve fibres, the terminals of which are widely spread and end in grape-like buttons (*en grappe*) and restricting the muscle contractions to small localities. However, the scattered effect can affect the whole muscle fibre. Often a palisade ending is characteristic of these nerve endings, where they bend back into the muscle endings and they feature in the global layer of the EOM. At each end the EOM merges with tendinous attachments. Tendon receptors appear not to be required for infant human binocular function. Bruenech and Ruskell (2001 reported that myotendinous nerve endings, found in adult specimens, did not feature in very young specimens, although some Golgi tendon (GT) organs appear to be present in neonates. Reports of such GT organs tend to vary in the literature concerning the EOM, and these organs may not operate very conventionally in young children.

Muscle insertions into the eyeball show a transition between myelinated muscle fibres and tendon material, with nerve endings that show many

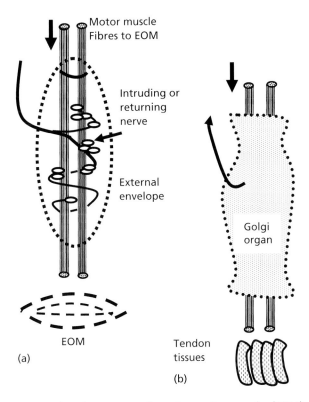

Figure 7.22 Encapsulated structures in extra-ocular muscle (EOM). **(a)** Muscle spindles, stretch receptors as in skeletal muscles. Sensory nerve fibres spiral around muscle fibres. Motor nerve fibres take similar courses, damping the host muscle activity. **(b)** Golgi organs are associated with tendons, possibly detecting changes in position, size and stretch, and sending sensory messages. The afferent nerve fibres twine around encapsulated fibres and leave through the wall of the enclosure.

encapsulated 'palisade' terminations with recurrent directions. The term 'myotendinous cylinders' was used by Ruskell (1978). Debate arose as to possible sensory functions, in addition to the likely motor activity (Ruskell, 1989, 1999). There were changes as age increased. Muscle spindles (favourite candidates for proprioception) were considered to be unlikely to have this function, perhaps augmenting spatial perception, and similar doubt was cast on the role of myotendinous cylinders. The issue is not really resolved, and Bruenech (1996) suitably indicated the need to reconcile retinal image displacements with eye movements, which should follow objects of regard. When receptors within the EOM fail to contribute to this requirement, how else can this be achieved? Thus, when the 'displacement–cancellation hypothesis' fails, one tends to turn to **efference copy** (also known as 'corollary discharge'). Efference copy is a memory of eye position that is used to facilitate oculomotor movements, and to recognise the location of visual percepts. Efference copy is part of the way that an internal mapping of a subject's surrounding physical space is obtained. It is present for willed movements of the eyes, and also reflex movements such as saccadic, smooth pursuit and the rapid element of optokinetic nystagmus (Leigh and Zee, 2006). It is responsible for the phenomenon of past-pointing in oculomotor paresis.

Efferent or afferent neural activity?

'Proprioception' was Sherrington's classical term for the reflex coordination of information from receptors in skeletal muscles, as the body moves and adjusts posture. Sherrington evidently tended to consider possible conscious sense of eye position. Assuming the EOM as a special type of skeletal muscle, rich in felder and fibrille fibres, sending afferent proprioceptive messages, information reaching the brain could influence refinements of motor control. Is it likely that extensive training can teach human subjects such skills? Cooper *et al.* (1955) provided information about the activity of muscle spindles in quadrupeds' extrinsic eye muscles. GT organs are attractive candidates for afferent sources in human EOM activity, as mentioned above.

Afferent and efferent routes might be working in tandem. In Southall's translation of his textbook (Helmholtz, 1924), Helmholtz considered muscular effort to lead to muscle tension, with contractions being 'felt'. He mentioned the 'feeling of' EOM innervation. Von Kries (1925), in his third appendix to Southall's translation, tended to discredit such EOM sensations; even Helmholtz appears to have concentrated on retinal clues related to innervation. Feelings from external palpebral areas have to be considered as possibly providing information about eye position.

In the modern literature, the importance of efference copy is found, for example, in Carpenter's (1977) extensive discussion of the possibilities of proprioceptive input. Fig. 7.23 illustrates the basic principle. The motor

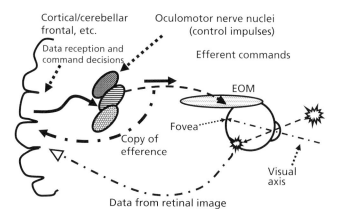

Figure 7.23 Possible 'efference copy' routes from the image on the inferior retina, requiring reflex eye movement upwards for eye fixation. 'EOM' merely represents the group of extra-ocular muscles involved.

instructions sent to the EOM might be adequately monitored to give clues as to eye position; this efference copy, or 'outflow', would require some special cortical interpretation. Various experiments were mentioned by Carpenter, who proposed that at least some movement of a retinal image is needed when sensing external movement; this would have to be interpreted in terms of a matching eye movement (Carpenter, 1977). Structures external to the orbit have already been mentioned.

7.6   Blood supply

The EOM have the greatest blood flow of body muscular tissue. Small branches of the ophthalmic artery, often with some variations, supply them. The lacrimal artery is involved for some of the muscles, usually including the LR and SR. Other muscles are supplied by terminations from the medial and lateral branches of the ophthalmic artery. Anterior ciliary arteries are frequently visible as they penetrate the tendons of the recti. Both superior and inferior veins are involved with drainage from the EOM in their vicinities, via muscular veins, the flow proceeding backwards and partly to the facial veins.

7.7   Extra-orbital activity

Unfortunately, normal human functions are often understood more easily after the study of their disorders. Also some applications to human function are derived from knowledge of animal physiology. It is useful now to consider activity that can supplement that of the EOM.

Normal eye movements may be influenced by eyelid position and movement. The contribution of Helmchen and Rambold (2007) included a review of an extensive literature concerning eyelid effects on vision and eye movement. Eye closure and blinking have links with the results of EOM activity. Bell's phenomenon is well known; it may allow some of the cornea to avoid trauma. In Bell's phenomenon the orbicularis muscle contracting as a reflex protective response tends to be accompanied by supraversion of the eyes. Normal binocular blinking, rather than monocular winking, is likely to induce eye movement, and the controls of the levator muscle are located close to the third nerve nuclei; vertical eye movement control is associated with Cajal's interstitial nucleus.

Ocular saccades are linked with supra-nuclear control that is co-coordinated with movement of the eyelids, via the medial longitudinal fasciculus. There are burst neurons associated with the para-median pontine reticular areas. Pontine omnipause neurons are also related to saccadic function, but their activity is somewhat inhibited by blinking. In addition, blinking brings complex influences on vergences and a variety of refined eye movements, some of which are useful, while others tend to reduce efficiency of the visual system.

Chapter 7: Revision quiz

(1) Which of these statements is most correct?
  (a) All but one of the EOM are controlled by the cranial nerve – called the 'abducens', as it has an important function in abducting the eyeball.
  (b) Felder muscle fibres are reported to have slower actions than the other main variety of fibres operating in the EOM.
  (c) It is the *fibrillenstruktur* muscle fibres that are innervated by nerve fibres with *en grappe* multiple terminations.
  (d) The superior rectus shares the same cranial nerve supply as the superior oblique muscle.

(2) A trainee surgeon intends to perform an operation for strabismus. His supervisor asks him to confirm which two rectus muscles are likely to be inserted **nearer** to the limbus than the lateral rectus. Thinking it through, rather confused, he manages to think of the correct reply, as follows. Which of his thoughts is most correct?
  (a) The LR is probably the nearest to the limbus, so any of the others should qualify.
  (b) All of the tendon insertions are over 7.5 mm from the limbus. Which do I say?
  (c) The two nearer than the LR must be the SR and the IR.
  (d) The MR is obviously nearest to the limbus. That is one, and the other is probably the IR, perhaps because the eye is so often looking downwards.

(3) Ocular movements can be around one of three main axes. Which of these statements is most correct?
  (a) Extorsion is caused either by the SO or the IO; also the IR rather than the SR.
  (b) The annulus of Zinn is related in some way to all the EOM, except the SO.
  (c) In adults the 'centre' of ocular rotation is always between 8 and 10 mm from the apex of the cornea.

(4) Over the last decade opinions about double insertions of human rectus muscles have been developed. In this connection, select the statement most likely to be acceptable:
  (a) It is most unlikely that during adduction, side slipping of the SR could be reduced, although pulley sleeves do contain some smooth muscle fibres.
  (b) In adults, pulley sleeves are usually located between 14 and 18 mm behind the ocular insertions of the SR, LR and MR.
  (c) The EOM have more *felderstruktur* fibres than *fibrillenstruktur* fibres, and the latter have much slower responses.

Answers
(1) b; (2) a; (3) a; (4) b.

Chapter 8
EYE MOVEMENTS

8.1 Monocular and binocular eye movements

The clinical name of monocular eye movements is **ductions**. They are classified as:

- elevation or supraduction – the eye moves up
- depression or infraduction – the eye moves down
- abduction – the eye moves temporally
- adduction – the eye moves medially
- excycloduction or extorsion – the right eye moves anticlockwise from an observer's point of view (or clockwise from the eye's point of view); the left eye rotates in the opposite direction
- incycloduction or intorsion – the right eye moves clockwise from an observer's point of view; the left eye rotates in the opposite direction.

For elevation the superior rectus and inferior oblique muscles contract, and the inferior rectus and superior oblique relax. For depression those muscles reverse their actions. For abduction the lateral rectus contracts and the medial rectus relaxes. For adduction those muscles reverse their actions. For excycloduction the inferior rectus and the inferior oblique contract, and the superior rectus and the superior oblique relax. For incycloduction those muscles reverse their actions.

Synonyms for individual eye movements:

- supraduction/sursumduction/elevation
- infraduction/deorsumduction/depression
- incycloduction/intorsion
- excycloduction/extorsion.

The **extent** of duction eye movements changes with age, and is most extensive in teenagers compared with the elderly. Schectman *et al.*, (2005) have given measurements of 58 (47) degrees for abduction, 47 (36) degrees for adduction, 50 (34) degrees for supraduction and 58 (44) degrees for infraduction, in subjects aged 14 to 19 years old (with the figures for 80 to 95 years old in brackets). There is no evidence for neuronal changes causing this reduction in eye movement. There is evidence of inferior displacement of the horizontal rectus muscles in old age causing reduced supraduction.

Normal Binocular Vision: theory, investigation and practical aspects. By David Stidwill and Robert Fletcher. © 2011 Blackwell Publishing Ltd

The clinical name for binocular eye movements is **versions**, where the eyes move together in the same direction (conjugate), and **vergences**, where the eyes make disjunctive movements of convergence or divergence. There are three classes of **binocular gaze position**:

- primary position of gaze: in which the eyes look straight ahead into the distance
- secondary position of gaze: in which the eyes move vertically (up or down) or horizontally (to left or right)
- tertiary position of gaze: in which the eyes move to an oblique position (e.g. up and to the right).

There are nine **positions of gaze**. These comprise the six **cardinal** (or diagnostic) **positions of gaze**, which are the diagnostic directions used in the motility test (see section 12.3 in Chapter 12), and supraversion, infraversion and the primary direction of gaze.

Note: different authors use the term 'cardinal' to refer to: (1) the six diagnostic positions of gaze for motility; (2) the diagnostic positions and the primary direction of gaze (making seven); (3) all nine positions of gaze; or (4) in relation to Listing's law, the primary direction of gaze and the four secondary positions of gaze not involving torsion – namely, up, down, left and right (making a total of five). It might best to avoid the use of the word 'cardinal'!

Versions are classed as:

- supraversion: the eyes move upwards together
- infraversion: the eyes move downwards together
- dextroversion: the eyes both move to the subject's right
- laevoversion: the eyes both move to the subject's left.

Vergences are classed as:

- supravergence: only one eye elevates
- infravergence: only one eye is depressed
- excyclovergence: the eyes rotate along the anteroposterior axis, right eye anticlockwise, left eye clockwise, seen from the front
- incyclovergence: the opposite rotation to excyclovergence
- convergence: both eyes adduct (positive vergence)
- divergence: both eyes abduct (negative vergence).

8.2 Neurological control and psycho-optical reflexes

The initiation of eye movements can arise from voluntary innervation, and from the psycho-optical reflexes, or from the postural reflexes. Cortical control of eye movements is found in the parastriate region: Brodmann anatomical areas 18 and 19 (functional area V2). The eye movement fields

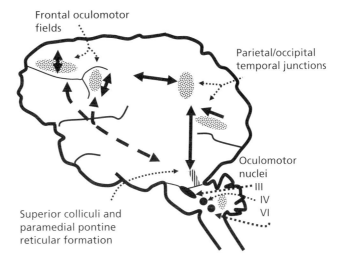

Frontal oculomotor
fields

Parietal/occipital
temporal junctions

Oculomotor
nuclei
III
IV
VI

Superior colliculi and
paramedial pontine
reticular formation

Figure 8.1 The brain areas associated with eye movement ('eye movement fields'). The eye movement fields are shaded, and arrows show the directions of eye movements involved.

here are closely related to retinal sensory representation: they are said to be 'retinotopic'. They are involved in initiating smooth pursuit, saccades and the optokinetic response. The motor control pathway leaves the visual cortex along the optic radiations via the **occipito-mesencephalic tract** to the **medial longitudinal fasciculus** and the oculomotor nerve nuclei (see Figs 8.1 and 8.2).

Secondary sensory/motor visual processing is found in the parietal-occipital area initiating the smooth pursuit following reflex based on visual detection of the three-dimensional direction and velocity of moving objects.

The fine control of gaze stabilisation and of all types of eye movement is mediated by structures within the cerebellum. There are oculomotor connections between the cerebellum and the frontal cortex and from there to the superior colliculus (see also section 2.2 in Chapter 2).

The frontal cortex controls voluntary limb and eye movements. Both visually initiated saccades and those that are triggered by memory have an input here from the frontal eye fields.

More detail is given in Leigh and Zee (2006).

The psycho-optical reflexes

The psycho-optical reflexes appear to be conditioned reflexes that are acquired soon after birth but then become immutable. They are:

- the **fixation reflex**: a new image falling on the peripheral retina creates a sensory stimulus in the visual cortex that triggers eye movements to move the retinal image on to the fovea

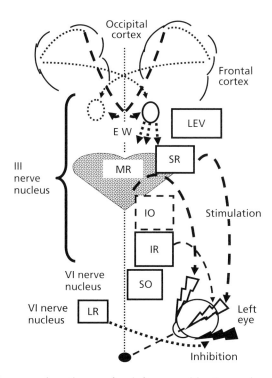

Figure 8.2 The neural pathways for left eye adduction; schematic view. The frontal and occipital cortex are involved, and also the Edinger–Westphal nucleus for other elements of the near triad. The nerve pathways for stimulation are shown, going to the medial rectus, the superior rectus and the inferior rectus; and for inhibition, going to the lateral rectus. IO, inferior oblique; IR, inferior rectus; LEV, levator; LR, lateral rectus; SO, superior oblique; SR, superior rectus.

- the **refixation reflex**: a shift in the lines of sight (visual axes) occurs to restore fixation to the original target
- the **version reflex or following reflex**: a conjugate eye movement to allow binocular foveal fixation on a moving target
- the **vergence reflex**: a disjunctive eye movement of convergence or divergence – this enables bifoveal fixation on an approaching or receding target
- the **fusion reflex**: this aligns the right and left eyes sufficiently precisely to allow binocular perception and stereopsis.

Reflexes may be and usually are combined, e.g. when looking from a near object on the left to a further object on the right. When a series of targets cross the visual field, the fixation and refixation reflexes organise the lines of sight to fixate each of the targets in turn. This effect is called **optokinetic nystagmus**, or **OKN**. The OKN consists of a fast **fixation reflex** followed by a slow **following reflex**. The fixation reflex is mediated by the **saccadic eye movement system**, and the following reflex by the **pursuit eye movement system**. Some of these reflexes occur with both eyes, or with one eye only if the change of fixation is along the line of sight of one eye. With both eyes involved, the reflexes may operate differently on each eye. For example, where a subject wears a powered spectacle lens in front of one eye and a zero power lens in front of the other and is presented with a visual target to one side of fixation, a fixation reflex occurs for both eyes. However, the amount of eye movement is different for each eye because of the prismatic effect of one lens when a change in fixation is made. This is an example of Hering's law being modified (see section 8.11).

Spatial localisation and motor control

Subjective localisation gives information of an object's position in space relative to us (egocentric localisation) and also in relation to other objects (relative localisation). Both require information about:

- the image's retinal location
- the orientation of the lines of sight (visual axes) relative to the head
- the direction in which the head and body are pointed.

Primary line of sight (visual axis) orientation appears to be adduced in part by oculomotor command memory, in part by visual cues, and also in some circumstances by ocular muscle proprioception. Thus spatial localisation is used to trigger the fixation reflex. Ocular muscle proprioceptors would use the ophthalmic division of the trigeminal nerve and the Gasserian ganglion to the trigeminal nucleus. It is possible also that proprioceptive data would have afferent transmission using oculomotor nerves. The proprioceptive data would then be provided to cortical visual motor and sensory processing areas (Leigh and Zee, 2006). Such pathways are particularly relevant to heterophoria compensation and heterotropia eye movement control, and in other circumstances when visual cues for controlling eye movements are not fully effective.

8.3 Gaze-shifting and gaze-stabilising eye movements

Eye (and head) movements are needed to use vision properly. An object of visual interest has to be relocated from the retinal periphery and held on the fovea. Drift away from the fovea of more than four degrees per second degrades visual acuity. There are two general categories of eye movement. Movements that **shift gaze** include the smooth pursuit system and saccadic eye movements. Gaze-shifting eye movements are under voluntary control from specific areas in the cerebral cortex. Eye movements that **stabilise gaze** include the optokinetic, vestibular and visual fixation systems. Vergence movements can be used to produce both gaze shifting and gaze stabilisation. When voluntary eye movements are made in response to a visual stimulus, the visual cortex encoding of object position is transformed into neural motor commands for the desired version or vergence. The cerebellum, superior colliculus and brain stem reticular formation are involved. The brain areas or eye movement fields associated with ocular movements are shown in Fig. 8.1. A useful review by Rowe (2003) stresses the clinical value of understanding neural anatomy and physiology related to eye movements.

Gaze stabilisation is an essential element of the visuum because: (1) it allows a reference between the position of the subject and physical space; and (2) it allows visual feedback when the subject is moving. The visual fixation system has a sensory and a motor element. The sensory element is the visual fixation reflex. The motor element to maintain gaze holding is called the **neural integrator**. Even in the primary position of gaze there is a tendency for muscle tonus to pull the eyes to a mutually divergent position. For non-primary gaze directions, the orbital contents have elastic tendencies to restore the eyes towards the primary position of gaze. Therefore muscular contraction is needed to maintain an eccentric direction of gaze. On extreme eccentricity of gaze there is some reduction in quality of fixation (Abadi and Scallan, 2001).

For version eye movements, a nerve signal containing a report of both velocity and position data is transmitted by oculomotor neurons for each muscle. Cortical cells in the medial vestibular nuclei and the nucleus prepositus hypoglossi mediate horizontal non-primary gaze. For vertical gaze directions, the interstitial nucleus of Cajal and other midbrain neurons are involved. See section 1.7 in Chapter 1 for visual feedback. Information from eye movement signals is also integrated by the vestibulo-cerebellum. A failure in this network forming the neural integrator causes gaze-evoked nystagmus, and anomalies of pursuit, vestibular and optokinetic eye movements. There is evidence that some children with developmental dyslexia show interruption of fixation with square-wave fixation losses (Currie *et al.*, 1986). Completely stable retinal images are subject to fading because sensory systems habituate (diminish) their response to constant stimuli. To avoid this there is a physiological instability of eye position during attempted fixation. The instability has three components:

1. micro-saccades of up to one-third of a degree occur in any direction, although they are reduced for some demanding visual tasks (Gowen *et al.*, 2005)
2. there is an ocular tremor of up to 0.01 degrees and at the rate of up to 150 Hertz
3. there are also slow drifts of fixation of up to 0.1 degree and at a rate of up to 0.25 degrees per second.

8.4   The five oculomotor subsystems

The five oculomotor subsystems are the saccadic, smooth pursuit, vergence, vestibulo-ocular and optokinetic nystagmus subsystems. Saccadic and smooth pursuit movements are made with two eyes moving in the same direction, and both therefore are **versions**. Versions may be involuntary in response to a visual stimulus, e.g. to the fixation reflex, to sound or to tactile stimulation. They may also be voluntary: under the control of the frontal cortex oculogyric centres. An example would be an eye movement made in response to a request during ophthalmoscopy.

Saccadic eye movements are used to place an image on the fovea. They consist of a series of lateral, oblique or vertical binocular eye movements. A **smooth pursuit** eye movement maintains the image of a moving object on the fovea. The **vergence system** provides precise bifoveal fixation and therefore stereopsis, even where the eyes may need to rotate at different speeds (asymmetrical convergence) or in different directions (e.g. divergence). The **vestibulo-ocular reflex** stabilises the primary line of sight during movement of the head by moving the eyes in the opposite direction to the head. **Optokinetic nystagmus** is the eye movement response to large moving visual fields when the head is stationary.

8.5 Saccadic eye movements

Versions triggered by the fixation and refixation reflexes (for example, when reading text) are called **saccades**. These rapid eye movements (REM) occur most notably in both involuntary and voluntary fixation changes but also in REM sleep and in the quick phase of optokinetic nystagmus (Catz and Their, 2007). The control of voluntary saccades is associated with the frontal eye movement field, found in the frontal cerebral region within Brodmann area 8. Voluntary saccade control is also associated with the dorsolateral prefrontal cortex, the anterior cingulate cortex and the supplementary eye movement field (see Leigh and Zee, 2006). The supplementary eye movement field arranges the sequence of saccades needed to achieve re-fixation. Involuntary saccades that occur as a reflex to the appearance of a new non-foveal image are triggered by the parietal eye movement field, in the parietal cortex.

Both the frontal and parietal eye movement fields send innervation to the right and left superior colliculi, which are situated anteriorly to the nuclei of the third, fourth and sixth cranial nerves. Representation from the contralateral visual field is received directly from each retina and also from the striate cortex and is topographically mapped onto the dorsal colliculus layers. So the dorsal layers report visual information. Their output is to the pulvinar and lateral geniculate nucleus (LGN), and also there are some connections to the ventral layers of the colliculus. The ventral layers have oculomotor functions: the selection of visual targets, the initiation of saccades and of eye, and combined eye and head, movements. The rotational movement of the globe during a saccade is between 100 degrees and 500 degrees per second, with duration usually under 100 ms. There is a delay of about 225 ms, varying with the respective stimulus intensity of the original and new fixation target. Although the image moves rapidly across the retina, the subject has no perception of movement or blur. This is a cortical monocular visual inhibition, also present in binocular vision, called **saccadic suppression**, and is accomplished by coordination of:

- midbrain-derived conjugate motor innervation to the extra-ocular muscles (EOM)
- retinal image feedback
- proprioceptive feedback from EOM **muscle spindles**, which might report the degree of contraction in each EOM (see section 7.5 in Chapter 7).

Saccadic suppression explains the absence of oscillopsia (visual awareness of image oscillation) in congenital nystagmus. Failure of saccadic suppression is said to occur in some cases of developmental (childhood-acquired) dyslexia. Both velocity discrimination and coherent motion detection of visual input have been shown to be deficient in some dyslexics (Wexler, 2005). The failure of saccadic suppression produces motion smear, a symptom occasionally encountered in clinical practice.

8.6 Smooth pursuit eye movements

Versions initiated by following an object moving in the visual environment are known as **smooth pursuit eye movements**. The movement of an image across the retina, and particularly the central retina, is the main trigger for smooth pursuit eye movements (Robinson, 1965). A more accurate response to target movement is obtained when the observed movement is predictable. However, even proprioceptive information from non-visual input, e.g. hand and arm movement, can initiate a smooth following eye movement. The actual accuracy of smooth pursuit is affected by concentration, and decreases in the elderly. It is likely that this class of eye movement arose from the need to keep an immobile object imaged on the fovea during self-movement of the individual.

The neural pathway for smooth pursuit is:

- the retina
- the parvocellular LGN layers
- the striate cortex
- the middle temporal and middle superior temporal area secondary visual areas (see Chapter 10), then involving the pontine and vestibular nuclei
- and finally the brainstem and the third, fourth and sixth cranial nerve nuclei.

This neural control pathway for maintaining fixation in a situation when either the target or the subject is moving (or both) appears to be separate from the neural integrator system, where both are stationary. Pursuit movements follow a moving target at 30 degrees per second: they are therefore much slower than saccadic movements. There is a delay, or latency, of around 100 ms, but the actual response is already programmed. Pursuit movements are usually investigated using first-order stimuli, such as a pen torch, or a moving laser spot on a tangent screen. For research purposes, second-order stimuli are used, such as contrast and flicker. These require higher-level cortical control systems.

8.7 Vergence eye movements

The function of vergence eye movements is to make disjunctive movements of the lines of sight (visual axes) in order either to track a gradually approaching or receding target, or to make a rapid change in fixation from a target at one distance to another at a different distance from the eyes. The speed of vergence movements is about 20 degrees per second, as opposed to 100–500 degrees per second for saccadic movements. In most practical situations, eye movements are a combination of both, and so vergence movements are faster than 20 degrees per second. The stimulus to vergence movements is either a retinal blur, with a latency of 200 ms, or a binocular disparity with a latency of 160 ms before the vergence movement starts. Blinking slows blur-induced vergence movements but appears to assist disparity-induced vergence movements. The neural control of vergence movements involves both saccadic and smooth pursuit systems. Possible pathways are discussed in Rowe (2004).

The normality (or otherwise) of vergence status may be defined in terms of both the motor and the sensory aspects of binocular fusion. The binocular motor status is defined by the presence of orthophoria, compensated heterophoria, decompensated heterophoria and intermittent or constant heterotropia. The normal binocular sensory status is indicated by the level of stereopsis (see Chapter 10). Stereopsis is optimal with orthophoria or compensated heterophoria, but declines with decompensated heterophoria. Where the motor status is intermittent or constant heterotropia, there is also an abnormal binocular sensory status, usually pathological binocular suppression or harmonious anomalous retinal correspondence (HARC), most commonly both: HARC with a central suppression area, for a constant heterotropia. An intermittent heterotropia is more likely to have pathological binocular suppression.

The classification of vergence status is as follows.

- Orthophoria: there is normal oculomotor balance with no fusional vergence operating.
- Compensated heterophoria: fusional vergence operates to maintain bifoveal fixation on the observed target. A small degree of fixation disparity is used to maintain fixation.
- Decompensated heterophoria (synonym: uncompensated heterophoria): fusional vergence operates, but larger amounts of fixation disparity are needed, and this can be identified using fixation disparity tests. Decompensated heterophoria may cause symptoms such as asthenopia, blurred vision, a pulling sensation on the eyes or intermittent diplopia; or it may reduce visual performance, such as reducing stereopsis, particularly in children within the sensitive period.

- Intermittent or constant heterotropia: only one eye fixates the observed target and so normal fusional vergence does not operate.

The sub-types of heterophoria are:

- exophoria: a tendency for either or both eyes to diverge (abduct)
- esophoria: a tendency for either or both eyes to converge (adduct)
- right hyperphoria: a tendency for the right eye to elevate and the left eye to depress
- left hyperphoria: a tendency for the left eye to elevate and the right eye to depress
- excyclophoria: a tendency for the right eye to rotate anticlockwise and the left eye to rotate clockwise, seen from the front of the subject.
- incyclophoria: a tendency for the right eye to rotate clockwise and the left eye to rotate anticlockwise, seen from the front of the subject.

The subtypes of heterotropia are the same as for heterophoria, but replacing a tendency for an actual deviation of one or either eye from binocular fixation on the observed target. The deviation may be intermittent or constant. If one eye deviates there is a unilateral heterotropia. If either eye deviates, there is an alternating heterotropia.

- Exotropia: a divergent deviation of one or either eye.
- Esotropia: a convergent deviation of one or either eye.
- Right hypertropia: a deviation of the right eye upward.
- Right hypotropia: a deviation of the right eye downward.
- Left hypertropia: a deviation of the left eye upward.
- Left hypotropia: a deviation of the left eye downward.
- Cyclotropia: there is some disagreement as to whether cyclophoria and cyclotropia exist as separate entities. Cyclodeviations are usually found in association with vertical deviations. Cyclophoria or cyclotropia is the name of a clinical condition. The scientific description of an individual cyclorotatory eye movement is intorsion or extorsion (see section 8.13).

Clinical anomalies of heterophoria and heterotropia (see Shin *et al.*, 2009) are classified as follows.

- Basic, where the distance and near deviations are the same.
- Divergence excess, where distance exo-deviation is larger than near exo-deviation.
- Divergence insufficiency, where distance eso-deviation exceeds near eso-deviation.
- Convergence excess, where near eso-deviation exceeds distance eso-deviation, which if untreated may lead to reduced stereopsis and amblyopia.
- Convergence weakness: where near exo-deviation exceeds distance exo-deviation. The term 'convergence insufficiency' is also used, but is generally reserved for cases in which the near point of convergence is poor. Both these conditions – convergence weakness, and a remote near point of convergence – can co-exist.

- Convergence spasm is actually an acute spasm of the **near triad**; excessive convergence, accommodation and miosis are all present. The term 'near triad' is used to recognise the fact that these functions normally operate together.

There are atypical forms of heterotropia, notably dissociated vertical deviation, where each eye may move up (or, less commonly, each eye may move down) upon covering, and dissociated horizontal deviation, where an asymmetrical cover/uncover test response is found, depending upon which eye is fixing.

8.8   Aetiology of vergence errors

Failure of the motor fusion system is a function of vergence control. For concomitant eso- and exo-deviations, the following scenarios may be responsible.

- For eso-deviations, uncorrected hypermetropia may lead to excessive convergence via the accommodative convergence to accommodation (AC/A) relationship. As a phoria, this may produce intermittent foveal suppression, and decreasing stereoacuity. This may then deteriorate into an intermittent or constant heterotropia, because of the presence of central pathological binocular suppression preventing sensory fusion, and therefore allowing the deviation to become manifest as a tropia. At this point, as the deviation angle increases, there is pathological binocular diplopia and confusion producing binocular rivalry. This may produce total suppression of the binocular field of the deviated eye, followed by the development of anomalous retinal correspondence (ARC).
- Also for eso-deviations, an alternative causation may be EOM or oculomotor nerve anomalies, or AC/A control errors (an abnormally high AC/A ratio) leading to a similar sequence of events.
- For exo-deviations, the initial trigger may be defocusing of one or both retinal images because of ametropia, leading to one of the eyes tending to move towards the physiological or anatomical position of rest. In this case, the resulting pathological binocular diplopia, confusion and binocular rivalry would generally be managed by large-scale suppression.
- Also for exo-deviations, an alternative trigger may be anomalous EOM, oculomotor nerve or AC/A error.

A further factor in motor fusion failure may be a defect in disconjugate heterophoria adaptation (see section 8.11). For incomitant deviations, there may be a congenital or an acquired failure of EOM or oculomotor nerve function.

The measurement of heterophoria and heterotropia is described in section 12.1 in Chapter 12. The detailed **investigation and management** of these conditions will be found in abnormal binocular vision textbooks. The measurement of **fusional reserves** or vergence amplitudes is described in section 12.10.

8.9 Associated eye and head movements: the postural reflexes

The postural reflexes are the **cervico-ocular reflex** (COR) (synonym: tonic neck reflex), and the **vestibulo-ocular reflex** (VOR). They are non-visual reflexes present at birth, which help to maintain fixation upon an object of interest despite head movements relative to the body or relative to the environment. The COR is the least important of the two and contributes to the stabilisation of gaze mainly in low illumination levels and when the VOR is defective (Barlow and Freedman, 1980). These reflexes are part of the **stato-kinetic reflex**, which produces appropriate movements of the limbs and eyes in response to a head movement (Plate 8.1).

To maintain foveal fixation when the subject is in motion, the optokinetic system corrects for both **translational** and **rotational** head movements. The VOR receives input relating to head movement from the otoliths (linear acceleration) and the semicircular canals (rotational acceleration). When the head is rotated in any axis, the centre point of the head rotation is normally behind the two eyes. There is a linear displacement of the two orbits. This translational head (and therefore eye) movement has three possible subtypes:

1. vertical head movement (as when jogging): a 'bobbing' movement
2. horizontal left–right head movement: a 'heaving' movement
3. horizontal anteroposterior head movement: a 'surging' movement.

If the object of regard is not in the median plane, or the head is turned or tilted, different translational corrections are applied to each eye by the **translational VOR** (t-VOR) system to each eye.

Similarly the **rotational VOR** (r-VOR) system stimulates eye movements that correct for the three possible head rotations:

1. pitch (vertical head rotation about the inter-aural axis, or x-axis)
2. yaw (horizontal head rotation about the rostrocaudal axis, or z-axis) (Figs 8.3 and 8.4)
3. roll (torsional head movements about the naso-occipital axis, or y-axis) (Fig. 8.5).

The t-VOR and r-VOR work best for short and rapid head movements. For longer and slower head movements, the otoliths and the semicircular canals have a declining vestibular response, and the **visual system** gradually takes over. The smooth pursuit eye movement system uses the fixation reflex to maintain gaze on a stationary object when the subject is in motion. In low light or contrast situations the fovea may not be sensitive enough, and then the optokinetic system stabilises gaze.

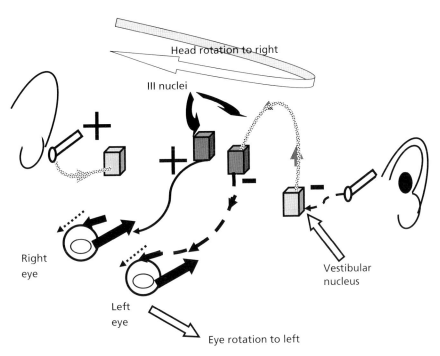

Figure 8.3 The stato-kinetic eye reflexes associated with head turning, i.e. horizontal head rotation about the rostrocaudal axis, or *z*-axis, also known as 'yaw'. Here the head turns to the right and only the left vestibular response is shown (in part) as third nerve stimulation to the right medial rectus and inhibition to the left medial rectus muscle. For additional effects see Fig. 8.4.

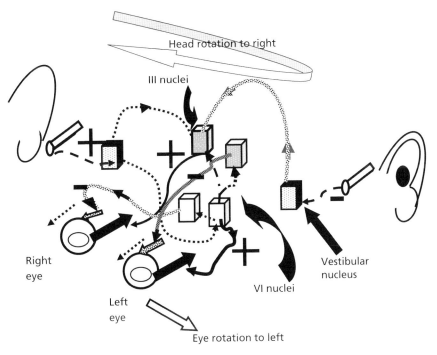

Figure 8.4 Further effects of a right head turn, as in Fig. 8.3. The sixth nerve nuclei provide stimulation to the left lateral rectus, and inhibition to the right lateral rectus, muscles. Both eyes rotate to the left.

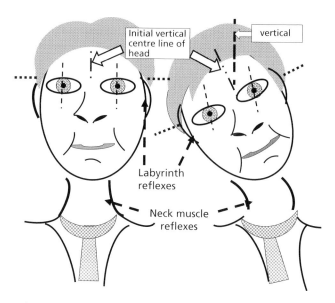

Figure 8.5 The stato-kinetic eye reflexes associated with head tilting, i.e. the rotational vestibulo-ocular reflex eye movement in response to a rotational roll movement of the head about the naso-occipital axis, or *y*-axis. Personal subjective demonstration is easy: in a room with a prominent vertical edge for a reference, and head held vertically, view (monocularly) a very bright vertical strip light for a short while: the retinal image giving a vertical after-image. Note the tilt of the after-image as the head is tilted and the eye cyclorotates. The after-image tilt is less than the head tilt.

A third category of VOR, **ocular counter-rolling VOR**, initiates excycloduction of one eye and incycloduction of the other eye in response to a sustained head tilt. The distinction between a head tilt and a head translation is made by an interpretation of otolith and semicircular canal efferents (Angelaki and Dickman, 2003).

The most disturbing effect of **VOR failure** is seen when head movements caused by vibrations when walking or running do not trigger corrective eye movements. Clear vision is lost until the subject stands still. Training by ballet dancers, using continuous body rotation but intermittent head rotation, tends to overcome such difficulties. The VOR reflex is partially or wholly cancelled during large gaze saccades, and also for head–eye saccades. The reason for this is that during a smooth pursuit movement of eyes and head in following a target moving to the left, the VOR would move the eyes to the right of the target, and fixation would be lost. The visual system is able to override the VOR in these circumstances. As a further example, consider a new **anisometropic spectacle** correction. This requires an unequal amount of eye rotation for each eye. This is caused by the different amounts of induced prismatic effect generated for each eye during version or vergence movements. There may be some disorientation at first, but this soon disappears.

Where there is damage to the vestibular system, a conflict may occur between the VOR and stable vision. Pathological nystagmus and a resulting apparent movement of the environment, oscillopsia, appear. VOR function may be assessed using an ophthalmoscope (preferably indirect) to view the optic disc of one eye while the subject fixates a target at 6 m with the other and rotates the head from side to side above two cycles per second. At this level the pursuit system is inoperative and maintenance of fixation indicates a normal VOR. An underactive VOR makes the observed optic disc move against the head movement. An overactive VOR shows the disc moving with the head (Leigh and Zee, 2006).

8.10 Optokinetic nystagmus eye movements

Optokinetic nystagmus (OKN), or the optokinetic reflex, is the eye movement response to large moving visual fields when the head is stationary. It consists of a combination of a slow compensatory eye movement followed by a fast re-setting saccadic movement. It produces the subjective impression of self-motion, rotating in a direction opposite to the visual field movement. There is a persistence of OKN after the stimulus of a moving visual field has stopped: the nystagmus continues briefly. This is optokinetic after-nystagmus and is caused by the **cerebral velocity-storage memory** mechanism. There is also a cortical control system to inhibit OKN, for example during following-head movements, when a moving object is being tracked by a head movement, and eye movement is not desirable. Apparatus for investigating OKN is described in Appendix 1 (section A12).

Note: in addition to OKN, other types of physiological nystagmus are voluntary nystagmus – the ability to produce horizontal nystagmus voluntarily – and end-positional nystagmus – where in performing the motility test, horizontal nystagmus is seen at the extremes of eye movement. Anomalies of OKN produce both visual anomalies, such as oscillopsia, and balance disorders. Pathological nystagmus is covered in texts on abnormal binocular vision.

8.11 Hering's law

For both pursuit and saccadic eye movements, the eyes move together, even if one eye is occluded, as the corresponding or **yoke muscles** receive the same amount of innervation. For example, the right lateral rectus and the left medial rectus are yoked for a change of fixation towards the right. Where two muscles in the same eye cooperate to produce an eye movement, they are known as **synergists**. For instance, the right superior rectus and right inferior oblique are synergists in elevating the right eye. Furthermore, a pair of synergists may be yoked with a pair governing the other eye. This occurs when the two elevators in one eye act together with those of the other eye to raise the binocular direction of gaze. Different muscles may be yoked together for different eye movements. For example, the medial recti are yoked for convergence but are **antagonists** for version movements. The co-contraction of yoked muscles in each eye obeys **Hering's law of equal innervation**. This states:

- that the equal movement of each eye during saccades occurs because of innate equal nerve stimulation for the muscles acting together
- that the explanation for apparently monocular eye movements, in asymmetrical convergence for example, is explained by the mathematical combination of version and vergence movements (Hering, 1879).

Hering's law applies to both voluntary and involuntary pursuit eye movements and also to vergence eye movements. Thus, in asymmetrical convergence there is evidence that the eye not required to move receives both an equal amount of yoked innervation and a cancelling innervation of its antagonist muscle. Deviations from Hering's law do occur when one eye is deeply amblyopic (Maxwell *et al.*, 1995), and in some saccade-vergence interactions (Sylvestre and Cullen, 2002). Additionally, when binocular eye movements are made looking through spectacle lenses of unequal power and therefore unequal magnification for each eye, the unequal prismatic effect will require one eye to move at a different rate from the other, if fusion is to be maintained (Lemij and Collewijn, 1991). This is called **disconjugate heterophoria adaptation**. It would have originated as a response to EOM strength asymmetry (not anisometropic spectacle correction). Such an asymmetry would occur with muscle underaction caused by disease or injury, but also with natural variations during childhood development and also during ageing. Indeed, there may be several adaptation motor programmes for use when needed in different directions of gaze, or varying fixation distances. Disconjugate heterophoria adaptation and disconjugate saccadic and pursuit adaptations can be gated in (brought into action) as needed. A failure of disconjugate heterophoria adaptation may be one element in the pathophysiology of strabismus (Bucci *et al.*, 1997).

8.12 Sherrington's law

The contraction of an individual EOM generally produces an eye movement, and in relation to this eye movement the muscle is called an **agonist**, from the Greek *agon* – 'angle'. The muscle in the same eye opposing the agonist is called the **ipsilateral antagonist**, e.g. the lateral rectus, with the medial rectus as the agonist. An **antagonist** muscle relaxes to facilitate the eye movement initiated by the agonist. These muscles reverse their actions for an eye movement in the opposite direction.

Disambiguation note: where muscles in either eye oppose each other's action, the opposing muscle is known as the **contralateral antagonist**, although von Noorden prefers the term '**antagonist of the yoke muscle**' (von Noorden and Campos, 2002).

Table 8.1 Monocular muscle agonist and antagonist actions

Duction	Agonist (Primary mover)	Secondary mover	Antagonist (opposite mover)
Supraduction	SR	IO	IR
Infraduction	IR	SO	SR
Adduction	MR	SR and IR	LR
Abduction	LR	SO and IO	MR
Excycloduction	IO	IR	SO
Incycloduction	SO	SR	IO

IO, inferior oblique; IR, inferior rectus; LR, lateral rectus; MR, medial rectus; SO, superior oblique; SR, superior rectus.

The pairing of agonist and antagonist for a single eye is known as **Sherrington's law of reciprocal innervation: when a neural impulse to contract is received by an agonist muscle, an equivalent impulse to relax is received by the ipsilateral antagonist: this is called 'reciprocal innervation'** (Sherrington, 1894, 1906, 1918). Table 8.1 lists the agonist and antagonist actions for specific directions of gaze. The truth of Sherrington's law has been demonstrated by using **electromyography (EMG)**. Using sensors, the increase in electrical activity in the agonist can be contrasted with the decrease in the antagonist muscle. Sherrington's law does not apply in Duane syndrome and other motoneurone misdirection syndromes. In Duane syndrome, the sixth cranial nerve is hypoplastic or absent, and an abnormal branch of the medial rectus nerve supply also serves the lateral rectus of the same eye, so both muscles contract on attempted convergence and the eye is retracted into the orbit.

8.13 Donders' law and Listing's law

Analysis of eye movements

It is convenient to analyse the possible movements of an eye by reference to x-, z- and y-axes passing **horizontally, vertically and anteroposteriorly** through the centre of rotation of the eye, respectively (Fig. 8.6), with the head in the primary, upright position.

Disambiguation note: here these three axes are applied to eye movements: a similar axis nomenclature can be used in relation to head movements. Leigh and Zee (2006) use a different nomenclature for eye movements, however, in which the x- and y-axes are swapped. This does not appear to be used in other literature, and is not used here.

The x-axis is called the **transverse axis**, and movements about this axis allow elevation and depression rotations of the eye. The angle through which the eye turns from the **primary** (straight-ahead) **position** is called the

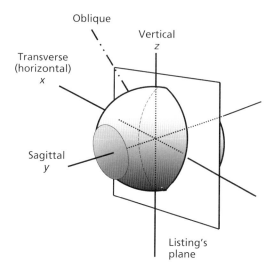

Figure 8.6 The oculo-motor reference axes and Listing's (equatorial) plane.

angle of elevation, or depression. The **primary position of gaze** is the motor equivalent of the sensory principal visual direction: the position of gaze when the fixation target is level with the eyes and on the medial plane, for a distant target. The primary position of gaze is also called the 'distance active position' (see section 9.1 in Chapter 9), the position of the eyes when there is a constant contraction of motor units in all the oculo-rotatory muscles, the tonic discharge.

- The z-axis is known as the **vertical axis**. Rotation medially (towards the nose) is called **adduction**, and rotation temporally is called **abduction**. The angle made by such an eye rotation from the primary position of gaze is called the **azimuth angle**.
- The y-axis is known as the **sagittal axis**. Movements around this anteroposterior axis create a cyclorotation of the eye. Rotation of the upper cornea towards the nose is 'intorsion', and away from the nose is 'extorsion'.

The x- and z-axes are located in a plane known as **Listing's (equatorial) plane**, which has a fixed position relative to the bony orbital walls (Fig. 8.7). Rotation of the eye along either of these axes is called **rotation to a secondary position**: the eye has moved from the primary position of gaze to a secondary position. However, if the eye is moved to a position requiring rotation of both x- and z-axes, this is **rotation to a tertiary position** and will also involve rotation about the y-axis: the anteroposterior, or sagittal, axis. Any rotation about the y-axis is called a **torsional movement**. Any oblique position of the eye will have involved **torsion**.

Donders' law states: **for a specific oblique (tertiary) position of gaze, there is always a particular amount of torsion present** (Donders, 1864).

This constancy of torsion for any specific tertiary direction of gaze allows corresponding retinal points in the right and left eyes to receive the same

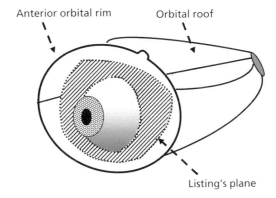

Anterior orbital rim   Orbital roof

Listing's plane

Figure 8.7 Listing's (equatorial) plane. This fundamental plane is shown extending to the walls of the orbit from the equator of the eye. This emphasises its fixed position relative to the bony orbital walls. The bold outlines represent the front and side limits of the orbit, extending as a bony conical cavity towards the optic foramen.

retinal image in a given situation, no matter how the eyes have arrived at that direction of gaze. In other words, the same rotational orientation of the eye is always found for a particular direction of gaze. You can test this by going into a room with fluorescent tube lighting at night. Turn all the lights off, close one eye, look at the middle of the fluorescent tube, and briefly switch it on and then off. In the darkened room, as you look up and to the right, and up and to the left, you will see the fluorescent tube afterimage tilting as you change your direction of gaze.

Note: there is no rotational torsion of the eye in the primary direction of gaze with the head upright, nor in any secondary direction of gaze (looking up, down or to the side), but only for tertiary directions of gaze.

The rotation angle of torsion (the cyclorotatory orientation of the eye) can be deduced from **Listing's law**, which states: **any eye position of gaze can be reached from the primary eye position by rotation about any given single axis lying in the equatorial (Listing's) plane of the eye.**

For the eye to be oriented in any non-primary direction of gaze, there are a maximum of four axes needed for the eye to rotate. They are, seen from the front: (1) horizontal (180 degrees, the x-axis); (2) vertical (90 degrees, the z-axis); (3) with the upper end of the axis at 45 degrees; and (4) with the upper end of the axis at 135 degrees. The axes are orthogonal to the primary direction of gaze (the y-axis). They are all located in the same plane: Listing's plane. The amount of torsion may thus be found by the equation:

$$\sin y = (\sin x \sin z)/(1 + \cos x \cos z)$$

where y = angle of torsional rotation, x = angle of elevation, z = angle of azimuth.

Listing's law is generally true for most eye movements, including smooth pursuit and saccadic eye movements. Deviations from Listing's law occur for movements from one tertiary position of gaze to another. Also in close convergence, Listing's plane is rotated temporally, probably by the agency of the extra-ocular pulley-sleeve system. The effect is to produce downgaze extorsion, and upgaze intorsional eye rotation, dependent upon the type of visual stimulus for convergence (Kapoula *et al.*, 1999). When the head is tilted, the eyes roll in the opposite direction and therefore are no longer in Listing's plane. This operation of the VOR contravenes Listing's law. Neither does it apply during vergence movements, but only when the eyes have finished the movement. Listing's law has mechanical advantages in producing the shortest route to a new eye position, and sensory advantages in minimising the threat to stereopsis that torsion produces. Proprioceptive and visual feedback of eye position is still needed to optimise control. In summary, Donders' law states that a fixed amount of torsion occurs for any specific tertiary direction and Listing's law quantifies this. A mathematical treatment is found at schorlab.berkeley.edu/vilis/whatisLL.htm (accessed 26 May 2010).

8.14   Torsion (true, incidental and false)

The EOM can move the eyes horizontally, vertically and obliquely. They can also produce a rotational movement, called **torsion**, around the visual axes. However, torsion cannot be produced independently of any other eye movement. Purely horizontally or vertical eye movements do not cause any rotational eye movement. Almost all tertiary eye movements, to oblique directions of gaze, do induce a rotational effect: this is called **incidental torsion**. The exception is where the eyes are converged and depressed into the direction of gaze normally used for close vision such as reading and writing. Here there is little or no incidental torsion (Rabbetts, 1972). The actual amount of incidental torsion produced by fixation in a tertiary gaze position never exceeds about 10 degrees. This is a small amount, particularly when you consider that the rotational misalignment of each eye is equal.

It has been shown that the amount of incidental torsion, in any given tertiary direction of gaze, will vary with the route the eyes have utilised to obtain the new direction of gaze (Porrill *et al.*, 1999). For example, to look up and to the right the eyes could move vertically upwards and then horizontally, or vice versa, or alternatively move obliquely to the new position. This torsional variability is corrected by the visual system. After correction, any remaining torsion is termed **false torsion**, because it is neither the variable **incidental torsion**, nor the **true torsion** (cyclofusion) that is being used to partially correct the incidental torsion. The constant amount of false torsion for any given tertiary direction of gaze complies with Donders' law and Listing's law. It may be calculated by formulae defined by Helmholtz (1924), Fick, and Listing (see Quaia and Optican, 2003).

The primary position plane that connects the distant object of regard with the base line (the line connecting the centres of rotation of the eyes) is called the primary plane of regard. With the eyes in the primary direction of gaze, the plane of regard is coincident with the **subjective horizontal plane**. When the eyes move into a tertiary direction of gaze, the angle between these two planes is called **the angle of torsion**. The subjective horizontal plane has moved away from the primary plane of regard.

Chapter 8: Revision quiz

Complete the missing words, perhaps in pencil.

Monocular eye movements are called ductions. The movement of one eye towards the nose is called _____ (1) and away is called _____ (2). Binocular eye movements made with both eyes moving in the same direction are called _____ (3) and moving in opposite directions are called _____ (4).

When the eyes move to a new gaze direction, the innervation given to one eye's muscles is _____ (5) to that of the other eye: Hering's law.

When a muscle in one eye contracts, the opposing muscle in the same eye _____ (6): this is Sherrington's law. For a particular oblique direction of gaze, there is always a particular amount of _____ (7) present: Donders' law.

Answers
(1) adduction; (2) abduction; (3) versions; (4) vergences; (5) equal; (6) contracts; (7) torsion.

Chapter 9
VISUAL RESPONSE TO NEAR OBJECTS

9.1 Vergence movements for near fixation

To explain near vergence movements, it is useful to discuss first the binocular motor relationship for distance fixation (Plate 9.1). The position that the eyes take up in the absence of innervation (i.e. in death) is called the anatomical position of rest: the lines of sight (visual axes) are somewhat divergent. Some degree of divergence may also occur under general anaesthesia, even when an esotropia is present when the individual is conscious. In most conscious situations, the eyes are at least under the effect of the postural reflexes (the vestibulo-ocular and cervico-ocular reflexes) even in darkness, and the eyes adopt the physiological position of rest, which is less divergent. When one eye fixates an object in the distance and the other eye is occluded, the non-fixing eye is in the distance passive position. The distance passive position is influenced by the postural reflexes and the fixation reflex derived from the non-occluded eye fixating a distant object. When the occluded eye is uncovered, binocular fusion produces bifoveal fixation, and the eyes are said to be in the distance active position. The active position is referred to as the primary position of gaze when the fixation target is level with the eyes and on the medial plane. When the passive and active positions are identical, in the primary direction of gaze, the subject is said to be orthophoric. If they differ, the subject has distance heterophoria. When the passive position is more converged than the active position, the subject has distance esophoria. When the passive position is more divergent than the active position, the subject has distance exophoria. The speed of cover/uncover test recovery in heterophoria is an indication of whether or not the heterophoria is compensated (see section 4.7 in Chapter 4).

Horizontal movement of the eyes from the anatomical position of rest towards a near target is subdivided into six stages of convergence. In order of increased convergence (for a subject with exophoria) they are:

1. **tonic convergence** – from the anatomical to the physiological position of rest
2. **initial convergence** – from the physiological position of rest to the distance passive position
3. **fusional convergence** – from the distance passive to the distance active position

Normal Binocular Vision: theory, investigation and practical aspects. By David Stidwill and Robert Fletcher. © 2011 Blackwell Publishing Ltd

4. **accommodative convergence** – from the distance active position as a result of the accommodation required towards the near passive position
5. **proximal convergence** – from the near passive position to the near proximal position
6. **near fusional convergence** – from the near proximal position to the near active position. If near exophoria is present (around 4 prism dioptres of near exophoria is physiological), positive fusional convergence will be needed. If near vision esophoria is present (as in convergence excess esophoria) then negative fusional convergence is required to obtain fusion.

Convergence measurement

Convergence ability is clinically measured in centimetres from the bridge of the nose to a target being fixated as closely as possible without producing diplopia: the **near point of convergence (NPC)**. For scientific purposes, the convergence angle for one eye may be recorded using a unit called the **metre angle**. The metre angle is defined as the angle of convergence that one eye makes to fixate an object 1 m away, in the median plane, from the **base line** connecting the centres of rotation of the two eyes. (The **large metre angle** is defined as the angle of convergence between the visual axes of both eyes looking at an object 1 m away.) The base line is conventionally assumed to be 2.7 cm behind the spectacle plane. So for one eye the convergence in metre angles is given by the formula:

$$\frac{\text{Convergence of one eye}}{\text{(in metre angles)}} = 100/\text{convergence distance in cm} + 2.7\,\text{cm}$$

The convergence angle also depends upon the size of the inter-pupillary distance. The convergence in prism dioptres, also known as the convergence stimulus, is given by:

$$\text{Convergence of one eye (prism dioptres)} = \text{half the inter-pupillary distance (cm)}/\text{convergence distance (metres)} + 0.027$$

where the convergence distance is measured from the spectacle plane to the object fixated. The convergence amplitude is a measure of the convergence between the far point of convergence and the near point of convergence. The far point of convergence is the most divergent position of the lines of sight (visual axes) consonant with binocular fusion. The convergence amplitude is used together with accommodative amplitude and other binocular motor measurements in graphical analysis of binocular vision stability.

- Abnormally poor convergence amplitude is known as **convergence insufficiency**.

- A lack of ability to sustain repeated convergence is known as **convergence infacility**. This may be investigated by making three consecutive NPC measurements. A normal result would be, say, 8, 10 and 7 cm, and convergence infacility would perhaps show 10, 15 and 20 cm. The management of convergence problems will be found in a clinical text.

Note: changes in convergence or divergence are associated with rotation around the anteroposterior axis of the eyes (torsion) and with cyclofusional eye movements (see section 1.7 in Chapter 1). Techniques for measuring convergence and other vergence functions are covered in section 12.7 in Chapter 12.

9.2   Vergence and accommodation

To obtain clear vision when changing fixation from a further to a nearer object, the (pre-presbyopic) eyes accommodate. For a near object situated 25 cm from an emmetropic subject, 4.00 dioptres of accommodation is required, although some 'tolerance' or 'lag' may introduce a smaller amount than that. This act induces accommodative convergence, also known as blur-induced convergence (see Appendix 1, section A8). The fine-tuning of convergence is provided by fusional convergence and subsidiary stimuli, also known as disparity-induced convergence. Where accommodation is not required, as for a –4.00 dioptre myope, convergence would be provided by the fusion reflex alone. The linkage between convergence and accommodation is not exact. If the amount of accommodation for a near object is deliberately varied by positive or negative lenses, accommodative convergence alters. For a given degree of convergence the amount of accommodative change consistent with maintenance of fusion is called the relative accommodation. For fusion to be maintained at a given fixation distance, the maximum amount of relaxation is called the negative relative accommodation (NRA), and the maximum increase in accommodation is called the positive relative accommodation (PRA). In a similar way, accommodative convergence can be kept constant, and the fusional convergence varied, while fusion is maintained. This can be achieved by varying the angle of a synoptophore (Fig. 9.1) or by placing prisms in front of the subject's eyes. Base-out prisms induce additional convergence. Base-in prisms reduce the amount of fusional convergence. The total range of convergence possible with a fixed amount of accommodation is called the amplitude of relative convergence. The maximum base-in prism consistent with maintaining fusion is the negative relative convergence (NRC). The maximum base-out prism while fusion is maintained is the positive relative convergence (PRC). The test distance should be stated for these functions, otherwise the assumption is made that the NRC and PRC are being measured from the distance active position.

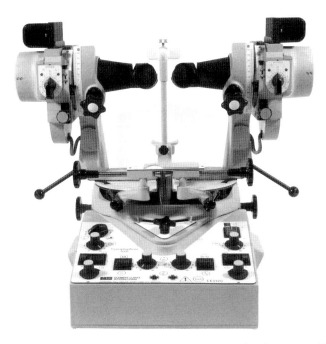

Figure 9.1 The synoptophore. This is a double mirror haploscope, which allows any image to be presented to each eye at any angle of convergence, divergence, vertical or rotational orientation. It can be used for assessing the angle of deviation in heterophoria and heterotropia, and for assessing the binocular sensory status, although with some limitations. Reproduced with kind permission of Haag-Streit UK Ltd.

9.3 Accommodation-induced convergence: the AC/A ratio

The stimulus AC/A ratio

The interactive connection between accommodation ('**A**') and convergence triggered by accommodating ('**AC**') is called the **accommodative convergence to accommodation ratio,** often abbreviated to **AC/A ratio**. The **stimulus AC/A ratio** is the amount of accommodative convergence in prism dioptres for each unit of stimulus to accommodation (dioptres of accommodation). This is a clinical measurement for which the accommodative stimulus (positive or negative trial lenses, for example) would be expected to result in the same amount of accommodative response. However, for near vision the response usually lags behind (is less than) the stimulus, and for distance fixation the accommodative response is usually greater than the stimulus. If the vergence associated with accommodation were the same as that needed for bifoveal fixation at any fixation distance, this ratio would be 6.0 Δ/1.00 D for an interpupillary distance of 60 mm (Leigh and Zee, 2006). However, the normal AC/A ratio is 4 prism dioptres (Δ) accommodative convergence to 1.00 D accommodative change with a standard deviation of 2 Δ. The AC/A ratio entails the use of vergence induced by binocular disparity to maintain binocular fixation on the visual target. Where the stimulus AC/A ratio is 6 Δ/1.00 D or more, clinical anomalies such as latent hypermetropia, or convergence excess, are likely. A low AC/A ratio may be associated with convergence weakness or convergence insufficiency (see section 8.7 in Chapter 8).

The **gradient method** (synonym: lens gradient method) is one way to investigate the relationship between accommodation and convergence. The Maddox wing test can be utilised. This is a method of dissociating the eyes for measurement of the near heterophoria. The Maddox wing test permits one eye to see a row or column of numbers, and the other eye can only see a pointer (an arrow). The numbers and arrow are positioned at 30 cm from the subject's eyes. The subject is asked to say which number the arrow points towards: this is the near heterophoria. Lenses then are placed in front of each eye in order to increase or to decrease the amount of accommodation required to clearly focus the near fixation target. This procedure demonstrates the effect of accommodation change on the near heterophoria. Near physiological exophoria is usually about 4 prism dioptres of exophoria. When +1.00 DS lenses are introduced, the heterophoria commonly increases to about 8 Δ of exophoria. So the reduction in accommodative demand increases the heterophoria by 4 Δ. This would indicate an AC/A ratio of 4 Δ to 1.00 D, which is within the normal range of 3 to 5 Δ/D. The full range is between 0 Δ and 12 Δ/D, and is constant until its utility ends with the onset of presbyopia. An alternative form of the gradient method is to measure the line of sight (visual axis) deviation for distance fixation, using a Maddox rod or the cover/uncover test, with and without trial lenses of different powers. The formula for the gradient method is:

$$AC/A \text{ ratio} = \frac{(\text{deviation without trial lenses} - \text{deviation with trial lenses})}{\text{trial lens power in dioptres}} \Delta/D$$

The **clinical method** (synonyms: heterophoria method, calculated stimulus AC/A method) is an alternative method of calculating the AC/A ratio. This compares the increase in convergence from the distance heterophoria value with the near heterophoria value. The result is divided by the change in focus in dioptres from distance to near fixation. The formula for the Clinical Method is:

$$AC/A \text{ ratio} = PD - (\text{phoria at } 33 \text{ cm} - \text{phoria at } 600 \text{ cm})/DA$$

where PD is the interpupillary distance in cm and **DA** (dioptres of accommodation) is the dioptric difference between 6 m and 40 cm (based on Jennings, 2001). As an example, for a PD of 60 mm (i.e. 6 cm), a near phoria (at 33 cm) of 6 Δ, and a distance phoria of zero Δ (at 6 m):

$$AC/A \text{ ratio} = 6 + (6 - 0)/3 = 8 \text{ (a high AC/A ratio)}$$

Although this is also called the heterophoria method, it can be used with caution for heterotropia, too. It would be necessary to ensure that normal retinal correspondence was present during the measurement.

The stimulus AC/A ratio is used clinically to investigate and manage anomalies of binocular vision such as **convergence excess**, where the ratio may be 6, 9 or 12 prism dioptres to 1 dioptre of accommodation and is associated with near esophoria or near esotropia.

A difference between the gradient method with an AC/A ratio of 2:1, and the clinical method with a ratio of 5:1 has been found (Jackson and Arnoldi, 2004).

The response AC/A ratio

The response AC/A ratio is the amount of accommodative convergence in prism dioptres for each unit of accommodation (dioptres of accommodation), as measured by an infrared optometer. The response AC/A ratio is mainly used in research. The response AC/A ratio is more accurate than the (clinical) stimulus AC/A ratio and generally gives a value almost 10% higher.

9.4 Convergence-induced accommodation: the CA/A ratio

Convergence can be considered to be the most prominent feature during binocular fixation of a near object, involving foveal fusion of the two retinal images. Accommodation is also involved, somewhat in proportion to convergence (Fig. 9.2). There is some tolerance to slight blurring of what is seen,

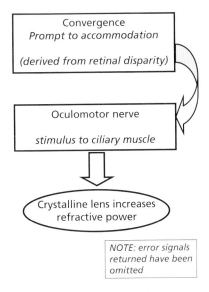

Figure 9.2 The role of convergence as a factor in accommodation; the sequence resulting in accommodative effort. Note error signals returned to the central brain control have been omitted here.

often involving a **lag of accommodation**, so convergence and the expected amount of accommodation are not always strictly matched. This is despite very definite associations with the third cranial nerves, including associated pupil contraction as part of the near triad of response to near vision.

Paradoxically, even when binocular vision is good, accommodation tends to increase almost 1.00 D to a resting state in low ambient illumination; this 'dark-focus' or 'dark-accommodation' bias also appears in some empty visual field conditions at high luminance levels. There is evidence to attribute altered tonic accommodation to low-contrast conditions combined with a lack of high-frequency stimulation.

Thus the complement of accommodative convergence is the function of convergence ('C') initiating accommodation: i.e. **convergence-induced accommodation ('CA')**, sometimes called vergence accommodation. Increased convergence stimulates increased accommodation. For each prism dioptre of convergence, about 0.07 to 0.15 dioptres of accommodation is induced. With decreasing accommodative amplitude in the older person, this ratio (**CA/C ratio**) reduces from the theoretical 0.16 dioptres that is theoretically required (Leigh and Zee, 2006). The theoretical response is actually likely in typical normal pre-presbyopic subjects. In exophoria, with excessive innervation required for a near object, greater accommodation is induced, except in older subjects (Fig. 9.3). The decrease in accommodation with age results in reduced accommodative response to convergence. The response reaches a plateau when maximum accommodative effort is operating.

The reflex neural paths operating normally are described as operating under 'closed-loop' conditions, applicable to most AC/A measurements. Tsuetaki and Schor (1987) adopted an approach enabling rapid measurements of the CA/C ratio and the adaptation of tonic accommodation, by

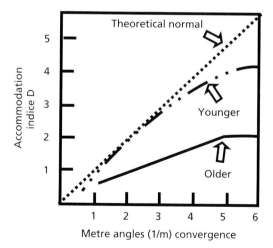

Figure 9.3 Accommodation stimulated by convergence, in average normal subjects and younger and older people, showing the plots of accommodation induced by convergence effort. The convergence is plotted on the horizontal axis, in the reciprocal of the convergence distance, i.e. in metre angles.

opening the accommodative loop. This involves a low spatial frequency difference of Gaussians (DOG) pattern as a stimulus, about 0.1 cycles per degree. Such a band-pass filtered bar resembles one cycle of a sine wave, essentially a bright vertical strip as a plateau flanked on each side by dark strips, all set on a field of median luminance. Such a contour virtually devoid of any spatial frequency is considered to provide minimal accommodative stimulus, resulting in an 'empty field' accommodative state. Convergence and fusion can be involved, with evaluation of the CA/A ratio. Prisms are used to stimulate disparity vergence, and the resulting change in accommodation is measured by an electronic optometer or by dynamic retinoscopy. Values of 0.4 dioptres/metre angle (D/MA) are found in pre-presbyopes. Convergence excess would give values of around 0.1 D/MA, and 0.8 D/MA for convergence insufficiency. However, it appears that accommodation is less important than the vergence reflexes as an aid to fusion. The clinical use of the CA/C ratio has shown little advantage over other methods of distinguishing symptomatic from symptom-free subjects (Daum *et al.*, 1989). An apparatus for investigating convergence-induced accommodation is described in Appendix 1 (section A8).

9.5   Graphical analysis of normal AC/A ratio

A graph, called the Donders' diagram, can be plotted to include positive and negative relative convergence and accommodation (Fig. 9.4). This graph is used clinically to establish the zone of clear normal binocular single vision. This is the area enclosed by the total amounts of positive and negative

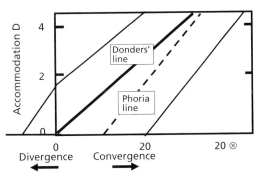

Figure 9.4   Donders' diagram. The graph plots the zone of clear binocular single vision as an enclosed area. The positive (adduction or convergence) fusional reserve is plotted on the right side of the graph, for each dioptre of accommodation actively used, beginning with zero accommodation at the bottom of the graph. The negative (abduction or divergence) fusional reserve is plotted similarly on the left side of the graph. The Donders' line shown is the plot of the amount of convergence induced by each dioptre of accommodation utilised. The accommodation is stimulated by looking through negative lenses (this technique is called the gradient test). The phoria line is plotted as the amount of convergence or divergence present when the eyes are dissociated, for each level of accommodative effort.

relative convergence available. On the Donders' diagram it is possible to plot convergence against accommodation, using the formula:

$$\text{Convergence} = 2 \times (\text{PD}) \times 100/[(100/\text{Acc}) + 2.7]$$

where PD is the interpupillary distance in cm, Acc is the accommodation in dioptres and 2.7 cm is the assumed distance between the base line connecting the centres of rotation of each eye (from which convergence is measured) and the spectacle plane (from which accommodation is conventionally measured). The plot of this formula produces a line on the Donders' diagram of accommodation/convergence called the Donders' line (Fig. 9.4). The convention is to measure stimulus values rather than response values. The accommodative stimulus is provided by varying the test distance or the dioptric strength of the lenses through which the subject looks. The stimulus to converge is achieved by reducing the test distance from 6 m or by using base-out prisms in front of the eyes. Additionally, the phoria line may be plotted on the graph. This is the plot of the heterophoria: the angles in prism dioptres between the dissociated lines of sight (visual axes), for increasing amounts of accommodation. It is measured by gradually decreasing the fixation distance from infinity (in practice, 6 m) to 20 cm and measuring the heterophoria at each successively closer fixation distance. There is an extensive literature on the use of graphical analysis for assessing anomalies of binocular vision: for example, Goss (1995).

9.6 Abnormal AC/A ratios

For an abnormally low AC/A ratio the Donders' diagram might look like Fig. 9.5. It can be seen that the Donders' line is only within the zone of comfort (the middle third of the total range of the fusional reserves), where the accommodation demand does not exceed 2 dioptres. The zone of comfort is discussed in section 9.7. The Donders' line is sometimes referred to as the demand line, as it is where the lines of sight (visual axes) are required to fixate, in contrast to the phoria line, which is where the visual axes are found when the eyes are dissociated. The Donders' line is the graphical plot of the convergence needed for gradually increasing accommodation while clear binocular single vision is maintained. The phoria line represents the position the eyes drift towards when they are dissociated, and no longer maintaining clear binocular single vision. In this example the Donders' line could be shifted to the edge of the zone of comfort for, say, 4 dioptres accommodation, by the use of base-in prisms totalling (20 − 15 = 5 Δ) shared between the eyes. This would ensure comfortable binocular vision.

For an **abnormally high AC/A ratio**, refer to Fig. 9.6. In this example the Donders' line is outside the zone of comfort for any accommodative demand. At 3 dioptres of accommodative demand, the Donders' line could be shifted to the edge of the zone of comfort by prescribing (+3.00) − (+2.00) = +1.00

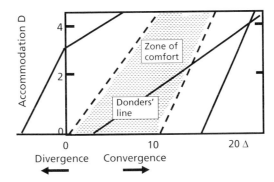

Figure 9.5 Donders' diagram. Low AC/A ratio, diagrammatic. The Donders' line leaves the zone of comfort for any accommodative effort beyond 2 dioptres. To resume comfortable binocular vision, either positive lenses would be prescribed to limit accommodative effort to 2 dioptres, or base-in prisms prescribed equal to the difference between the Donders' line and the zone of comfort for the amount of accommodation in use.

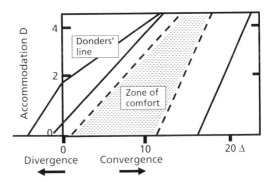

Figure 9.6 Donders' diagram. High AC/A ratio, diagrammatic. The Donders' line is outside the zone of comfort for any level of accommodative demand. Prescription of R and L +1.00 lenses would drop the Donders' (or 'demand') line into the zone of comfort.

lenses, which reduce the accommodative demand on the subject. In this example, for any level of accommodative demand, R and L +1.00 lenses would drop the Donders' line onto the edge of the zone of comfort.

9.7 Sheard's criterion and Percival's criterion

Sheard and Percival in the early twentieth century suggested empirical rules (criteria) to establish the zone of comfortable (symptom-free) binocular vision within the total zone of clear normal binocular single vision. These rules can be applied to lateral fusional imbalance for both distance and near fixation.

Sheard's criterion: the vergence reserve should be twice the vergence demand

The vergence demand is the dissociated heterophoria position of the lines of sight (visual axes) expressed usually in prism dioptres. The dissociated heterophoria is the angle between the lines of sight in heterophoria when the eyes are dissociated, e.g. by occluding one eye: the passive position for distance or for near fixation. The vergence reserve is the opposing limit of the zone of clear normal binocular single vision: the fusional reserve to the blur point in the opposite direction to the direction of the heterophoria. Sheard's criterion is sometimes expressed as: **the fusional reserve should be twice the amount of the heterophoria.**

Percival's criterion: the Donders' line should lie within the zone of comfort (Figs 9.5 and 9.6)

The **zone of comfort** is the middle third of the range of positive and negative relative convergence. This approach is also known as the **middle third technique**. Where Sheard's and Percival's criteria are not fulfilled in a clinical situation, then a change in spherical lens power, prescription of prisms or orthoptic exercises is indicated. Evans (2007) suggests that Sheard's criterion is valid only for distance exophoria, and Percival's criterion for near vision only. Since the middle of the twentieth century the measurement of fixation disparity has also been used to assess the likelihood of problems with binocular fusion control. This concept was suggested by Mallet (1964), following Lord Charnwood's seminal paper (Charnwood, 1951). Both fixation disparity assessment and Sheard and Percival's criteria are subject to the criticism that they offer a snapshot of the subject's fusion control at the time of the examination and may not relate to control at other times when the subject may be tired or operating in a difficult visual environment, such as night driving. However, Sheard and Percival's criteria do introduce measurement of relative convergence and divergence, often called the fusional reserves (see section 12.10 in Chapter 12). Measurement of fusional reserves together with the fixation disparity assessment give information that is more robust than an isolated fixation disparity finding. Further guidance in assessing normality of binocular vision is to be found in the **norms for binocularity** developed by Morgan (Morgan, 1983), Goss (Goss, 1995) and Hayes (Hayes *et al.*, 1998).

Chapter 9: Revision quiz

Complete the missing words, perhaps in pencil.

The position that the eyes take up relative to each other in the absence of innervation is called the _____ (1) position of rest. When one eye fixates a distant target and the other eye is occluded, the non-fixing eye is in the _____ (2) position.

The near point of convergence is measured from the nearest point that can be fixated binocularly, up to the b_____ of the n_____ (3). To look from a distant object to a close object (in a pre-presbyope) induces _____ (4) convergence. The normal AC/A ratio is _____ (5) prism dioptres to 1 dioptre of accommodation. Sheard's criterion for comfortable binocular vision states that the convergence reserve should be _____ (6) the amount of the convergence demand.

Distance negative fusional reserves may be measured by increasing the strength of prism base-_____ (7) until single vision is lost and diplopia occurs.

Answers
(1) anatomical; (2) passive; (3) bridge of the nose; (4) accommodative; (5) 3.5; (6) twice; (7) in.

Chapter 10

THE BINOCULAR INTEGRATIVE ACTION OF THE VISUAL SYSTEM

This chapter concentrates on a basic outline of a complex and extensive subject. The main features hinge on visual cortex responses to binocular stimuli that are described in more detail in extensive texts such as Davson (1990a) and by Chalupa and Werner (2004), and also on spatial aspects of neurophysiology (Davson, 1990b). The depth of objects in physical three-dimensional space is assessed from both monocular and binocular information. The different view of the world seen by each eye creates the binocular appreciation of depth. Where objects are situated further or nearer than the fixation point, a horizontal displacement in the direction of the same feature as seen by each eye produces a binocular disparity. Binocular percepts develop from the interactions of varied cortical cellular activities, situated in a few parts of the cortex and cerebellum. For the present, relatively simplistic, survey it is reasonable to pay most attention to the visual cortex, anatomically related to distinctive striated (banded) appearances in cross section, lying in the occipital region of the brain.

The information from each eye is first combined in the striate visual cortex, **visual area V1**. The term 'striate' is obtained from the notable pale *stria of Gennari*, the visible cortical surface striation taking medullated nerve fibres to cortical layer 4 from the lateral geniculate nucleus (LGN). Ideas as to human cortical function are based upon extrapolation from cat and monkey investigations as well as human clinical situations such as strokes and tumours affecting the visual cortical region; visual field defects and pupil anomalies contribute extra information. The LGN sends signals of immediate interest to parts of the visual cortex, principally in the area known as **visual area V1, layer 4C**, via the optic radiations. Sensory regions of the cerebral cortex contain six distinct 'layers', numbered **1** to **6** with some subdivisions. Large and small retinal receptive fields have reasonably good representation in the cortex, as receptive areas, provided by parvocellular tracts and magnocellular fibres, respectively.

Cortical **area 17** (after Brodmann's anatomical description, a century ago) lies within the thickness of the cortex in the calcarine sulcus of each brain hemisphere, the two sides facing each other across the medial calcarine fissure. The important and relatively large representation of the foveas lies posteriorly. Fibres conveying sensory signals from corresponding 'points' of the two retinas remain close to each other. Communication exists anteriorly between these two sides, and there are widespread connections to other

Normal Binocular Vision: theory, investigation and practical aspects. By David Stidwill and Robert Fletcher. © 2011 Blackwell Publishing Ltd

regions within the two hemispheres of the brain. Oculomotor nerve nuclei are necessarily provided with links so that sensory input can produce a motor response where appropriate. Cells of different types exist – some simple and others more complex in function. This region contains columns of cells having complicated functions, such as binocular integration, eye dominance and colour discrimination. Also there is activity providing stereoscopic vision based upon binocular disparity. Brodmann area 17, the striate cortex, sometimes referred to as the 'primary' visual area, has near neighbours such as the prestriate cortex and the corpus callosum, which connects the hemispheres; the terms 'parastriate cortex' (area 18) and 'peristriate cortex' (area 19) were previously applied to adjacent regions, although modern usage is to class areas 18 and 19 together as the 'extrastriate visual cortex'. In primates the anatomical areas 17, the striate cortex, and areas 18 and 19, the extrastriate cortex, are approximately the same as the functional areas **V1** (striate cortex) and the extrastriate cortex: visual areas **V2**, **V3**, **V4** and **V5/MT**.

10.1 Receptive fields of the retina

The rod and cone receptors feed information to retinal ganglion cells. Bipolar, horizontal and amacrine cells modify the information. Several retinal receptors may stimulate one ganglion cell; this is called **cellular convergence**. In addition, some retinal receptors send **excitatory** stimuli, and some send **inhibitory** stimuli, to ganglion cells. The retinal area producing stimuli affecting a single ganglion cell is called the **receptive field** of that ganglion cell. Receptive fields in monkeys and cats are of two types. The **ON-centre** receptive field stimulates ganglion cell response if a light spot falls on the centre of the receptive field, but inhibits the response if the light spot falls on the annulus surrounding the centre of the receptive field (Fig. 10.1). An **OFF-centre** receptive field has the opposite effect. Diffuse elimination over both centre and surrounding stimulus areas produces a weak response for both ON-centre and OFF-centre receptive fields. The **mapping** of the retina is maintained through the optic nerves, the chiasm, the dorsal LGN and the visual cortex. This is known as **retinotopic mapping**. There is, however, a neural magnification effect, so that the central few degrees of the retina is represented by the most posterior third of the visual cortex.

10.2 Function of the optic chiasm

In lower vertebrates the right retina is represented in the left visual cortex and the left retina in the right cortex. Because of this **full decussation**, the frog has binocular vision with two separate visual fields, which meet but do not overlap in the median plane after full decussation. In mammals some right eye retinal neurones cross to the left visual cortex and some go to the

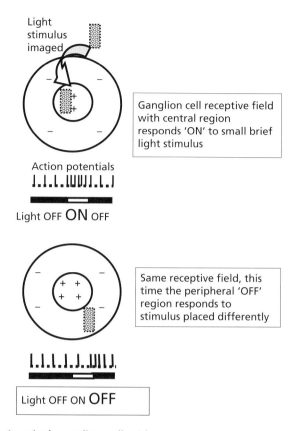

Figure 10.1 A retinal ganglion cell with an 'on-centre' receptive field. When a light stimulus falls on retinal receptors that provide the ganglion cell central field, the ganglion cell sharply increases its resting state discharges. When the light stimulus falls on retinal receptors that provide the ganglion cell peripheral field, the ganglion cell reduces its resting state discharges, until the stimulus is switched off, and then there may be an increase in response. (The reverse situation occurs with an 'off-centre' retinal ganglion cell.) Uniform illumination stimulating both the peripheral and the central part of the receptive field cancels out the 'on' and 'off' responses, leaving the resting state discharges.

right visual cortex, called **hemi-decussation**, or partial decussation. For a horse with almost 360 degrees of visual field, the binocular overlap is about 5 degrees, as only a small proportion of neurones partially decussate. For humans 53–57% of retinal neurones (the nasal retinal fibres) cross over to the opposite lobe of the visual cortex. Temporal retinal fibres travel to the ipsilateral visual cortex (see Plate 4.1). Hemi-decussation allows the same object to have a dual cortical representation, in the sense that the object is imaged on corresponding points of each eye, and neurones from each retina take information to the right and left monocular cells of V1, before feeding in to a binocular cortical cell. An object to the left of central fixation is imaged on the nasal retina of the left eye and the temporal retina of the right eye. Both images reach the right visual cortex lobe.

10.3   Function of the LGN

The retinal neurones synapsing at the dorsal LGN arrive at six neural layers with an interlaminar region between each layer. **Layers 1 and 2** have **magnocellular neurones** (larger or M neurones), most sensitive for faster movement, low spatial frequency and high temporal frequency of visual stimuli. They identify 'where' things are in visual space. The other layers have smaller P neurones – the **parvocellular neurones** responding most to slow movement, colour detection and high spatial frequencies. They identify 'what' the visual stimuli comprise.

Layers **1, 4** and **6** of each dorsal LGN receive fibres from the opposite eye, which cross over at the chiasm. **Layers 2, 3 and 5** receive ipsilateral fibres. Thus nerve fibres from corresponding points on each retina meet in the LGN. There is a feed-forward inhibitory interaction between the right-eye- and left-eye-specific LGN neurones (Blitz and Regehr, 2005). This occurs at the border between each LGN layer. This may be of value in situations of binocular rivalry or binocular suppression (Varela and Singer, 1987). The main LGN function is to approximate nerve fibres relaying similar images from each eye before their pathway to the visual cortex, where binocular integration occurs. The LGN brings together the magnocellular (the motion pathway) and parvocellular (the pattern pathway) data from the same point in physical space. These pathways continue through the visual cortex and are known as the **parallel pathways**.

10.4   Receptive fields of the LGN

These resemble retinal receptive fields, with both ON-centre and OFF-centre types. Each LGN cell receives stimulation from only a few retinal ganglion cells of the same ON-centre or OFF-centre type. When the LGN interocular inhibitory interaction is active, there are changes in the ON and OFF parts of the resulting cortical receptive fields, and the centres of the monocular receptive fields are different. The inference is that the LGN interocular inhibition contributes to cortical binocular disparity function (Kikuchi *et al.*, 2008). However, there is no response by LGN cells to diffuse illumination of both the centre and the surrounding annulus of their receptive fields. The LGN receptive fields are therefore more sensitive to contrast than retinal receptive fields. The LGN cells also maintain a constant output of activity whenever retinal input is a constant level of light or darkness.

10.5   Receptive fields in the primary visual cortex: visual area V1

Cells in the primary visual cortex (**area V1**) respond best to a line stimulus such as a bright or dark stripe, rather than to spots of light as with retinal and LGN receptive fields. There are three types of cells in V1 with different receptive fields: **simple cells**, **complex cells** and **hypercomplex cells**.

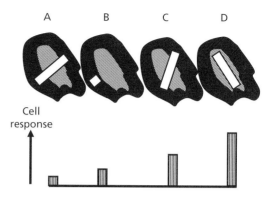

Figure 10.2 The receptive fields of simple visual cortex cells. About 80% of these simple cells have a monocular input, and 20% a binocular input. The visual stimulus is shown in white. The cortical cell receptive field excitation region is shown in grey, and the inhibition region is shown in black. For **visual stimulus A** with a bar of light orientated at 90 degrees to the excitation field, there would be a minimal response by the cell. For **visual stimulus B** with a spot of light in the inhibition field, there would be a slight inhibitory response by the cell. For **visual stimulus C** with a bar of light orientated at 45 degrees to the excitation field, there would be a sub-maximal response by the cell. For **visual stimulus D** with a bar of light orientated parallel to the excitation field, there would be a maximum response by the cell. Note: a diffuse illumination stimulus affects both excitatory and inhibitory regions equally, and so there is no response to this stimulus.

A **simple cell** responds minimally to a spot of light: as an excitatory response if falling on an ON-centre area, as an inhibiting response if the light spot falls on a surrounding OFF-area. There is no response to diffuse light stimulation simultaneously over both ON and OFF areas. Hence there is no assessment of the absolute illumination level of the retina. A slit or bar of light produces no response if orientated across ON-and-OFF areas, some response if at an angle, and maximal response if aligned with an ON-centre strip. There are a variety of simple cell receptive fields (Fig. 10.2).

Complex striate cortex cells may respond either to a line ON-stimulus (a light bar) or to a line OFF-stimulus (a dark bar). There is only an ON-response or an OFF-response for each complex cell, so that a stimulus anywhere within the receptive field will produce a response. Some complex cells require a particular orientation of the positive or negative stimulus in order to respond (Fig. 10.3). Other complex cells respond to lateral position of the light or darkness, or to specific lateral movement.

Hypercomplex striate cells have the same range of responses as complex cells except that they are all orientation-sensitive. They all respond only, or maximally, to a line stimulus of a specific length for individual cells. They are therefore right-angle (orthogonal) area detectors. Some duplicate this property to act as width-detectors provided the stimulus is moving at the correct orientation and correct direction – three separate properties of the stimulus are required (Fig. 10.4). It would appear that the three types of

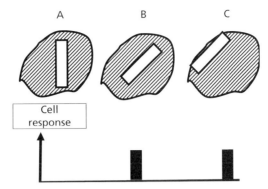

Figure 10.3 The responses of a complex cortical cell relative to orientation of stimulus. About 30% of these cells have a monocular input, and 70% a binocular input. They do not have excitation and inhibitory regions in the receptive field, as simple cells do. They give an identical response to a bar stimulus so long as it is orientated at the same angle as the receptive field, wherever the stimulus is received within the receptive field. No response is given for misaligned bars of light. **Visual stimulus A** is not orientated at the same angle as the receptive field, so only a minimal response will occur. **Visual stimuli B and C** are in line with the receptive field axis and a similar response will be given for each presentation. There are other complex cells that react similarly, but to a dark bar at the correct orientation. Other complex cells respond to an orientated bar only if it is moving in a certain direction, e.g. left to right.

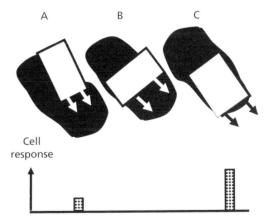

Figure 10.4 The response of a hypercomplex cortical cell relative to movement direction/location, including fitting into angles/corners. About 15% of these cells have a monocular input, and 85% a binocular input. They react in the same way as complex cells, except that they only respond for a correctly orientated bar of a specific length. This property allows the detection of corners. There are other hypercomplex cells that respond only for movement of a bar of a certain width, moving in a certain direction. **Visual stimulus A** is approximately the correct length and orientation, so a low level response occurs. **Visual stimulus B** is the wrong length although correct orientation of movement: no response occurs. **Visual stimulus C** provides the optimal stimulation and response.

striate cortical cells – simple, complex and hypercomplex – form an ascending hierarchy, allowing recognition of increasingly complex attributes, with increasing binocular input. Many visual cortex areas with specific neural properties serving different visual functions are retinotopic. Hypercomplex striate cells have receptive field centres that map the visual fields. The mapping can be investigated by functional magnetic resonance imaging (Warnking *et al.*, 2002).

10.6   Area V1 – binocular integration: summation

It has been shown that the combination of monocular inputs into binocular cells first occurs in visual area V1 (Holmes, 1945; Hubel and Wiesel, 1962; Barlow *et al.*, 1967): monocular neurones from the LGN project to layer 4 of visual area V1. Neurones from the left and right eyes alternate in successive ocular dominance columns of layer 4. A synapse here takes the visual stimulus to **binocular cells** in the cortical layers 1 to 3, above layer 4; and to 5 and 6, below layer 4. (The layers are numbered downwards from the cortical surface.) Thus the binocular cells receive connections from adjacent right and left monocular neurones in layer 4 (Fig. 10.5).

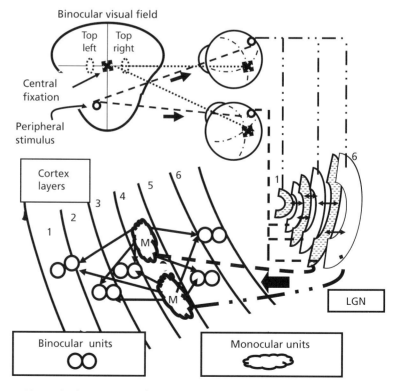

Figure 10.5   The integration of monocular retinal stimuli via the lateral geniculate nucleus (LGN) to the monocular cells, and then the binocular cells in layer 4 of the visual cortex.

Individual binocular cells respond by increasing their firing rate to visual stimulus orientation: to motion either to or from the subject, and to increased or decreased contrast. In particular, they respond most to stimuli specific to the individual cell, i.e. the direction of orientation, the direction of motion and the preferred contrast polarity. They respond to the preferred stimulation from either eye, but much more strongly where it originates in receptive fields of both eyes. This is therefore a site of **neural binocular summation**. In some cases **binocular facilitation** occurs and the binocular cell's response is greater than the sum of its two monocular inputs. This is found in clinical situations, such as where binocular visual acuity is greater than monocular visual acuity. Binocular summation can also be confirmed objectively by comparing monocular and binocular visually evoked potential (VEP) recording. The binocular VEP will generally show a greater response if binocular visual summation is present. A more sophisticated form of VEP is described below, in section 10.7.

Note: the terms 'V1', 'V2', 'V3' and so on relates to the fact that V1 was identified before V2 and does not indicate tiers of visual processing.

10.7 Area V1 – binocular integration: inhibition

If the lines of sight (visual axes) are not both aligned on the object of regard, the monocular inputs to V1 layer 4 binocular cells differ. There could be a mismatch of stimulus **orientation**, or **location** or **width**. This would reduce binocular summation gradually to the point where there is **absence of binocular summation**, or even **binocular inhibition** of the binocular cells' output. This occurs in the clinical conditions of physiological binocular suppression and pathological binocular suppression. Persistent high activity from one monocular cell driving a binocular cell, combined with persistent low activity from the monocular cell for the other eye, results in loss of the weaker connection. A sophisticated VEP test for the degree of binocular summation is used clinically by recording VEP response using a uniform visual field with sinusoidal varying flicker, presented at different rates for each eye. Where there is inhibition, i.e. no summation, the VEP graph shows only the two input frequencies. With summation, the graph shows peaks at frequencies equivalent to the sum of the two frequencies and to the difference between the frequencies: this is called **binocular beat VEP** (see Baitch and Levi, 1988). Thus the presence or absence of binocular summation, or of binocular inhibition, can be demonstrated.

10.8 Area V1: absolute binocular disparity detection

As part of binocular summation activity, around 50% of area V1 simple and complex cortical binocular cells can also detect **binocular disparity**. Where the right and left inputs into V1 layer 4 binocular cells are less conflicting than in section 10.7 above (causing binocular inhibition), but merely consist of a disparity difference, the degree of disparity is detectable by certain cortical binocular cells tuned for this purpose. A disparity-selective cell is called a **disparity detector**. Its **disparity tuning function** relates to the frequency of firing of the cell in response to the stimulus it receives. Its **preferred disparity** is the binocular disparity to which the cell responds most strongly. The cell's **disparity selectivity** relates to the spread of the disparity tuning function. A more selective cell would show a narrower tuning function, i.e. a smaller range of firing frequencies. Binocular disparity occurs when a single object is imaged on non-corresponding right and left retinal points, because the eyes are not fixating that object. The **absolute binocular disparity** of an object is the (fixed) difference between the external longitudinal angles made by the object in physical space in relation to each eye (Fig. 6.25 in Chapter 6). The binocular disparity can be crossed, or uncrossed, in each case to varying levels of disparity, or the disparity can be of zero value. In the latter case, the visual system has recognised that the two images are in fact falling on corresponding retinal areas.

Binocular disparity results in the perception of depth (see section 11.7 in Chapter 11). Schumer and Ganz (1979) showed an adaptation after-effect related to depth perception. To create the after-effect, the visuum is experimentally adapted to specific binocular disparity. This adaptation then causes a quantifiable error in disparity detection. The adaptation is a similar process binocularly to the monocular interocular transfer tilt after-effect (see section 4.5 in Chapter 4). This experimental effect is explained by temporary changes (i.e. adaptation), in this case of cortical binocular disparity processing cells. From this experimental adaptation it is possible to identify the range of disparities to which a chosen adapting disparity detector can cause adaptation. In fact, there appears to be a small number, three or possibly slightly more, of **disparity channels**, each of which covers a broad range of disparities, e.g. for crossed disparities, and for uncrossed disparities. **Relative binocular disparity**, the difference between two objects' absolute disparities, is described in section 10.12.

10.9   Area V1 – methods of disparity detection

There are two methods by which cortical neurones detect binocular disparity. Position encoding binocular cells respond maximally to an individually given amount of lateral shift of the monocular retinal receptive fields. These are high spatial frequency parvocellular neurones (Barlow *et al.*, 1967). Phase difference encoding binocular cells identify different amounts of disparity by recognition of a given misalignment of the excitatory central regions of monocular receptive field profiles (Anzai *et al.*, 1997).

Each binocular cell is pre-set for a specific amount of disparity with a maximal (summation/stereopsis) response for the preferred disparity, and a gradually decreasing response for disparities further away from the preferred one, eventually becoming less than the monocular input (binocular inhibition/suppression) and then returning to the monocular input response (diplopia).

It is possible to plot the **neurophysiological equivalent of the horopter** and Panum's fusional area. To do this, a light stimulus is produced, which can be moved to stimulate the fixation point of one eye, and increasingly disparate retinal areas of the other eye: the light is moved along the line of sight/visual axis of one eye, but increasingly further from the binocular fixation point. Single cell cortical recordings are made of the response of cortical binocular cells at sequentially more lateral distances from the cell representing the fixation point. More peripheral locations have a larger number of monocular cortical cells synapsing with the disparity-detecting binocular cell representing the fixation point. This is because Panum's fusional areas are larger in the retinal periphery. In addition, for each cortical location in area V1 there will be more binocular cells tuned to zero disparity (the horopter) and fewer tuned to increasingly uncrossed or crossed disparities. This corresponds with the highest stereoacuity level being adjacent to the horopter.

10.10   Area V1 – the four main types of binocular-disparity-processing cells

There are four main sorts of **true binocular-disparity processors** involved in visual area V1:

- type 1 – excitatory tuned cells for zero disparity
- type 2 – inhibitory tuned cells
- type 3 – near stimulus untuned cells
- type 4 – far stimulus untuned cells.

They assess depth perception by comparing a group of receptive fields. Poggio and Fischer (1977) first described them, in terms of **absolute disparity**. The responses of an absolute-tuned disparity cell remain constant even with a change in background disparity (see section 10.12) (and see Bishop and Pettigrew, 1986). A binocularly driven neurone shows summation if its response is equal to the monocular inputs, but shows facilitation or suppression if the neurone's response is greater or less, respectively, than the monocular inputs.

Type 1: excitatory tuned cells for zero disparity

When right and left monocular corresponding receptive fields are simultaneously stimulated, their input into **type 1** cells causes maximal response; hence the term 'excitatory tuned'. This stimulation occurs for an object situated exactly on the horopter and stimulating corresponding retinal points. The effect of shifting an object in front or behind the horopter is to produce a lateral shift of the retinal image. Alternatively, a prism could be used to the same effect. As the image starts to move away from a corresponding retinal point, the **binocular summation** by the type 1 cell starts to diminish and is replaced with **binocular inhibition** at about 10 minutes of arc separation. Further lateral shift of the retinal image stops binocular inhibition, and the type 1 cell responds at the level equivalent to stimulation from one eye only, i.e. zero summation. At this point, the subject would experience diplopia.

Type 2: inhibitory tuned cells

When the right and left monocular receptive fields are simultaneously stimulated, i.e. for an object exactly on the horopter, their input into type 2 (inhibitory tuned) cells causes only minimal response. Moving the object in front of or behind the horopter (by separating the retinal images laterally) increases the response of type 2 cells. This indicates that the object has moved off the horopter, although these cells are not specifically sensitive as to whether movement is in front or behind the horopter: they do not distinguish between crossed and uncrossed disparities. The recognition of position of an object as being in front or behind the horopter aids stereoscopic appreciation.

Type 3: near stimulus untuned cells

These detect whether an object is **closer** than the fixation point on the horopter: that is, in crossed disparity.

Type 4: far stimulus untuned cells

These detect whether an object is more **distant** than the fixation point on the horopter, in uncrossed disparity. It is noteworthy that the range of disparities detected by both near and far stimulus untuned cells is greater than is normally used in depth perception, and is similar to the range of disparities found in vergence eye movements (Westheimer and Mitchell, 1969). It is therefore likely that this information is also used for vergence motor response.

In summary, where one visual stimulus is detected by type 1 cells (on the horopter), and another by type 2 cells (off the horopter), the presence of a stereoscopic percept will emerge. Stimulation of type 3 and type 4 cells will qualify the stereopsis as to whether the percept is in front or behind the horopter. Ohzawa and Freeman (1986) showed that V1 disparity-selective cells also respond to the differential phase of sinusoidal gratings. Cumming and Parker (1997, 1999) demonstrated that about 80% of V1 neurones are tuned for **absolute binocular disparity** of random dot stereograms. They also found that some V1 binocular-disparity-selective cells also respond to binocular inputs that do not produce depth perception. They respond to **anti-correlation**: the association of random dot stereo pairs, in which the dots for one eye are opposite compared with those for the other eye. Anti-correlation assists in identifying corresponding-area information from each eye, rather than in stereopsis perception.

Binocular visual processing in the cortex is carried out in the primary visual cortex area V1 as described, and also in area V2, adjacent to V1 on the occipital lobe cortical surface, and also area V3. In addition, area V5 (the middle temporal (MT) cortex), the middle superior temporal (MST) cortex and the parietal and frontal cortex also process binocular vision. These further structures and their functions are now described.

10.11 The visual pathways after visual area V1: ventral and dorsal visual processing streams in extrastriate areas

Visual area V1 transmits two streams of visual information to the extrastriate visual cortex. The streams have different contributions to stereopsis perception, and to other visual functions (Neri *et al.*, 2004). The lower, or **ventral, stream** has neurones that specifically respond to and help to analyse three-dimensional binocular-disparity input (Uka *et al.*, 2005). So the recognition of three-dimensional shapes is a major function of the ventral visual processing stream. This stream continues to area V4 and to the inferior temporal cortex. The ventral stream is concerned with object representation and also visual memory storage. Ventral stream V2 neurones gain input from V1 narrow adjacent receptive fields, which allows relative disparity sensitivity to be processed in V2.

The upper, or **dorsal, stream** passes from V1 to V2, to the dorsomedial area (including V3), to V5/MT and to the posterior parietal region. This pathway is related to the analysis of the location of objects, and with stereo-motion perception (motion-in-depth), and with hand–eye coordination and control, including saccadic eye movements. Dorsal cells obtain input from broad adjacent and overlapping receptive fields in V1 and process the analysis of the slant or tilt of a visual surface. Dorsal stream neurones do not respond to relative depth stimuli as required for three-dimensional-surface analysis (Uka and DeAngelis, 2006). The dorsal stream seems responsible for analysing depth structure during movement of the subject (self-motion) and in the perception of extended visual surfaces. The activities of the ventral and dorsal streams are sometimes summarised as the 'what/where', or the 'perception/action', pathways.

10.12 Area V2: relative binocular disparity detection

Although disparity-detecting binocular cells comprise about 50% of the cells in area V1, this increases to 70% for area V2 cells. Cortical visual areas in V2 stained with cytochrome oxidase, a metabolic marker stain, show non-staining layers (interstripes) alternating between thin-stripe staining layers and thick-stripe staining layers (see Table 10.1). The thin stripes process low temporal frequency and high spatial frequency stimuli, and chromatic stimuli. The thick stripes detect coarse binocular disparities (and motion) and receive

Table 10.1 Binocular-disparity-processing areas in visual cortex area V2 (for fine stereopsis, gross stereopsis and motion stereopsis)

From v1	Received by v2
Magno	Thick stripe regions: low spatial frequency disparity detection, and motion processing = gross stereopsis
Parvo	Interstripe regions: high spatial frequency disparity detection, and chromatic stimuli processing = fine stereopsis
Parvo	Thin stripe regions: high spatial frequency disparity detection, and luminance level and chromatic stimuli processing = fine stereopsis

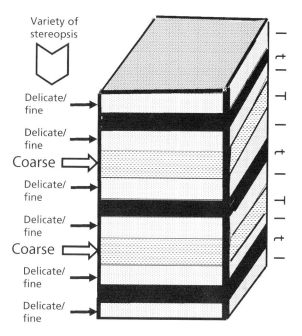

Figure 10.6 Primary visual cortex area V2 (after Steinman *et al.*, 2000). Cortical cell layers within visual area V2 can be differentially stained with cytochrome oxidase, a metabolic marker. These layers are referred to as thick and thin staining layers, and non-staining interstripe layers. Coarser binocular disparities for stereopsis, based upon magnocellular input, are processed in **thick layers, T**. Between these and **thinner layers, t**, lie the **interstripe layers, I**; these are associated with parvocellular disparity data based upon high spatial frequencies. These layers are indicated on the right of the figure.

input from area V1 magnocellular complex cells. The thick stripes of V2 have been shown to have a topographical mapping for disparity response (Chen *et al.*, 2006), which does not occur in V1. It appears that the V2 thick stripes contain maps for orientation of disparities. Cells in the interstripe layers detect high spatial frequency signals, equivalent to fine stereopsis, and are innervated by area V1 parvocellular simple cells (Fig. 10.6). The parvocellular and magnocellular pathways combine to produce full binocular disparity processing utilising all three types of stripe layers (Li and Guo, 1995).

The visual area V2 has ventral and dorsal representation in both hemispheres, which together provide a retinotopic picture of visual space. V2 receives and also sends information back to V1, and transmits to V3, V4 and V5/MT (Shipp and Zeki, 1985; Rockland, 1995). Early work on the binocular-disparity tuning function was based on **absolute binocular disparity**, and V2 cells were described as obligatory binocular for absolute disparity (Hubel and Wiesel, 1970). Qiu and von der Heydt (2005) found V2 cells were selective for absolute binocular-disparity-defined contours (and also for contour orientation and differentiation from the background). However, Westheimer (1979) showed that binocular depth assessment in humans depends more on **relative binocular disparity**, the difference between the absolute disparities of two objects. Here, one object is fixated by the two foveas, and relative disparity measures the relative depth between it and the second, non-fixated, object (see section 11.7 in Chapter 11).

Thomas *et al.* (2002) demonstrated relative binocular disparity tuning in V2, although the tuning was not quite equal to the full background disparity shift. A relative binocular disparity tuned cell alters its tuning to match the change in background disparity. For a shift of the background disparity away from the subject, the tuning is moved backwards. If the background disparity moves forward, so does the tuning of the relative-binocular-disparity-tuned cell. Because the relative binocular disparity is the difference between two absolute binocular disparities, the fovea is removed as a reference point. Relative-binocular-disparity detection is found mainly in cortical cells beyond the V1 area. Thomas *et al.*, (2002) demonstrated a mechanism in area V2 where summation onto a complex cell is provided by absolute-disparity-receptive-fields in pairs of fields, each sensitive to an absolute binocular disparity. An estimate of the monocular inputs can be subtracted, and the final output is effectively a summation of two pairs of complementary absolute binocular disparity neurones, providing relative binocular disparity. What is happening is that the cortical circuitry that works at the V1 level to produce absolute binocular disparity is being copied at the V2 level to produce relative binocular disparity.

10.13 Area V3: velocity, colour, orientation and disparity

Visual area V3 responds to fixed stereopsis but not to changes in depth (i.e. not to **motion-in-depth** perception). The full functions of area V3 are still unknown, although about half the cells respond to disparity between right and left perceptive fields. It is thought that there are both ventral and dorsal elements of V3. Area V3 also contains cells, which respond to orientation, and to planar motion, which is motion across the horopter (Montaser-Kouhsari *et al.*, 2007). In the last decade it appears that, certainly in the monkey visual cortex as a whole, there are around 35 separate visual locations with an interconnecting network of perhaps 350 pathways. This arrangement allows basic 'building blocks' such as velocity of moving images, the colour of surfaces, the orientation of visual information ('contours') and binocular disparity to be combined to make more sophisticated assessments of binocular vision – e.g. as to when and where a target moving around a subject's head is likely to re-appear. V3 would certainly contain some of these discrete cortical visual areas. V3 has a high proportion of binocular-disparity-tuned neurones and is a source, with V2, of such information going to V5/MT.

Note: in humans, the visual area V3 is more correctly referred to as the 'third visual complex, including area V3', as there are different opinions as to its exact location, extent and functions.

10.14   Area V4: simple shape recognition and attention

In the macaque monkey, the third visual area in the ventral stream is called V4. The anatomical name of this area is the pre-lunate gyrus. The position of the human equivalent has not yet been located. V4 has inputs from the frontal eye movement fields involved in eye-movement control, which are situated in the frontal cortex. V4 cells are tuned for spatial frequency, orientation and colour, providing functions of simple shape recognition, and V4 shows plasticity and receptive field changes associated with attention.

10.15   The inferior temporal cortex: complex shape recognition

The ventral stream continues to the inferior temporal cortex. This area is tuned for complicated targets, such as the recognition of faces.

10.16   Area V5/MT: functions and plasticity for adaptation and learning

Visual area V5, the middle temporal cortex, sometimes referred to as V5/MT, is located within the dorsal stream only, and receives directly some signals originating from layers 4B and 6 in V1, and originally from the extra-foveal (i.e. non-central) visual field. These signals are used for velocity tuning of V5/MT cells. A lesion here creates a scotoma for motion. In this case, in the adversely affected part of the visual field, the speed of a moving object cannot be evaluated. There is a second, indirect, pathway from layer 4B of V1 to the thick stripes of V2, then to V3 and finally to V5/MT. These signals are used for binocular disparity tuning of V5/MT cells. Albright *et al.* (1984) showed that V5/MT is topographically mapped for direction selectivity. Thus selective integration of the basic building blocks of both binocular disparity and of direction of motion takes place in V5/MT. Cells with similar direction sensitivity are arranged in columns in the same way as ocular dominance columns, and adjacent columns have a consecutive rotation (column by column) of the preferred direction sensitivity. DeAngelis and Newsome (1999) also found a columnar arrangement here for binocular disparity.

Motion-in-depth

Dynamic depth perception requires a combination of sensitivity to disparity and to motion. The direct and indirect pathways converge, as mentioned above, so that most neurones in V5/MT are selective for both direction of motion and for binocular disparity (Maunsell and Van Essen, 1983). Indeed, there is simultaneous:

- mutual inhibition by opposing groups of neurones, maximally sensitive to the same binocular disparity, but tuned also to opposite directions of movement
- facilitation between other twin groups of neurones, also tuned to opposite directions of motion, but in this case maximally sensitive to different levels of binocular disparity (Bradley *et al.*, 1998). This sounds complicated, but it just means that V5/MT can recognise two independently moving surfaces, at two different depths, the essence of motion-in-depth perception. Interestingly, there is some evidence also for response in V5/MT to **monocular clues** to depth perception created by **motion parallax**.

In the macaque monkey all V5/MT cortical cells have binocular input. This is shown by almost 100% interocular transfer (see section 4.5 in Chapter 4) for global stereopsis random-dot motion images in V5/MT, compared with the visual area V1 partial transfer of about 70% for moving-grating images (Raymond, 1993).

Stereopsis grades

By using a variety of experimental methods to evaluate stereopsis detection in V5/MT for fine depth perception and higher levels of stereopsis (needing sensitivity to small differences in relative disparity), it has been found that V5/MT neurones do not perform particularly well. However, there is a much better response to discrimination between far and near absolute disparities (Uka and DeAngelis, 2003, 2006). Such coarse depth discrimination is achieved at the maximal level anywhere in the cortex, in area V5/MT.

Multiple functions

The widespread representation of binocular disparity detectors in a variety of cortical areas suggests that different visual cortex areas use this information **locally** for specialised functions, such as whether an object is beyond or within the horopter, high-level stereopsis, the analysis of three-dimension shape orientation and rotation, and the assessment of the visual effects of self-motion. However, it is also likely that disparity and depth perception rely on **simultaneous processing** in several cortical regions.

In addition to direction selectivity, motion-in-depth and fine and coarse depth discrimination, there is evidence in V5/MT of **plasticity of function**, allowing adaptation and learning skills in the individual – e.g. training in fine depth discrimination, and possibly utilisation of other areas such as V4 to aid such tasks (Umeda *et al.*, 2007). It appears that learning, whether by experience or training, or in response to cortical damage, can modify pathways for assessment of sensory information, e.g. as to whether a ventral or dorsal pathway is used. In doing this, the actual representation of the sensory information is not itself affected. Nevertheless, such plasticity is likely to be involved in the development of **anomalous retinal correspondence** (in the author's opinion). At the level of V5/MT, the dorsal stream also has functions in relation to **extended visual surface disparities** – in effect, disparity gradient and disparity curvature, described in section 11.7 in Chapter 11 (Nguyenkim and DeAngelis, 2003). The dorsal stream continues with recognition of extended visual surface disparities in the parietal area (Shikata *et al.*, 1996). So there may be disparity receptive fields, with central areas responding to disparity, and surrounding areas that suppress a response to disparity. Finally, it should be noted that V5/MT has **outputs** towards the frontal eye movement areas, and towards the eye-movement fields of the parietal cortex, so that plasticity in oculomotor control also may be involved.

10.17 Area MST: complex surface rotation and optic flow

Visual area MST (the middle superior temporal area) receives innervation from area V5/MT. This area responds to the **rotation** of three-dimensional targets. It is also sensitive to **optic flow**, the sensation of movement through the environment – e.g. when travelling on a moving stairway.

10.18 Parietal and frontal cortex: binocular vision functions

The posterior parietal cortex has functions providing **visual attention**, **spatial memory** and the **triangulation** of objects in visual space. It aids assessment of their **location relative** to each other and to the subject. It may have functions in delivering the fixation and refixation reflexes. Parietal and frontal cortex areas have recently been shown to have regions in which disparity-selective neurones apparently relate to **visuo-motor control**, such as the ventral inter-parietal (VIP) area (Colby *et al.*, 1993), the frontal eye (move-

Table 10.2 Summary of neural processing in LGN and cortex

Lateral geniculate nucleus layers	Layers 1 and 2 → Magnocellular neurons (the **'where'** pathway)
	Layers 4 to 6 → Parvocellular neurons (the **'what'** pathway)
Cortex areas	Cortical area V1 50% monocular + 50% binocular, mapped to retina
	Cortical area V2 receptive fields larger, 70% binocular and respond to disparity and motion; process gross and fine stereopsis
	Cortical area V3 processes disparity, motion and orientation
	Cortical area V4 processes spatial frequency, orientation, colour and shape recognition and has inputs from frontal eye movement fields
	Cortical area V5/MT (middle temporal cortex) processes motion-in-depth
	Cortical area MST (middle superior temporal cortex) processes rotation of three-dimensional targets, and optic flow
	Parietal cortex processes visual memory, spatial memory and relative location of objects in visual space
	Frontal cortex processes visuo-motor control

ment) field (FEF) (Ferraina *et al.*, 1993), the lateral parietal (LIP) area (Genovesio and Ferraina, 2004) and the caudal inter-parietal (CIP) area (Sakata *et al.*, 2005). See Table 10.2 for a summary of neural processing in the LGN and cortex.

10.19 Association and gnostic areas

Adjacent to the primary visual cortex there is a unimodal association cortical area, which connects visual sensory cortex with the infero-temporal cortex and the polymodal and supramodal association areas: these are concerned with perception, attention and judgement. The higher association areas receive input from the motor and sensory cortical regions: see Appendix 2. The higher association areas are also known as gnostic areas, as they are involved in knowledge, memory, emotions and consciousness.

10.20 The mechanism of integrating retinal hemi-fields

The left-hand side of each retina is represented in the left cerebral hemisphere, and the right-hand side in the right hemisphere. An image large enough to cover the binocular visual field of each eye is split into right and left halves and is located in the right and left hemispheres. The two half images are separated in the visual cortex. Integration of the right and left binocular half visual fields is provided by the **corpus callosum** (see Fig. 10.7), and also by the higher-level gnostic areas (Brodmann areas 5, 7, 39 and 40), which provide integration of input from all senses, and a suitable response.

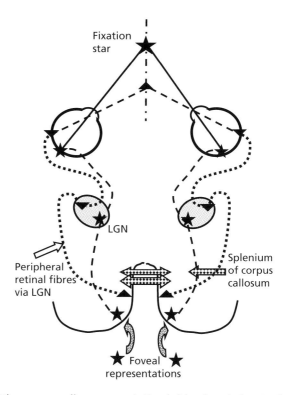

Figure 10.7 The corpus callosum association bridge in relation to the visual pathways (according to Davson, 1990). LGN, lateral geniculate nucleus.

Additionally, there is a unique foveal (and retinal medial plane) dual representation in the visual cortex. To provide high-level binocular perception from the fovea and the retinal midline of each retina there are **two separate systems**. These both provide **overlapping representation** from each eye from a vertical strip of retina including the fovea and extending approximately one-degree subtense either side. In monkeys, this strip varies between 1 and 3 degrees wide. In humans at the fovea the overlap is of the order of 0.4 degree or almost 1 prism dioptre, i.e. a target 1 cm wide at 1 m (Walsh and Hoyt, 2004). The central 1.0 degree foveal retinal area is about 0.01% of the total retinal area, but occupies about 8–10% of the striate cortex.

The **first system** operates by allowing retinal ganglion cell input from both sides of the median line of that retina to be included in the post-chiasmal pathway of that eye. The same thing happens also for the other eye (Plate 10.1). This results in the vertical strip of retina incorporating the fovea of each eye being represented in both the ipsilateral and contral-ateral striate cortex (Blakemore, 1969). So the (similar) images falling on both foveas are duplicated in the striate cortex of each cerebral hemi-sphere. This system allows for **fine foveal stereopsis**. The **second system** operates by utilising the cross-linkage between the right and left visual

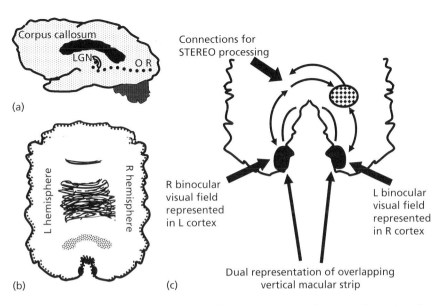

Figure 10.8 The binocular connection for coarse stereopsis processing using the corpus callosum connection. (**a**) Location of the corpus callosum relative to the optic radiations and the visual cortex; sagittal plane view. (**b**) The structure of the corpus callosum connecting the right and left cerebral hemispheres; axial plane view. (**c**) The suggested area for stereopsis processing in the right hemisphere is shown. L, left; R, right.

cortical lobes through the corpus callosum. This system allows for **coarse stereopsis** (Fig. 10.8).

Table 10.2 summarises the functions of the lateral geniculate nucleus and the visual sensory areas of the brain.

Chapter 10: Revision quiz

Complete the missing words, perhaps in pencil.

The retinal area receiving stimuli affecting a single retinal ganglion cell is called the _____ (1) field of the ganglion cell. Visual cortex cells respond best to a _____ (2) stimulus rather than a spot stimulus, as with retinal and lateral geniculate nucleus fields. Hypercomplex visual striate cells respond to light or dark bar stimuli, but at this higher level the cells are _____ (3) specific.

Striate cortex layer 4 cells receive _____ (4) input but pass this to layers 1 to 3 and to layers 5 and 6, which thus accumulate _____ (5) input from right and left eye stimuli from layer 4 cells.

The vertical strip of each retina including the fovea has enhanced stereopsis input, because its representation in the visual cortex is _____ (6) on each hemi-cortex. There is also a cross linkage between each hemi-cortex via the c_____ c_____ (7).

Answers
(1) receptive; (2) line; (3) orientation; (4) monocular; (5) binocular; (6) duplicated; (7) corpus callosum.

Chapter 11

DEPTH PERCEPTION

11.1 Monocular depth perception

Classification of monocular depth perception

In real life, depth perception is an amalgam of binocular and monocular clues. In predators such as snakes, a rapid to-and-fro movement of the head is used to assess the location in depth of their prey. The image of the prey is then transferred to either side of the snake's retina, assuming the snake has no fixation reflex! (Only tree snakes have foveas and stereopsis). When the angular displacement either side of the retinal centre is equal, the snake has measured a fixed striking distance and then attacks.

Other (human) monocular depth assessment factors include the following.

- **Aerial perspective** – relatively distant objects are seen less clearly, with reduced contrast, and have a blue tint as a result of light scatter from dust and water vapour mist; also objects seen in hues towards the red end of the spectrum tend to be seen as closer.
- **Hue attenuation** – distant objects have reduced colour brightness.
- **Texture gradient** – near objects are spread out more than similar distant objects.
- **Linear (geometric) perspective** – an example of geometric perspective is first seen in paintings by Brunelleschi and later by Canaletto, and more prosaically with railway lines apparently converging into the distance.
- **Overlapping** – a distant object is partially covered by a nearer one; this is also known as interposition.
- **Motion parallax** – analogous to spatial horizontal disparity detection in binocular vision, this is a temporal or dynamic monocular depth perception faculty. Here, the image displacement across the retina of, say, a nearer object is compared with the image of a further fixated object when the subject moves laterally. Motion parallax is used clinically to identify the depth of objects, such as floaters, in the ocular media. A level of threshold sensitivity similar to that of binocular stereoacuity is possible (Fig. 11.1). The faster apparent lateral movement of closer objects passing the moving subject, compared with the slower apparent movement of further objects, gives an indication of relative distance.

Normal Binocular Vision: theory, investigation and practical aspects. By David Stidwill and Robert Fletcher. © 2011 Blackwell Publishing Ltd

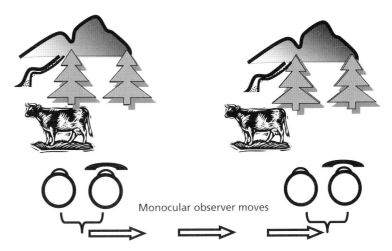

Figure 11.1 Motion parallax. The monocularly occluded observer moves from left to right. An apparent relative movement of the foreground against the background is seen. No – it is not the cow that moves!

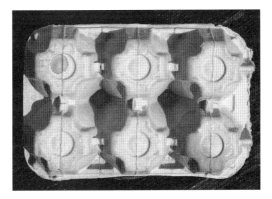

Figure 11.2 Light direction. The human visual system expects objects to be illuminated from above. The egg box appears to have the egg-containing areas projecting, unless the picture is rotated through 180 degrees.

- **Light direction and shading** – in the natural world, most objects are illuminated from light sources higher than themselves. So a concave depression on a vertical surface will have the upper half in shadow, and the lower half in higher illumination (Fig. 11.2). Similarly a convex protrusion on a vertical surface will cause shading or a shadow on the flat surface beneath it.
- **Non-pictorial information** – ocular accommodation gives an (imprecise) assessment of depth, based on the amount of third nerve innervation required to produce a sharp retinal image (Fisher and Ciuffreda, 1988).
- **Retinal image size** – a cognitive assumption is made that a smaller retinal image relates to a distant target and a larger image to a nearer

target, particularly for familiar objects. This is an acquired skill, and so an adult may have a completely different ability from that of a child, who may have both unfamiliarity with the distance object, say a motorcycle, and inexperience in assessing its distance based upon retinal image size. Even for adults, if the object is less familiar, the depth assessment may be quite poor. Judgments of distance derived from retinal image size are complicated by the effect of size constancy (see the section below). Seen through a telescope, a person will appear to be closer, rather than magnified.

Monocular depth perception: constancy of size

By contrast to the last point above, objects with different retinal image sizes may be judged as having the same physical size if the objects are perceived to be located at different distances from the subject (Fig. 11.3). Here a familiar object is incorrectly perceived to have a constant size despite changes in retinal image size. This effect is most pronounced when there are other objects in the visual field. The experimental procedure is to present a **test object** at a fixed distance, but where the apparent size of the object can be adjusted by the subject, and a **standard object** presented at different distances but with its size adjusted by the investigator so that it always subtends a constant visual angle, whatever distance it is from the subject. When there are no other objects in the visual field, the subject correctly matches the size of the standard object; size constancy is absent. However, if the test procedure is carried out in a normal visual environment with other objects visible to the subject, size constancy appears: the test object size is hardly altered by the subject.

Another example of size constancy is seen when increasingly strong base-out prisms are put before a subject's eyes when viewing a target at a fixed

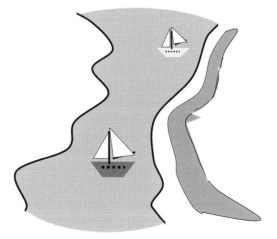

Figure 11.3 Size constancy. Similar objects appear to be the same size, even though their angular subtense is different.

distance. As the prism strength increases, the subject has to increasingly converge the eyes. The effect of this is to make the target appear smaller and closer as the prism strength increases. Thus the prescription of prisms in a visual correction is likely to alter the judgment of distance for a while. The effect of size constancy is to diminish the accuracy of monocular depth perception.

Monocular depth perception: constancy of shape

A familiar object is seen as having the same shape even though presented at different angles. For example, a book rotated from initially presenting its maximal retinal image size to appearing almost edge-on tends to retain its original apparent shape. Similarly, round plates on a table appear to preserve their shape at whatever angle they are viewed. Shape constancy therefore adversely affects monocular depth perception. Constancy of shape is reduced in the absence of other visual cues, which would more accurately help with the assessment of changes in shape.

11.2 Binocular depth perception

Convergence

'Convergence' is a term meaning both the position of the lines of sight for near fixation, and the act of altering the angle between the lines of sight from a distant to a nearer object of regard. The act of converging is normally a reflex to a near target but can also be produced voluntarily. The nearest point of convergence varies between individuals but is generally between 5 and 12 cm. 'Infacility of convergence' describes an inability to repeat the same near point of convergence.

The level of innervation required to converge the eyes gives an approximation of the distance of an object fixated (Erkelens and Regan, 1986). This is a relative estimation of distance, not absolute, as an individual wearing horizontal prisms will be more or less convergent than someone not wearing prisms. Some adapt to the prismatic effect on the lines of sight (visual axes), and so no abnormal sensation of depth is appreciated. During adaptation to a new prism prescription, however, there may be disturbances of depth perception. In general, accommodation and convergence are associated with micropsia: the observed object appears to be closer and smaller. The perceived direction of the near target is along the line that bisects the angle of convergence of the lines of sight (visual axes) measured at the object of regard.

Apparent depth perception: pseudo-chromostereopsis

The use by artists of 'warmer' (more red, or 'advancing') colours to enhance an illusion of depth in a flat painting has been known since the early

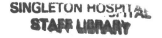

nineteenth century. Sundet (1976) and others attribute descriptions to Goethe and Bruecke. Most subjects agree that a red object appears nearer than a blue or green object (equally 'bright') in the same plane. Some report the opposite appearance. The clinical duochrome test usually shows the phenomenon. A common explanation, based on ocular transverse chromatic aberration and slight temporal displacement of the pupils from the eye's optical axis, is often named the Bruecke–Einthoven chromostereopsis effect; this holds up better with small pupils. Longitudinal chromatic aberration may produce wavelength-related blur in large pupils. Ye *et al.* (1991) investigated the influence of pupil diameter in detail. Vos (1960) and Sundet (1976) stress how asymmetry of the Stiles–Crawford directional effect can contribute. Viewing binocularly through small pinholes, separated variously, gives a simple demonstration. The retinal image of a green object will be displaced nasally relative to the image of a red object. The green image has less crossed disparity than a red one, the latter appearing nearer. Note, however, that some subjects may report a related appearance monocularly.

Induced binocular depth perception: temporal disparity

When, during binocular fixation, one eye views a moving object such as a pendulum through a neutral density filter, a delay in visual processing speed occurs in that eye's impression compared with the other. This results in the binocular cortical image receiving information simultaneously from non-corresponding retinal points. The pendulum appears to be swinging in an elliptical path, clockwise (from above) if the filter is over the left eye. The faster the pendulum moves and the larger the swing, the greater is the apparent disparity. The oscillation should be less than five cycles a second. The pendulum speed will be greater when it is vertical and least as it reaches the end of its swing on each side. A very large bob displays illusory changes of size as convergence varies. This is the **Pulfrich phenomenon**. It can be used to recreate true stereopsis when filming with a single home video camera. The camera has to be kept moving relative to the scenery in a clockwise or anticlockwise path around the scene. The viewers then watch with a neutral density filter in front of the appropriate eye (right or left) and the original stereopsis of the scene is reproduced. Greater neutral density filter absorption increases the effect, and differently coloured filters for each eye may induce it, i.e. when not expected. Fig. 11.4 demonstrates the illusion.

Weale (1954a,b) described practical and theoretic aspects, including variations from conventional elliptical tracks, with many references. Lit (1978) compared apparent depth displacement effect features of the Pulfrich and Mach–Dvorak phenomena. The Mach–Dvorak effect is similar to the Pulfrich effect but produced by intermittent stimulus presentation, the stimulus for one eye being delayed slightly. Such spatiotemporal parallactic appearances could involve monocular lateral displacements attributable to different variations in stimulus exposure and latency. There are some resemblances to the Fröligh effect, which has connections with apparent reflex

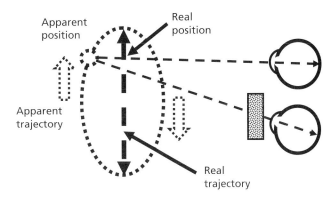

Figure 11.4 The Pulfrich phenomenon. With a neutral density filter in front of one eye, a pendulum oscillating in one plane appears to be swinging in an elliptical path. This is caused by a delay in visual processing for images received by the affected eye.

movement in retinoscopy of astigmatic eyes as well the beta variety of the phi phenomenon. As pointed out by Regan and Cyanader (1979), cells in the ocular dominance columns of the visual cortex, which are binocularly activated, can enjoy different interocular latency; directionally sensitive cells may have a stereoscopic role.

True binocular depth perception: stereopsis

The two pre-eminent advantages of binocular vision are the presence of a spare organ if one eye is not functioning and the accurate perception of depth if both eyes are operating normally. Supplementary benefits of stereopsis are:

- an enhanced ability to locate and to avoid approaching targets
- the facility to move through a congested environment without collision – for example, walking in a crowded street
- the ability to identify important data within a confusing background – **figure–ground separation**, also known as camouflage breaking.

The binocular perception of depth is called **stereopsis**, which is actually disparity sensitivity. It is most precise when a comparison of the position of two objects is made. One object is situated on the horopter at the intersection of the lines of sight (visual axes), and the other object is either in front of or behind the horopter, and is close enough to be within Panum's fusional area but not imaged on corresponding retinal points. In this case, the relative separation of the two retinal images in each eye is called the 'horizontal retinal binocular disparity' (see section 1.6 in Chapter 1). This disparity allows the assessment of the depth separation of the fixated and non-fixated objects (see Fig. 11.5). The images of each object are both fused, because the objects lie within Panum's area. The threshold for best stereoacuity is about 2–8 arc seconds in humans under optimal conditions. Clinical

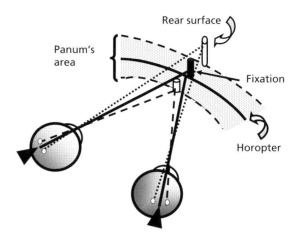

Figure 11.5 A three-dimensional object straddling Panum's fusional area in depth fails to elicit diplopia. Black arrows indicate the foveas in each eye. Small white spots indicate non-corresponding retinal areas stimulated by objects for which minimal disparities fail to elicit diplopia but do produce a stereoscopic percept.

tests usually accept a reading of 30 arc seconds as normal for local stereopsis, and 60 arc seconds for global stereopsis.

The assessment of the direction of the depth of the non-fixated object – in front or behind the fixated object – is given by the direction of displacement of the retinal images, given below.

- **Crossed disparities** relate to objects nearer than the horopter. They are 'crossed' because a target nearer than the horopter (which the eyes are fixating) will be seen to the left by the right eye, and to the right by the left eye.
- **Uncrossed disparities** relate to objects situated beyond the horopter. Here the unilateral image seen by the right eye will appear to the right of its visual axis; and to the left of the left eye's visual axis. The fixated object has **zero disparity**, and will appear to be in its true location because it is imaged on corresponding retinal areas.

The distance between a viewer and a target within his/her visual field (in physical space) is called the **absolute depth** and is found by the difference in the external longitudinal angles (Fig. 11.6), i.e. the angle between binocular fixation at infinity and the horizontal angle subtended by the object. The difference in the external longitudinal angles is called the **absolute disparity**, and is used mainly to initiate vergence eye movements (Pobuda and Erkelens, 1993). Although absolute depth is derived from the absolute disparity, this assessment is modified by monocular information such as geometric perspective, aerial perspective and apparent size.

The difference in depth of two or more objects in physical space is assessed (using binocular information) by their **relative disparity**, which is the difference between their two absolute disparities. This means that stereopsis detects the depth difference between the fixated object and another

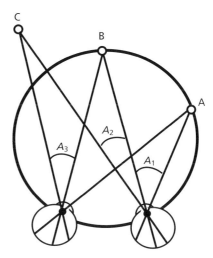

Figure 11.6 The distance between the subject and an object within the visual field is found by the difference in the external longitudinal angles i.e. the angle between binocular fixation at infinity and the horizontal angle subtended by the object. Here both eyes fixate object B, and the external angles A_1 and A_2 are equal. This is because both objects A and B are on the Vieth–Müller circle (VMC). Object C is not on the VMC, and the external longitudinal angle A_3 does not equal A_1 and A_2.

object, rather than their exact location in depth. This difference in depth is called the **relative depth**. So relative depth informs the viewer which of the two objects is nearer, but without giving the absolute depth of either. The assessment of relative depth is also modified by monocular information such as motion parallax, light, shadow and overlap. The maximum range of stereoscopic vision is the distance at which the interocular base line subtends an angle equal to the best stereoscopic acuity.

Stereopsis is poor at assessing absolute disparity, because the visual system uses **depth constancy** to judge apparent distance. Depth constancy relates to judgement of the distance of an object independently from the actual distance at which it is located. It results from distance scaling arising from information such as the amount of ocular convergence and accommodation present, the intrinsic information presented by an object as to its shape and size, and also memory of the size of a well-known object, and linear perspective clues. Depth constancy may misinterpret the actual distance of an object. In addition, the memory of known objects may contaminate depth information obtained from retinal disparity. Retinal disparities may themselves be distorted by viewing objects through prisms or lenses. Depth constancy is a subdivision of perceptual constancy, which affects the perception of shape, colour and location, so that the appearance tends to conform to experience rather than the stimulus itself (see text about constancy of size and shape in section 11.1). Under extreme conditions depth constancy collapses, so that, for example, scenery seen from an aircraft looks unnaturally small. Where a series of objects are placed on a surface, which is tilted with respect to the horopter, the change in disparities – the **relative binocular**

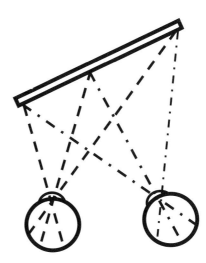

Figure 11.7 Relative disparity gradient. A series of binocular disparity assessments by the visual system gives an indication of a tilted surface.

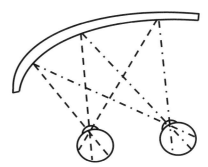

Figure 11.8 Relative disparity curvature. A series of increasing binocular disparities give an indication of the curve of a surface.

disparity – along the surface produces a **relative disparity gradient**, which is recognised by the visuum (Fig. 11.7). If the surface is also curved there will be an identifiable rate of change of disparities. This is known as **relative disparity curvature** (Fig. 11.8).

Classification of stereopsis

There are three types of stereopsis: local stereopsis, global stereopsis and stereopsis adjacent to Panum's fusional area.

Local stereopsis

Local, or contour, stereopsis is demonstrated by stereoscopic targets containing monocularly identifiable contours or lines, having different disparities for each eye. An example is one of the tests on the **Randot stereotest**, which includes a series of stereoscopic images containing four circles, one of which has different disparities for each eye. Unfortunately, a monocular individual can see one of the four circles shifted to the right and may recognise this circle as the odd one out, although not seen in depth compared with the other three circles, as intended.

This effect is even more apparent when single line stereograms are viewed. The difference in horizontal separation between two vertical lines seen in one eye compared with the other gives the depth effect, e.g. the Bradford stereogram series. However, such line stereograms are useful for orthoptic exercises and in carefully controlled experimental measurements of threshold stereopsis disparities.

Global stereopsis

Global stereopsis is measured with stereoscopic targets in which monocular clues are not evident. Julesz first achieved this with the **random-dot stereogram**. First a computer-generated series of black-and-white spots is produced where the chance of being black or white is random. The pattern is duplicated to produce an identical image for each eye. Next, for the picture seen by one eye only, a thin vertical rectangle of black-and-white spots is stripped from one side of a square area within the pattern and replaced on the other side of the square, which has been shifted laterally. There is now a disparity between the shifted square seen by one eye and the non-shifted area seen by the other eye: see Fig. 11.9a for the design of a random-dot stereogram. Fig. 11.9b illustrates the appearance of a random-dot stereogram. The square is seen in depth against the non-shifted background. However, there are no monocular clues to stereopsis, and the stereoscopic percept can only appear when there is binocular fusion.

The interpretation of a random-dot stereogram requires cortical matching of similar right and left spots and the recognition of their disparity to give **local stereopsis**. The cortex then matches larger areas sharing the same disparity and assigns the same depth for the area for which **global stereopsis** operates. These two processes are independent. Exchanging right and left eye visual input with a suitable optical device, the local stereopsis is seen reversed or in fluctuating depth, but global stereopsis is unaffected (Shimojo and Nakajima, 1981). Such an optical device diverts the right eye visual input to the left eye, and vice versa. This device is called a 'pseudo-stereoscope' (or 'pseudoscope') (Fig. 11.10). Global stereopsis produces cyclopean vision, in which there are no monocular clues present; the outline of a cyclopean (random-dot) stereoscopic object is determined solely by the change in depth at its circumference, and not by any change in colour, luminance or overlap.

Stereopsis adjacent to Panum's fusional area

Although accurate stereopsis is restricted to objects lying in Panum's fusional area, depth perception does not end suddenly at the edge of Panum's area.

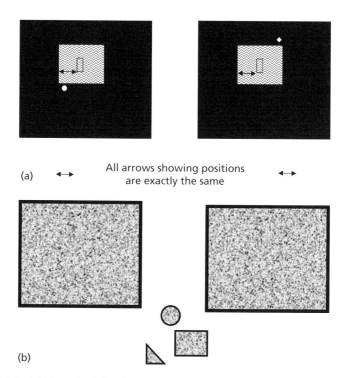

(a) ↔ All arrows showing positions
are exactly the same ↔

(b)

Figure 11.9 (a) The principle of a random-dot stereogram is presented, the central rectangle in the picture for one eye being shifted laterally. This shift may be observed with a monocular loupe looking at each picture in turn. (b) A stereoscope, base-out prism(s) or suitable unaided binocular viewing reveals three objects displaced in depth, resembling those shown separately below the stereoscopic pair.

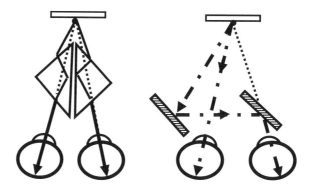

Figure 11.10 The principle of two types of pseudoscope, presenting horizontally reversed images to each eye. To achieve the desired percept of reversed depth, the right and left stereograms must be rearranged.

There is a further zone of depth perception where diplopia occurs but the visual system is able to detect whether crossed or uncrossed diplopia is occurring. A gross assessment of the position of the diplopic images is possible. Crossed diplopic images relate to an object nearer the fixation point, and uncrossed diplopic images relate to a point further than the fixation point. Eventually, at about 1000 minutes of arc disparity, diplopia only is seen but without any depth perception. The accuracy of depth perception gradually decreases as the object seen in diplopia has increasing disparity.

The spatial limit of stereopsis within or beyond Panum's area can be subdivided into a region of **patent stereopsis** and one of **qualitative stereopsis**:

- Patent stereopsis is present for objects that are not on the horopter but are still within Panum's area. When the objects move just outside Panum's area, they are seen double but still with a strong impression of depth. This is known as 'patent stereopsis with double images'. Within these two areas a subject can be aware of changes in depth derived from an increase in binocular disparity. There is, however, an exponential reduction in stereoscopic acuity as the target is positioned further from the horopter. It should be noted that patent stereopsis may explain the discovery of gross stereopsis in a small angle heterotropia without anomalous correspondence being present. Indeed, it might act as a trigger for anomalous correspondence.
- Qualitative stereopsis describes the uncertain perception of relative depth changes in the area still further from the horopter (either beyond, or within, the horopter). Compared with a fixed reference target, the subject will locate a moveable test target either in front or behind. The target is seen double, and the strong sense of depth is lost. The subject is still able to identify the double images as being either in front of or behind the fixation point, but cannot say how far in front or behind. Eventually, as binocular disparity increases, the subject is unable to quantify any change in apparent depth, with an upper disparity limit of about 1000 arc minutes of disparity (Fig. 11.11).

Anomalies of stereopsis processing

In 1971 Richards proposed the existence of **disparity channels** that separately allow the perception that an object is in front, behind, or either in front or behind, the horopter. However, individual channels may not function in as many as 30% of the normal population. This reduction in normal disparity detection is sometimes called 'stereo blindness'. Thus it is possible to be stereo blind to different extents:

- suppression of one eye, with all stereopsis markedly reduced or absent
- stereo blindness for crossed disparity
- stereo blindness for uncrossed disparity
- stereo blindness for disparity type – disparity is detected but crossed disparities cannot be distinguished from uncrossed disparities; the object is recognised as not being on the horopter but the subject cannot tell whether it is in front or behind the horopter.

Details of these and related anomalies, e.g. defective stereo-motion percept, should be sought in clinical texts (such as Steinman *et al.*, 2000).

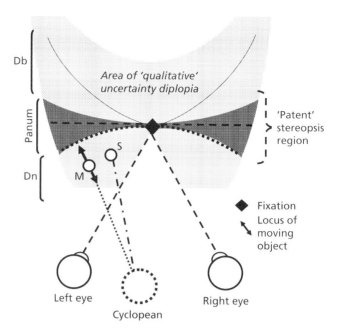

Figure 11.11 Thresholds of stereopsis bordering Panum's fusional area. Panum's fusional area is indicated in dark grey: patent stereopsis occurs here. Patent stereopsis with double images extends just outside Panum's area. Further away, the light grey regions show qualitative stereopsis, where double images are seen, and whether static or moving, can be identified only as being in front or behind the fixation point. Db, diplopia beyond fixation; Dn, diplopia nearer than fixation; M, moving object; S, static object.

It is possible for the visuum to adapt over time to a given disparity value, which then causes transient reduction in depth perception (Blakemore and Julesz, 1971; Mitchell and Baker, 1973). For adjacent varying disparities, **depth averaging** can occur. Here a group of image points seen together in depth have their disparities pooled or averaged so as to eliminate depth perception errors owing to ambiguity. This can result in fine differences in depth being ignored; the tilt of a surface might be less apparent.

Important influences on stereopsis

Refractive errors: degradation of stereopsis

Equal blur on each eye lowers stereopsis less than monocular blur. Individuals with congenital nystagmus may have better stereopsis than is usually associated with the same level of visual acuity in monocular amblyopia.

Contrast sensitivity

Reduction in contrast sensitivity will lower stereopsis levels rapidly. Stereopsis thresholds increase by the square root of the target brightness

(Cormack, *et al.*, 1991). Monocular contrast sensitivity reduction lowers stereoacuity more than binocular reduction.

Motion-in-depth

This degrades stereoacuity and does so more for objects receding than approaching. This involves testing **dynamic stereoacuity**: sensitivity to oscillations in depth. Dynamic stereoacuity can be measured using a computer programme in which a stereoscopic target appears to move towards the subject. The target is observed with red and blue glasses to separate the right and left images. The disparity of these two images increases as the target approaches. The apparent depth of the moving target is compared with fixed targets of varying stereopsis that are also present on the computer screen. Dynamic stereoacuity is a useful test for visual performance in sports.

Lateral motion

Lateral motion of targets at speeds of up to three degrees per second does not reduce stereoacuity (Westheimer and McKee, 1978).

Increased lateral separation

Greater separation between adjacent stereopsis targets decreases stereoacuities. The best stereoacuities are found with target separations between 20 and 60 minutes of arc.

Extra-retinal eccentricity

Greater eccentricity of a target seen in depth decreases stereoacuity. Foveal receptive fields are smaller and have higher depth perception than peripheral fields.

Limiting distance

The furthest distance at which stereopsis operates depends upon the interpupillary distance of the subject, and their level of stereopsis. The distance (d) can be found using the formula d = (interpupillary distance)/(stereoacuity in radians), so for an exceptionally good stereoacuity of 10 arc seconds, stereopsis would disappear at 1.2 km.

Additional aspects

Comparing the depth of a second (test) target to a primary (reference) target is more difficult when both targets have a disparity. The best result is found when the reference target has **zero disparity**, i.e. it is located on the horopter (Ogle, 1953). Experimentally, using a technique of binocular perimetry with stereoscopic targets, anomalies such as **stereoscopic scotomata** have been found, (i.e. in addition to those at the physiological blind spots). It is also possible to have a **scotoma for stereo-motion**, in which the movement of any object towards or away from the subject is not perceived (Regan *et al.*, 1986).

Temporal and spatial characteristics of stereopsis

The duration of a disparity affects perception. For brief durations, only large disparities are detected, although sensitivity is increased if the target is moving in depth. Over a longer viewing period, fine disparities are recognised, particularly if the targets are static. There is a delay in the region of 150 ms in the recognition of random-dot global stereopsis in the case of a subject with normal binocular vision. With experience, a subject can speed up the recognition of stereopsis, although this skill is specific for a particular orientation, e.g. of lines forming the stereo-pair (Ramachandran and Braddick, 1973). This delay in perception, **stereo-latency**, has been used as a test of stereoscopic perception (Larson and Faubert, 1992).

A second component of binocular perception, in addition to stereopsis, is called **figure–ground recognition**, and has a latency of around 250 ms (Miyawaki *et al.*, 2002). This is the identification of a target against its background. The **size** (i.e. area) of a disparity stimulus affects stereopsis sensitivity. Large retinal disparities are associated with low spatial frequency (large) receptive fields. As the area of the disparity stimulus decreases, more sensitive stereopsis is possible, as high spatial frequency (small) receptive fields are then involved. This process is called **size-disparity correlation** (Ohzawa *et al.*, 1996). It appears that the magnocellular (M) system processes low stereopsis thresholds and the parvocellular (P) system relates to high levels of stereopsis. The size-disparity correlation differentiates between **peripheral stereopsis** at eccentricities of 1.0–10 degrees from the fovea, and **central stereopsis** (detecting stereopsis disparities of 60 seconds or less) over the 1.0 degree central foveal area. Peripheral stereopsis, which utilises stereopsis disparities of the order of degrees of arc, helps to maintain **peripheral fusion** even in the presence of a central organic or functional scotoma.

Measurement of stereopsis

For stereopsis measurement head movements are usually prevented, although sometimes such movement aids the gradual awareness of relative depth in a clinical test. The stereoacuity of an individual person is defined as the smallest resolvable distance in depth when measured by the minimum discernable difference in binocular parallax. It is in fact the minimal resolvable binocular disparity between two objects in physical space. For stereopsis values at around the threshold the stereoacuity may be found from the approximate formula: **stereoacuity (the angular stereo-disparity in** radians) = (distance between centres of rotation of the eyes) × (gap between two targets just resolvable in depth)/(distance between the mean nodal point to the nearer object)^2, or:

$$n = 2ad/D^2$$

where n is the angular measure of stereoacuity, and is the angle subtended between the two objects from the mean nodal points. The stereoacuity is measured in radians, and the other measurements are in units of length, e.g. metres. a is the distance between the centre of rotation of one eye and the median plane, so $2a$ is the interpupillary distance; d is the smallest resolvable distance in depth in anteroposterior position in the median plane between the two objects; D is the distance between the mean nodal point to the nearer object. The position of the mean nodal points changes when the eyes converge, but the effect is too small to affect measurement of stereoacuity. To convert the stereoacuity in radians to stereoacuity in arc seconds, multiply by 206,265. (**Note**: This conversion factor is given incorrectly in some textbooks). For stereopsis levels that are not near the threshold the exact formula should be used, which is:

$$n = 2ad/(D^2 + dD)$$

For **research purposes**, stereopsis is measured by the **method of constant stimuli**. This uses a statistical analysis applied to the three-needle test (see below). A less rigorous method is to use a haploscope or Holmes stereoscope with line stereograms. A slide presenting two laterally separated vertical lines is presented to each eye. For both eyes one of the two lines is presented at the same place in physical space. For one eye only, the second line is shifted laterally to introduce a small binocular disparity. Stereoacuity can be measured with line stereograms because the disparities are smaller than the limit of resolution of the eye. The lateral shift for fine disparities will not be appreciated subjectively, but the depth effect will be seen. High levels of stereoacuity are also found with experimental apparatus using small light flashes such as electrical sparks for stereoscopic stimuli. Recently a method for measuring stereoacuity at 6 m using a real depth distance stereoacuity test has been described by Young *et al.* (2009).

For **clinical assessment** a number of methods are available.

The three-needle test

Two vertical lines are presented in the fronto-parallel plane and a third vertical wire between them is moved nearer or further from them. The subject's head must be still to avoid parallax artefacts. The top and bottom of the wires are screened from view, and a comparison in the angular subtense of the thickness of the wires can be removed by replacing the lateral wires with the edges of two flat surfaces. This provides a fine measurement of stereopsis, but is time-consuming for clinical use.

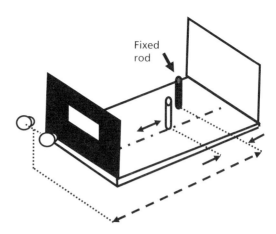

Fixed
rod

Figure 11.12 The Howard–Dolman, or two-rod, method for stereoscopic acuity measurement. Extraneous cues are removed by viewing through the narrow aperture. The moving rod is adjusted appropriately, perhaps by a staircase series of movements, judged to be at the same distance as the other rod. The rod is then moved until a difference in depth is just perceived. These two measurements are then used to calculate the stereoacuity.

The Howard–Dolman test

Two rods (the test and the reference rods) are placed in the fronto-parallel plane and their upper and lower extremities hidden by a viewing aperture (Fig. 11.12). The test rod is moved until it appears to be aligned with the reference rod: the point of subjective equality. The subject then moves the test rod until a difference in depth is perceived and this gives the value of the stereoacuity. The same formula is used as above:

$$n = 2ad/D^2$$

Where n is the **angular stereoscopic disparity** in radians, $2a$ is the inter-pupillary distance, d is the distance between the test and the reference rods and D is the fixation distance to the reference rod. Apparatus for performing the Howard–Dolman test is described in Appendix 1 (section A10).

Anaglyph stereopsis tests

These tests use filters of different colours such as red and green, or red and blue, to separate the images of each eye. The subject views a page printed in both colours with the test target having a fixed disparity. The target may have local or global disparity. In the **TNO stereotest** (Plate 11.1), both local and global disparities are used. The local stereopsis is used to familiarise the subject with the test technique. Global stereopsis is used to measure stereoacuity in this test. The TNO stereotest measures stereoacuities from 2000 to 15 seconds of arc. Stereoacuity of 60 seconds TNO is regarded as normal. Levels of 30 degrees and 15 seconds are difficult to observe on this test, possibly because image contrast is reduced by the light absorption of the filter used.

Most stereoscopic vision tests assess crossed disparity. However, uncrossed disparity stereopsis can be measured by holding the TNO and other book-type stereopsis tests upside down. Improvement of amblyopia and of decompensated heterophoria is associated with a gradual improvement in stereopsis. Decompensated exophoria is associated with decreased uncrossed disparity stereopsis and esophoria with crossed disparity stereopsis. The presence of stereopsis gives a good prognosis for amblyopia therapy.

Vectographic stereopsis tests

These tests use viewing filters in which the right and left eye filters are cross-polarised at 90 degrees. The same polarisation is used for cross-polarisation of the right and left eye targets printed on plastics sheets, which are superimposed. Only the target details are polarised and not the sheets on which they are printed. The **Randot Stereotest** (Stereo Optical Co., Inc.) uses this method and presents global stereopsis random-dot targets at 500 and 250 seconds. It also presents two other tests using local stereopsis. Smaller levels of disparity (i.e. higher thresholds) are also presented but only for the local stereopsis tests. Even if global stereopsis is not evident (e.g. on a TNO test), the two local stereopsis tests on the Randot test may indicate that binocular fusion is being attempted by the visuum. This is important for assessing the prognosis – for example, in a child with amblyopia. Vectographic stereopsis tests are also produced with separate plastics sheets for each eye so that orthoptic vergence exercises may be undertaken. There are also computer programs, which assess and exercise pursuit, saccadic, and vergence functions, using random-dot stereoscopic targets.

Free fusion

The presence of stereopsis may also be observed by the techniques of **free fusion**. A pair of stereogram pictures side by side can be fused into a single percept, either by inhibiting convergence, or by overconverging (Fig. 11.13).

A version of this technique is used in the **auto-stereogram** (Tyler and Clarke, 1990), which produces autostereopsis. The two disparate images are interlaced for the right and the left eye. Generally the subject has to inhibit convergence so that the visual axes are parallel. If this is not possible, then overconvergence can be used, but the stereoscopy will be reversed. The exact binocular convergence used is not critical, as several different vergence values will produce a similar effect. A further variation is seen in the panographic **Lang stereopsis tests**. Here the test card presentation of random-dot images for right and left eyes is sliced into a large number of vertical strips.

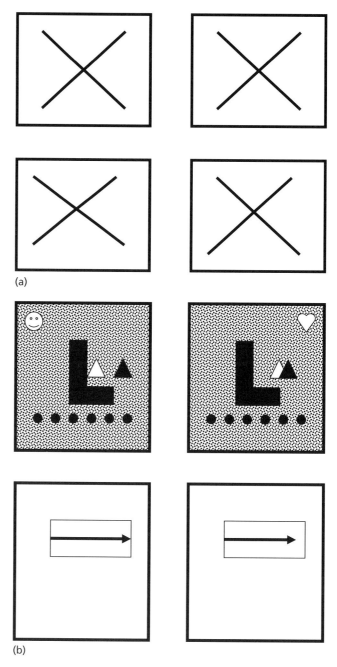

(a)

(b)

Figure 11.13 (a,b,c) Free fusion stereopsis stereograms, used without a stereo-scope by the observer either overconverging or inhibiting convergence.

A pair of strips for right and left eyes is located behind a high-powered vertical plastics cylinder, and several hundred such cylinders are arranged vertically on the front of the test card. The vertical cylinders project the right and left images to the appropriate eye. The Lang tests do not require

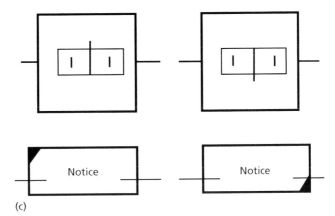

(c)

Figure 11.13 *Continued*

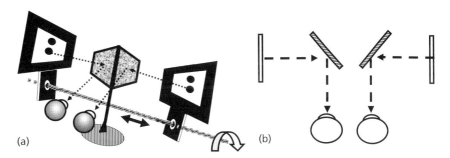

(a)   (b)

Figure 11.14 The Wheatstone mirror stereoscope, circa 1838–1843. **(a)** Impression of the original device, with screw adjustments allowing alteration of the distance between the eyes and the stereograms. **(b)** Basic light-ray paths. For some purposes each mirror should rotate around the ocular centres of rotation.

filters, glasses or instrumentation. The disparities range from 200 to 1200 seconds of arc and can be used to elicit and measure a response in children from around 9 months old (Stidwill, 1990).

Mirror stereoscope of Wheatstone

Historically the first stereoscopes were the **mirror stereoscope of Wheatstone** (Wheatstone, 1838; Wheatstone, 1852) and the **1849 lens stereoscope of Brewster** (Figs. 11.14 and 11.15), (Brewster, 1856). Wheatstone's stereoscope allows the targets for the right and left eyes to be presented by reflection through mirrors placed at 45 degrees to the line of sight. The mirror for the viewer's right eye reflects a target on the viewer's right, and the mirror for the left eye reflects a target on the left. The targets are situated 50 cm or so away and would require active accommodation. Using this instrument, Wheatstone, a medical practitioner, was the first to appreciate the binocular disparity origin of stereopsis.

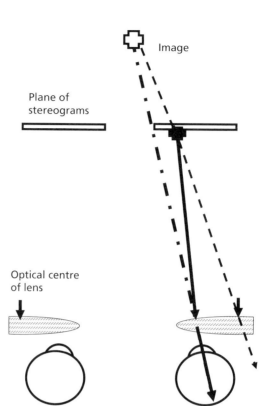

Figure 11.15 The Brewster lens stereoscope (modified by Holmes). The light-ray paths show that the effects of both convergence and accommodation are provided by the instrument, unlike the Wheatstone stereoscope.

Scottish physician Sir David Brewster's lens stereoscope used a positive lens cut in half and separated laterally to provide both a focused and fused binocular image, using the base-out prismatic effect of the decentred lens halves. The prisms base-out in front of each eye allowed the two targets to be placed side by side in front of the subject. The positive spherical lens increased the depth sensation caused by binocular parallax and convergence. The **Holmes stereoscope** added adjustable positive lenses to allow for individual adjustment. A later version was the **Brewster–Holmes stereoscope**, which is still used for assessment and orthoptic exercises using sets of stereograms such as the Bradford series. A Brewster–Holmes stereoscope is described in Appendix 1 (section A7) and also a **Pigeon–Cantonnet stereoscope** suitable for therapeutic use. A **Worth amblyoscope (1890)** is shown in Fig. 11.16. This had a series of slides for each eye, including stereoscopic slides. In the 1950s stereoscopes were developed that allowed varying accommodation and convergence demand, for therapeutic purposes: notably the **Asher–Law stereoscope** (Asher and Law, 1952).

Currently stereopsis is needed for aerial map making, geology, checking coinage and currency notes for forgery, in engineering and in many scientific uses. Stereopsis is used constantly in most normal life situations, often aiding

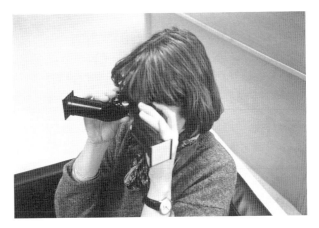

Figure 11.16 The Worth amblyoscope of 1890–1910. This instrument had a series of slides for each eye, including stereoscopic slides. The right and left eye images were fused by altering the angle between the two tubes. The tubes had a positive lens at the viewing end, and a plane mirror just beyond the lens, allowing fusion at different angles of convergence or divergence. Reproduced with permission.

hand–eye coordination. Drug development often requires three-dimensional imaging of a molecule. Seismic data from oil and gas exploration are similarly best shown in stereopsis. The remote control of mechanical equipment, including Mars rovers, is enhanced by stereoscopic displays. For these purposes, digital stereo-plotting systems produce a polarised image for each eye alternately, seen on a computer monitor with an alternating polarising screen and corresponding polarising spectacles. Alternatively, two monitor screens can be viewed with mirrors. A sophisticated form of complex depth (and motion in depth) assessment can be achieved with multiple television cameras. This is known as structure from motion.

Rotating sector, semi-silvered mirrors and liquid crystal alternating occlusion

Experimentally, rotating sector, semi-silvered mirrors and liquid crystal alternating occlusion devices may be used to present the disparate images to each eye.

Synoptophore

The synoptophore is a clinical stereoscope (a haploscope) that allows the image intended for each eye to be presented along the primary line of sight, even in the presence of a heterophoria or heterotropia (see Fig. 9.1 in Chapter 9). It consists of two tubes, which may have the angle between them altered horizontally, vertically and rotationally. A series of pairs of slides for each tube allow stereopsis testing and measurement of the angle of the deviation from orthophoria. Different slides are used to assess the degree of sensory fusion of the right and left images, and also to provide exercises to improve both the motor and sensory function of an individual. The low illumination level, the small field of view and the apparent proximity of the targets seen through the tubes all limit the practical utility of the instrument. An experimental version is described in Appendix 1 (section A16).

Some of these objections are removed by the **single mirror haploscope** (Earnshaw, 1962). One eye looks directly at a target 1 m ahead, and the other eye at a similar target on an adjacent wall at a right angle to the first wall, through a calibrated rotating mirror. The mirror is rotated until the primary lines of sight (visual axes) are each directed at the targets, which are identical or nearly so, for each eye. A stereopair can be used. In addition to stereopsis testing, the motor status may also be measured. The angle between the lines of sight is read from the calibration; this represents the angle of heterophoria or heterotropia. An uncalibrated version simply consists of a small mirror attached to a small ruler held vertically. An example is described in Appendix 1 (section A15). This can be used to exercise fusional reserves, or indeed for the student of binocular vision to investigate their binocular motor control!

Stereoscopic acuity norms

Stereoscopic acuity as measured by experimental methods with trained subjects has been found to be around 5 seconds of arc. There are clinical tests, such as the TNO stereotest, which measure down to 15 seconds of arc – such a result would be excellent, if time-consuming, to achieve. In clinical practice, a TNO result of 60 seconds is regarded as 'normal', i.e. there is then no evidence of binocular suppression, and the visual acuities are likely to be normal. There is also a reduction in stereoacuity for eccentric targets, imaged away from the fovea, down to absence of stereopsis at 16 or more degrees peripherally. Stereoscopic acuity diminishes as the observed target becomes more remote. The absolute limit of any stereopsis is between 800 and 1300 m, depending upon the distance between the subject's eyes: the interpupillary distance, which is usually between 60 and 70 mm in adults. Where either the target is moving to or from the subject, or vice versa, stereoscopic acuity (dynamic stereoacuity) is around 50 seconds of arc when measured in experimental conditions.

Chapter 11: Revision quiz

Complete the missing words, perhaps in pencil.

The relative depth of objects can be assessed monocularly by comparing speeds of movement for near and far objects as their images move across the retina. This is called m_____ p_____ (1). When a pendulum swinging in one place is viewed with a neutral density filter in front of one eye it appears to move in three dimensions. This is called the _____ (2) phenomenon. The ability in binocular perception to identify one target against a confusing background is called f_____–g_____ (3) separation. Global stereopsis involves perception of stereoscopic targets in which _____ (4) clues are not present. The region where Panum's area gives way to minimal diplopia, but is still capable of allowing depth perception, is called the area of p_____ s_____ (5). The area beyond this with frank diplopia does not immediately lose the function of depth perception; this region is that of _____ (6) stereopsis.

Answers
(1) motion parallax; (2) Pulfrich; (3) figure–ground; (4) monocular; (5) patent stereopsis; (6) qualitative.

Chapter 12

MEASUREMENT OF BINOCULAR MOTOR AND SENSORY STATUS

Without extending the coverage of this text to abnormal binocular vision, it may be useful to review the methods of establishing the binocular vision status of an individual. These methods are described in principle; the details of the investigation of anomalies will be found in clinical texts. It is recommended that the motor function of the eyes is examined in the primary position of gaze first, to check both any deviations from orthotropia and orthophoria, and also to check the stability of fixation. Next, the peripheral eye movement system is tested, i.e. the muscles, tendons and orbital fascia and pulley sleeves, using the motility tests. Then the central apparatus of eye movement is assessed: pursuits, saccades, vestibulo-ocular reflex (VOR) and vergence control. This chapter then discusses fixation disparity, and finally evaluation of sensory binocular integration.

12.1 Motor status tests: the cover/uncover test and alternatives

The **objective cover/uncover test** (synonym and abbreviated form 'the cover test') is used:

- to distinguish between orthotropia and heterotropia
- to distinguish between orthophoria and heterophoria.

It is also the only method commonly available for differentiating between heterophoria and heterotropia (but see also the line of sight objective heterotropia test below).

The cover/uncover test can be used in heterotropia and in heterophoria to estimate or to measure the angle between the right and left visual axes. Where both eyes are fixating the same target, normally this angle is zero: a condition technically called 'orthotropia'.

Method

The subject is directed to look binocularly at a detailed target capable of resolution by each eye. Where the eye with the lesser visual acuity sees about 6/18 or better, a letter or symbol is chosen so that accommodation, if present, may be stimulated, and thus an accommodative strabismus may be

---

Normal Binocular Vision: theory, investigation and practical aspects. By David Stidwill and Robert Fletcher. © 2011 Blackwell Publishing Ltd

detected. Where the lesser acuity is worse than 6/18, there is a risk that the subject may change fixation from one side of the symbol to the other, and confuse the test. In this case a spotlight should be chosen as a fixation target. The cover test is performed with, and also without, any refractive correction at the usual test distances of 6 m, and then at 40 cm. An opaque or semi-opaque occluder is used to rapidly cover one eye. Occlusion removes the fusion reflex so that neither sensory nor motor fusion can operate. Sufficient time should be allowed for dissociation to occur, up to 1–2 seconds. It is crucially important to determine whether the subject has binocular diplopia before performing the cover/uncover test, because in this case, firstly the patient has strabismus, and secondly the test will not give a definite result. The alternating cover test will be necessary (see below). In orthotropia no movement of the non-occluded eye is then seen, when the other eye is covered and then uncovered: each eye in turn is tested in this way. If, on covering one eye, a movement (to obtain foveal fixation) of the non-occluded eye is seen, the condition of **heterotropia** is present.

The direction of the abnormal movement is noted – horizontal, vertical or oblique (a rotational movement is difficult to see) – and the amount of the movement can be measured in prism dioptres (Δ) or, less commonly, in degrees. A prism bar is placed in front of the deviated eye and the amount of prism altered so that there is no movement of the deviated eye when the fixing eye is (again) covered. The amount of deviation can also be estimated by comparison with version eye movements of known extent. To do this, the subject is directed to make a saccadic eye movement from one letter on a visual acuity chart to another, say 18 cm laterally. For a fixation distance of 6 m, this would be a horizontal eye movement of 3Δ. The cover/uncover test is then performed and a comparison made between the saccadic movement and the cover/uncover test fixation reflex movement. The heterotropia may be present in either eye, or may alternate between the eyes. The **total angle** of the deviation is measured by gradually increasing the strength of the prism in the prism bar, using the cover test each time the prism strength is increased, until the investigator can see no movement of the deviated eye to move to take up fixation. The repeated dissociation involved by this technique tends to give a larger deviation angle than may be present initially. The **habitual angle** is measured by the simultaneous prism cover test. The fixating eye is covered with an occluder, and at the same time the other eye has a prism of the estimated angle of the deviation placed in front of it. If correctly estimated, there will be no movement of the now uncovered eye. The habitual angle will be equal to or less than the total angle.

If orthotropia is present, the cover/uncover test is next repeated to examine whether orthophoria is present. In this case the investigator looks for a recovery movement of the covered eye when the occluder is removed from it (to regain fixation of the test target). It is convenient for the investigator to be in the monocular field of the subject's occluded eye and to view the eye while the occluder is removed, preferably without also occluding the investigator: the occluder is removed vertically rather than horizontally. If there is no recovery movement, then the subject is orthophoric (as well as orthotropic). If a recovery movement occurs in either or both eyes, the condition of heterophoria is present.

In heterophoria, when the occluder is removed a skilled observer will see an ocular **recovery movement** when the previously occluded eye moves to regain foveal fixation of the test target. A recovery movement nasalwards indicates exophoria, temporalwards indicates esophoria, vertically downwards indicates a hyperphoria and vertically upwards indicates a hypophoria. A rotational recovery would indicate a cyclophoria. About half of all vertical heterophorias are associated with a vertical muscle paresis, and as these muscles have both vertical and horizontal components of their main muscle action, a weakness in a vertical muscle would be expected to produce both vertical and horizontal heterophoria, i.e. oblique heterophoria. Cyclophoria is uncommon but is associated with hyperphoria. The amount of heterophoria can be measured with loose prisms, or with a prism bar for horizontal, vertical and oblique deviations. Sufficient prism strength is placed before the occluded eye so that when the occluder is removed, no recovery movement occurs. A skilled investigator can detect an eye movement of 1.5Δ with the objective cover/uncover test. However, using a standard prism bar with two prism dioptre steps, the resolution is 2Δ, and the precision has a standard deviation of 0.4–1.0Δ (Han *et al.*, 2010). The units of measurement are normally prism dioptres, but degrees are used for cyclophoria.

The objective **alternating cover test** is used in the presence of binocular diplopia, and also where the deviation amount of strabismus or heterophoria is so small as to be questionable. The subject is directed to look at the target, and the occluder is placed before one eye. The occluder is directly transferred to be in front of the other eye, without allowing any binocular stimulation in between: that would be the normal cover/uncover test. The effect of the repeated alternating cover test may be to convert the habitual angle of deviation into the larger and more easily seen total deviation angle. The alternating cover test is used also in conjunction with the motility test, to establish whether there is any variation in the deviation angle between the six diagnostic positions of gaze.

Although it is little used clinically, it is also possible to perform a **subjective cover test**. On the one hand, subjective tests have the disadvantage that the result is dependent upon the reliability of the subject's response. On the other hand, small amounts of eye movement, particularly non-horizontally, may be difficult to observe objectively. In this situation a subjective test is more likely to give a positive response: an observant subject may see an image shift of under 1Δ, where the investigator does not notice any eye movement. For the complete range of deviation amounts (large and small), the inter-subject repeatability of both the objective cover/uncover test and of dissociating tests, for 98% confidence limits, is the same: about 2–3Δ (Rainey *et al.*, 1998). Han *et al.* (2010) give a resolution of 1Δ for the Maddox rod, with the standard deviation of precision between 0.3 and 0.6Δ. The subjective cover test is performed by moving the occluder alternately from one eye to the other, as in the alternating cover test. The subject with heterotropia or heterophoria will subjectively see an apparent movement of the test target in the opposite direction to any eye movement. The amount of the deviation can be measured by neutralising the apparent movement with a prism. If the subject fixates a target consisting of a vertical bar, any cyclophoria present will be evident by a change in the orientation of the target. Any vertically acting muscle paresis will produce this effect in the affected gaze position. It is important clinically to note any significant change in deviation angle that appears over a period of time, and to assign a reason for this – for example, the under-action of an extra-ocular muscle (EOM).

An alternative subjective test, for heterophoria, is the **Maddox rod (dissociating) test** (see Han *et al.*, 2010). Originally a single high-powered cylindrical lens (a rod), the current Maddox rod consists of a number of high-powered negative cylindrical grooves that produce a thin streak of light when a spot of light is fixated, normally at 6 m from the subject. As the Maddox rod is placed before only one eye, the eyes are **dissociated,** i.e. binocular fusion is impossible. If heterophoria is present, the eyes move effectively to the **distance passive position.** The heterophoria is measured with prism strength chosen to align the streak with the spotlight. Ideally the test is carried out in normal visual conditions so that the surrounding details maintain the normal accommodation stimulus. To avoid suppression of the red streak, it may be necessary to lower the room illumination minimally, or to rotate the Maddox rod slightly. If the Maddox rod has a one prism dioptre prism mounted in front of it, and both are placed in a crossed-cylinder lens holder, the Maddox rod can be twirled to produce a deflection of the red streak above, below and left and right of the spotlight, thus rapidly confirming that the lines of sight (visual axes) are within 1Δ of orthophoria. A Maddox rod can be used to measure horizontal, vertical and oblique heterophoria, using a prism bar or loose prisms. Alternatively the distance between the spotlight and the streak position can be observed by the subject on a graduated tangent scale: the **Thorington test**. For near fixation heterophoria measurement the **Maddox wing test** can be used. This subjective test measures horizontal and vertical heterophoria, and also cyclophoria. An alternative version with better stimuli for accommodation, the Mills test, is currently not in production. It is advisable to use more than one method of assessing a deviation angle. Cyclophoria can be measured by a Maddox wing test for near vision deviations, and may be associated with oculomotor paresis of a muscle with cycloduction as its primary action, such as the superior oblique muscle. For distance vision deviations, this is carried out with two Maddox rods in a trial frame, one in front of each eye. The streaks appear to be tilted away from each other, to the right and to the left, in the frontal plane. The rods are rotated until the light streaks they produce appear parallel. The angle of rotation can be read from the trial frame. Two **Bagolini striated lenses** can be used similarly, with vertical light streaks before each eye, although in this case the effect of cyclophoria may be to create an apparent tilt of a single streak so that the top of the streak is tilted away from or towards the subject's frontal plane. The Bagolini striated lenses then are rotated to produce an apparently vertical light streak, and the angle between the Bagolini striations marks indicates the amount of the cyclophoria.

Alternative tests for assessing binocular motor status, particularly in young children, or in subjects who have deep amblyopia in the heterotropic eye, and who therefore may not respond to a cover/uncover test include the following.

- The **Brückner test**. This is a comparison of the right and left eye's retinal red reflex seen when the fixation reflex is stimulated using an ophthalmoscope. The brighter reflex belongs to the non-fixing eye in heterotropia. The deviation is not quantified. However, there are several other possible causes for the brightness difference, so this test should not be used in isolation.
- The **Hirschberg test**. This compares the position of the (first) corneal reflex in relation to the pupil centre. A comparison is made of the reflex position in each eye with binocular fixation, and then with monocular fixation. The heterotropic eye will have a difference between the binocular and monocular corneal reflex locations. A difference of 1 mm is said to equal 15Δ of deviation in heterotropia in adults and 22Δ in children. This gives a very approximate indication of the deviation angle.
- The **line of sight objective heterotropia test**. This measures the approximate angle between the right and left lines of sight/visual axes in unilateral heterotropia (Stidwill, 2009). It is necessary first to measure the angle lambda in each eye. This is the angle between the line of sight and the pupillary axis. To measure the angle lambda, the investigator holds a ruler horizontally 50 cm in front of the subject's eye (the other eye being occluded). The subject fixates the end of the ruler. A pen torch is then moved horizontally along the top of the ruler until its reflection is seen in the centre of the subject's pupil. The distance in centimetres from the end of the ruler to the position of the pen torch represents the angle lambda in prism dioptres when multiplied by two. This is repeated for the second eye, and the angle lambda is recorded for each eye. It is usually about 3Δ, the line of sight being nasal (medial) to the pupillary axis. Now the subject fixates the end of the ruler binocularly, and the position of the corneal reflex is again measured for each eye. Where the second measurement for one eye only differs from the angle lambda, then a heterotropia is present in this eye, and the deviation angle is the difference between the binocular measurement and the angle lambda in that eye. Where the angle lambda is different for each eye, but there is no difference between the angle lambda and the binocular measurement for each eye, pseudo-tropia is present. It is of course possible to have both pseudo-tropia and an actual heterotropia in the same subject! Neither the cover/uncover test nor the line of sight objective heterotropia test can be relied upon in the presence of eccentric fixation. However, fixation can be checked and measured with an ophthalmoscope first. If the

assumption is made that the angle lambda in the eye without central fixation equals that of the other eye, then the heterotropia angle can be assessed even in the presence of non-central or unsteady fixation, using the line of sight test.

Disambiguation note: the angles describing the position of the eye are:

- angle alpha, between the optic axis and the visual axis (the visual axis is strictly the line connecting the object of regard and the anterior nodal point, a continuation of this line from the second nodal point to the fovea is not readily measurable)
- angle gamma, between the optic axis and the fixation axis (which joins the object fixated with the centre of rotation of the eye)
- angle kappa, between the optic axis and the line of sight, which is strictly the line between the entrance pupil centre and the object of regard
- angle lambda, between the line of sight and the pupillary axis (this axis is the line normal to the cornea through the centre of the entrance pupil).

It is possible to measure the deviation angle in heterotropia and heterophoria with a haploscope such as the **synoptophore** (Fig. 9.1). This instrument does not distinguish between these two conditions, however. The small field of view, low illumination level and apparent proximity of the visual targets may produce a tendency to overestimate eso-deviations and to underestimate exo-deviations. The instrument is more suited for comparing deviation angles between one occasion and the next, and for therapeutic use.

12.2   The gaze stabilisation system

To examine the quality of fixation, the **gaze stabilisation system** is assessed. This is the function of the neural integrator (see section 8.3 in Chapter 8). In some cases, while performing the cover/uncover test, and asking the subject to look at a target, it is obvious that fixation is defective, e.g. when there is a visible constant flicker in fixation, usually horizontally, called 'nystagmus'. In longstanding cases the subject will be unaware of the eye tremor, although the visual acuity is generally below normal. In recent-onset nystagmus, the subject may be aware of an apparent movement of the environment: oscillopsia. Alternatively, fixation may be checked using an ophthalmoscope. The subject is asked to look at the ophthalmoscope fixation target. Abnormal unsteady fixation, drifts, nystagmus or saccadic intrusions may be seen in a subject with good acuity.

Note: saccadic intrusions (irregular micro-saccades) may be seen in normal elderly people, and gaze will be less precise with preschool children. The presence of non-central fixation, or unsteady fixation associated with amblyopia, is an orthoptic anomaly and not a defect of the stabilisation system.

Next, the subject is directed to look straight ahead but without a fixation target, e.g. in darkness; no eye movement should be seen with the ophthalmoscope. Finally, in normal lighting conditions, with the observer looking at the subject's eyes from the side, the subject is asked to gaze up, down, left and right with a white paper sheet in front of both eyes to remove the fixation reflex: no gaze-evoked nystagmus should be seen, nor when the subject is directed to look straight ahead again. In this case the gaze stabilisation system is normal.

12.3   The motility test

The objective motility test is used to check the normal function of each of the 12 EOM and therefore of their nerve supply and cerebral control areas. The subject is directed to follow an illuminated pen torch, at a distance of about 40 cm, into the main direction of action of each EOM (Fig. 12.1).

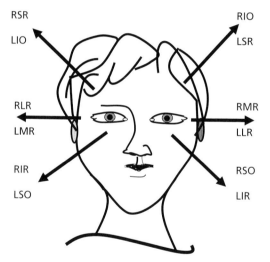

Figure 12.1   The extra-ocular muscle motility test. A target is moved in each of the directions shown, and an alternating cover test is performed. A greater cover test movement in any one (or more) directions of gaze will indicate any underaction of one (or more) muscle(s), and also show the accompanying overaction of the yoked muscle in the other eye. For underaction of a horizontally acting muscle, there will be a horizontal underaction seen. For underaction of a vertically acting muscle, an oblique underaction will be seen. The test can also be performed subjectively, checking for diplopia, and in particular the direction(s) of gaze with the widest diplopic separation. For horizontally acting muscles, the outermost image will belong to the affected eye. For vertically acting muscles, the higher image for elevators, and the lower image for depressors, will belong to the affected eye. Any horizontal element of underaction for these muscles should be ignored. LIO, left inferior oblique; LIR, left inferior rectus; LLR, left lateral rectus; LMR, left medial rectus; LSO, left superior oblique; LSR, left superior rectus; RIO, right inferior oblique; RIR, right inferior rectus; RLR, right lateral rectus; RMR, right medial rectus; RSO, right superior oblique; RSR, right superior rectus.

The pen torch should be kept within an angle of 50 degrees to the primary direction of gaze, so that it is within the binocular field of view: the corneal reflexes should always be present. The test distance may need to be greater than 40 cm for the lateral rectus muscles to explore their full action. With the eyes fixating the pen torch in each of the six **diagnostic directions of gaze**, an opaque or semi-opaque occluder is used to cover each eye alternately: the alternating cover test. If the eyes respond by moving (during the cover test) only when gazing in one direction of action, or alternatively more in one direction than any other, the condition of **incomitancy** is present, for one direction of gaze. This would generally involve the underaction of one muscle and the overaction of the yoked muscle in the other eye. It is possible for more than one direction of gaze to show incomitancy. For the alphabetical syndromes: V, A, X, Y and inverted Y, and for isolated overactions, a clinical textbook should be consulted. Generally the alphabetical syndromes will be seen only with an objective motility test: diplopia only occurs if they break down into a heterotropia. Paresis of two or more EOM is known as ophthalmoplegia. Internuclear ophthalmoplegia (INO) is seen as limited adduction of one eye, with simultaneous jerking abducting nystagmus in the other eye, caused by a lesion between the third and fourth nerve nuclei, in the medial longitudinal fasciculus. Unilateral ptosis is associated with superior rectus underaction. Where there is an abnormal head posture (AHP) the motility test is performed both with and without the AHP. If the eye movements are normal, the condition of **concomitancy** is present and will not require any further investigation. Where there is a large underaction of an EOM, the full extent of the limitation may not be apparent, as the normally acting eye will be fixating and may reach the limit of its movement before the underacting muscle has fully arrived in its field of action. In this case, a monocular motility test should be employed. This is sometimes referred to as investigating ocular ductions. The monocular motility test will indicate a mechanical rather than neurological paresis aetiology if the underaction is similar to that found in the binocular motility test. To further distinguish between mechanical restriction and neurological deficit, tests involving forced duction, variations in intra-ocular pressure, and magnetic resonance imaging may be used. A Hess screen plot may show absence of secondary sequelae; that is, effects on muscles other than the paretic muscle and its contralateral antagonist, where mechanical restriction is present.

The subjective motility test may identify smaller amounts of incomitancy that may be difficult to identify objectively. It also can be used to confirm an objective finding. The subject is asked to report on any diplopia, starting with the primary position of gaze. They then follow the pen torch into each of the diagnostic directions of gaze, and are asked to report where any diplopia occurs and where it appears to be widest. An equal bright stimulus must be provided for both eyes if diplopia is to be reported, so a focused pen torch should angled away from the eyes otherwise a brighter image will be seen be one eye than by the other. The diplopic images may be horizontal, oblique or vertically apart. In the direction (or directions) of widest diplopia, an alternating cover test is performed. For the two horizontal diagnostic directions of gaze, the subject reports which eye's image appears to be placed most laterally. The most lateral image belongs to the eye with the underacting muscle, and the underacting muscle will be that normally operating maximally in that direction. For the four vertical diagnostic directions of gaze, the subject reports which eye's image appears to be placed furthest vertically from the primary direction of gaze, i.e. the highest image in upgaze, and the lowest image in downgaze. This image will belong to the underacting eye, and will be in the direction of maximal action of the underacting muscle. It is important to realise that the highest, or lowest, image may not be the furthest, as vertically acting muscle paresis produces a reduction in both vertical and horizontal movement, the diplopia being oblique. The horizontal element may be larger because of insertion and related idiosyncrasies, but the vertical element only is diagnostic. Incomitancy where the primary action of the affected muscle is a cycloduction may investigated as described in section 12.1, using a Maddox wing test for near vision and double Maddox rods for distance fixation. Comitancy may also be investigated using a Lees screen or a Hess screen test, and the latter is also available in a readily accessible form as a computer program, e.g. Thomson Software Solutions PC Hess Screen Pro. The presence and amount of double vision may be recorded using a **diplopia chart**. With the subject's head erect, and wearing red and green glasses, a linear light source is used to record the amount, direction and orientation of diplopia.

Note: none of the above methods strictly investigates or measures vertically acting muscle function in their main direction of action. This is because the main direction for the superior and inferior oblique muscles is in the region of 50 degrees from the primary gaze direction, and in the region of 23 degrees for the superior and inferior rectus muscles. The clinical tests use the same direction of gaze for both oblique and vertically acting rectus muscles.

It is worth noting that a failure in egocentric localisation is seen in recent oculomotor paresis, where the subject is asked to point in the direction of an object held in the field of action of the underacting muscle. Particularly if their pointing hand is hidden from view, the subject points laterally further than the object. This 'past-pointing' is thought to be explained by efference copy (see section 7.5 in Chapter 7). Recent motility anomalies of vertically acting muscles also may be diagnosed using the head tilt tests, e.g. of Bielschowsky. These are described in clinical texts and, interestingly, depend upon ocular counter-rolling. This is a 5-degree eye rotational movement about the line of sight produced in humans when the head is tilted 45 degrees to either shoulder. In recent vertical muscle paresis, the counter-rolling becomes asymmetrical as between tilts to the right and to the left. A subjective equivalent to the head tilt tests is the user-friendly Lindblom test (Lindblom *et al.*, 1997). This uses a horizontal metre rule to detect the cycloduction effects of acquired (rather than congenital) muscle paresis.

12.4   Pursuit eye movement tests

The motility test is a pursuit test, but it is primarily used clinically for investigating EOM and cranial nerve function. In addition to testing comitancy, the motility test also checks the **smooth pursuit** system. Any replacement of smooth pursuit by saccades, overshoot or undershoot would be abnormal. There may, however, be a normal **memory for stimulus motion**, which produces anticipatory drifts and predictive acceleration. Some normal subjects may show a smoother pursuit movement in an upward direction than downwards. The target for smooth pursuit assessment should be moved slowly initially and repeated more rapidly. The directions tested should be horizontally and then vertically. The target should also be stopped unexpectedly: the eye movement should continue briefly in the normal subject. Anomalies such as oculomotor dysmetria (overshoot), ocular flutter, opsoclonus, cogwheel eye movements and ocular bobbing are described in clinical texts (e.g. Stidwill, 1998). Smooth pursuit infacility, also fixation and re-fixation problems are seen in dyspraxia. It is also possible to perform a voluntary motility or pursuit test. Here the subject is asked to make eye movements in the diagnostic directions of gaze, also checking eyelid movements. The voluntary motility test confirms frontal cortex (willed) oculomotor and lid function. Abnormal lid movements, such as unilateral ptosis or lid retraction, can be associated with EOM anomalies.

12.5   Saccadic eye movement tests

Testing for normal saccadic function may be undertaken using electro-oculogram apparatus. This records eye movement in a practical situation, for example when reading text. Eye movements are detected either by light sensors recording reflected light from the eyes during movement, or by attaching electrodes to the skin adjacent to the eyes to record changes in electrical charge during eye movement. However, other factors (pursuit, vergence) in addition to saccadic function may be present. Alternatively, a skilled observer may assess reflex saccadic function. The subject is asked to look from one target to a second target requiring a 45-degree eye movement. The targets should be arranged horizontally, then vertically and then obliquely. The saccadic movement should be made promptly, accurately and equally by each eye. A response that is jerky, overshoots or undershoots would be abnormal. It is useful to ask the subject to make a voluntary saccade without a visual stimulus, although an auditory stimulus may be used. Failure of voluntary saccades, with retention of reflex saccades to visual stimuli, is a characteristic of ocular motor apraxia. Delayed saccades, and difficulty in making downward saccades, is a characteristic of progressive suparanuclear palsy. Clinical saccadic tests such as the New York Optometric Association King Devick test, and the developmental eye movement test, which use randomly spaced numbers in rows and columns, are available, but are alleged not to assess purely saccadic eye movements (Coulter and Shallo-Hoffmann, 2000).

12.6   The vestibulo-ocular reflex

The VOR can be demonstrated (with the subject's consent) by gently placing the observer's hands on each side of the subject's head and rotating the head to right and left, and then up and downwards. The presence of a fixation reflex can be removed using a sheet of paper just in front of the subject, or with Frenzel lenses. The normal VOR will maintain the eyes in the primary position of gaze. An abnormality of the VOR cause the eyes to move with, or against, the head movement. In neurological practice, the VOR is assessed by rotating the subject (or patient) in a clinical chair. It is vital to use a seat belt or other restraint: subjects can fall otherwise. After one or more rotations, the chair is stopped and the subject will exhibit optokinetic nystagmus or, more correctly, optokinetic after-nystagmus. True optokinetic nystagmus actually only occurs while the chair is rotating. The after-nystagmus will be damped rapidly by visual fixation. This test would generally be carried out in an ear, nose and throat or neurology department because, ideally, it is tested without visual stimuli being present, i.e. in darkness. In this case, upon ceasing rotation of the chair the optokinetic after-nystagmus persists for 20–40 seconds.

12.7   Vergence tests

To examine **vergence functions**, a near point rule may be used to measure the **near point of convergence** (NPC): that is the nearest point capable of being fixated binocularly. Convergence is part of the near triad of convergence, accommodation and miosis, which occur together in normal vision (see section 8.7 in Chapter 8). Measuring convergence function can be carried out in a number of ways.

- The target for measuring the **NPC** is a vertical line printed on a card mounted on a ruler (such as the Royal Air Force accommodation and convergence rule). The end point of measurement is when the target is seen as double, or one of the subject's eyes is seen to diverge.
  It is also possible to note the recovery position when the target is withdrawn from the subject, until single binocular vision is regained. The classical normal findings are 8 cm and 11 cm for break and recovery, respectively (or break at 6 cm: see Maples and Hoenes, 2007).
- A further test of adequate convergence control is the ability of the subject to **voluntarily diverge** from a target at the nearest point of convergence to parallel visual axes, as failure to do so may be associated with poor vergence control.

- Where the measured NPC seems normal, but the subject appears to report difficulty with convergence, the **jump convergence** can be assessed. Having the subject change convergence from a target at 50 cm to one at increasingly near fixation distances, typically from 30 to 10 cm, assesses jump convergence. The ability to jump-converge together with the smooth or jerky nature of the vergence movement is recorded. This may be more closely related to symptoms than the NPC alone and relates to the demands of normal near vision.
- **Convergence amplitude** can also be measured by increasing the convergence demand with binocular rotating prisms (base-out), fixating a binocular target, until diplopia occurs.
- **Specific convergence infacility** is a lack of ability to sustain repeated convergence. This may be investigated by making three consecutive NPC measurements. A normal result would be, say, 8, 10 and 7 cm, and convergence infacility would perhaps show 10, 15 and 20 cm. The management of convergence problems will be found in a clinical text.
- **General vergence facility** is tested using prism flippers with a fixation target of letters one size larger than the visual acuity. As divergence (abduction) is less powerful than convergence (adduction), a combination of 1.5 Δ base-in each eye is followed by 6 Δ base-out each eye (Gall *et al.*, 1998). The normal subject should be able to retain binocular fixation when these prisms are alternated (flipped) at 12 cycles per minute (cpm) for fixation at 6 m and 15 cpm for fixation at 40 cm.
- **Measuring the fusional reserves also assesses vergence function** (see section 12.10). The management of vergence problems such as convergence and divergence excess, convergence and divergence weakness, and convergence insufficiency will be found in a clinical text.
- Measurement methods for the **accommodative convergence to accommodation ratio** are discussed at section 9.3 in Chapter 9.

12.8 Fixation disparity tests

Fixation disparity tests are used to establish whether a heterophoria is compensated and unlikely to cause any problem to the subject, or decompensated (see section 4.7 in Chapter 4). These tests use the dichoptic principle, where part of the target is seen by both eyes, and part by each eye. Where the elements seen separately by each eye are not aligned with each other, the presence of abnormal fixation disparity is shown. The Mallett distance and near units indicate the aligning prism (previously known as the associated heterophoria*)*, which is an indication that a correcting prism, refractive adjustment, or orthoptic exercise is needed. The aligning prism is the minimum amount of prism needed to bring the fixation disparity test nonius bars into alignment. Horizontal alignment may also be achieved by using the minimum amount of spherical lens power binocularly. The tests also indicate any vertical and torsional fixation disparity. The aligning prism measurement is correlated with symptoms of heterophoria decompensation (Jenkins *et al.*, 1989, Yekta *et al.*, 1989). The Mallett distance and near units with central fusional locks allow measurement of the aligning prism. Alternative versions of the Mallett system have also been produced, including some for computer monitor display, but these may not have been validated as the original has been.

Evans (2007) suggests that heterophoria decompensation is indicated by:

- an aligning prism in excess of 1Δ on the Mallett units for pre-presbyopes and over 2Δ for presbyopes, or
- low opposing fusional reserve rapidly leading to diplopia, or
- excessive fixation disparity/aligning prism readings for the particular fixation disparity test equipment being used.

Disambiguation note: In optometric practice, decompensation of a heterophoria may produce symptoms of asthenopia, blurred vision, reduced stereopsis, or intermittent diplopia. In neuro-ophthalmological terms, a heterophoria may 'decompensate' into a heterotropia, with constant diplopia, but it will revert to a heterophoria by closing the eyes for a few minutes.

The Sheedy disparometer and the Wesson fixation disparity card are used for near fixation to measure the full amount of the abnormal fixation disparity and are used to complete a graphical analysis (see section 9.5 in Chapter 9) to establish the diagnosis (Sheedy and Saladin, 1978). The Zeiss Polatest fixation disparity test has a peripheral binocular lock and shows a larger degree of aligning prism than the Mallett units.

12.9   Fixation disparity curves and prism adaptation

As an abnormal amount of fixation disparity may be rendered normal by an aligning prism, it is possible to reverse this process, and to make a graph of the amount of fixation disparity induced in a subject by looking at a target through increasing amounts of prism base-in and also base-out. Such a graph shows a fixation disparity curve (Ogle, 1950) (Fig. 12.2). The induced fixation disparity is related to adaptation to the prism powers: prism adaptation (see section 4.8 in Chapter 4). To measure the induced fixation disparity it is necessary to use a Sheedy disparometer, or a Wesson fixation disparity card. The Sheedy disparometer presents cross-polarised vertical and horizontal nonius bars for each eye. The bars for one eye are fixed, and those for the other eye can be moved left or right horizontally, and up and down vertically by means of a rotating knob behind the instrument. This is rotated until the nonius bars for each eye appear to be in line, and the amount of fixation disparity can be read off the instrument. The Wesson fixation disparity card has a single black vertical nonius bar for one eye and a series of coloured vertical bars to the right and the left for the other eye. The right and left targets are cross-polarised. The subject is asked

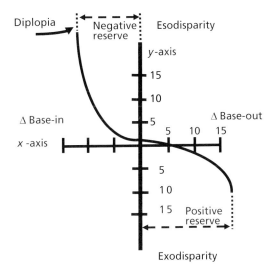

Figure 12.2 The fixation disparity curve. The amount of fixation disparity (on the vertical, *y*-axis, in minutes of arc) is plotted for increasing amounts of base-out and then base-in prisms (on the horizontal, *x*-axis). The prisms are placed before the eyes to induce the fixation disparity. The subject's natural fixation disparity without any added prism is indicated where the fixation disparity curve crosses the *y*-axis. The positive and negative fusional reserves are indicated. Beyond the limit of the reserves, diplopia will be present.

to state which of the coloured bars is aligned with the black bar, and the horizontal fixation disparity is found from a reference table.

Note: there is no evidence that the amount of fixation disparity found by the Sheedy disparometer and the Wesson fixation disparity card is directly related to symptoms of asthenopia. These devices are best used to establish fixation disparity curves to aid diagnosis and management.

To obtain fixation disparity curves, prisms of 2, 4, 6 and 8Δ are placed first base-in and then base-out before one eye. The amount of induced fixation disparity for each prism strength is then recorded and plotted on the graph. The prism power is plotted horizontally in prism dioptres on the graph's *x*-axis, and the induced fixation disparity for each strength of prism is plotted in minutes of arc vertically on the graph *y*-axis. In the resulting fixation disparity curve, Ogle *et al.* (1967) recognised four categories or shapes of curves. The most common, type I, is found in about 60% of individuals (Fig. 12.3). The central part of a type I plot is relatively flat, showing small changes in induced fixation disparity in this area. The plot is steeper either side of the central area, showing increasing amounts of induced disparity, and beyond that the fusional system fails and diplopia occurs. Where a heterophoria is decompensated, there will be a horizontal shift of the plot. The appearance of the plot in types II and III is shown in Figure 12.3. The effect of prescribing an aligning prism will be to shift the plot back to the normal position. This may also be achieved by fusional reserve exercises or by prescribing positive or negative prescription lenses.

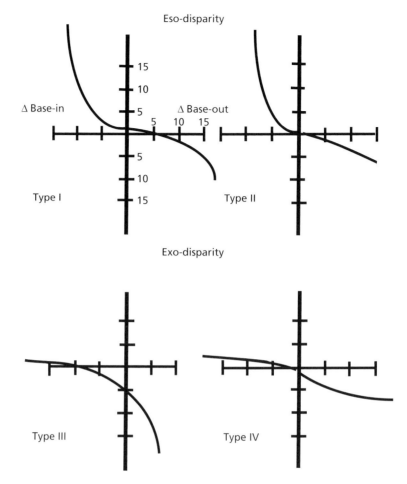

Figure 12.3 The type I fixation disparity curve is flatter in the central area. A flattened curve indicates that the vergence system is able to compensate for the induced fixation disparity, which is shown on the vertical axis. Further from the origin, the curve is steeper, and the added prisms decompensate the heterophoria. In this example of a type II plot, the subject has orthophoria. The fixation disparity is low and would remain low should the subject develop esophoria. The type III curve shown here illustrates an exophoria, which is close to decompensation. The steeper the slope of the fixation disparity curve, the less able is the fusional system able to manage the disparity. With the (rare) type IV curve, the subject will have symptoms, even though the curve is flat.

For example, the effect of a negative lens will be to cause accommodation-induced convergence: this will correct a decompensated exophoria.

12.10   The fusional reflex system

The fusional reflex system may be assessed by measuring fusional reserves. 'Fusional reserves' refers to the adduction (convergence) and adduction (divergence) ability of a subject with reference to a given fixation distance, with synonyms 'vergence amplitudes', 'relative vergences', 'prism vergences', 'fusion amplitudes', 'positive and negative fusional vergence' (PFV and NFV) and 'binocular ductions'. Fusional reserves may also be measured for vertical and rotational eye movements.

The term 'reserve' implies that the full amount of this capacity is not normally needed to maintain binocular fusion. It is possible, however, to have a condition in which the heterophoria is minimal and the fusional reserves are theoretically adequate but very limited in extent, and symptoms consonate with inadequate reserves are present. This is binocular instability, sometimes found in developmental dyslexia (Evans, 1998), and is described in clinical texts.

Fusional reserves are the value (usually expressed in prism dioptres) of the maximal fusional vergence available to maintain normal single binocular vision. Measurements may be taken for positive reserves (adduction/positive relative convergence), negative reserves (abduction/negative relative convergence) and for vertical reserves, both at 6 m and at 40 cm. Although these measurements may be evaluated using a rotatory variable prism stereoscope, a synoptophore or a single mirror haploscope, the usual practice is to use a prism bar. The convention is first to measure:

- distance negative fusional reserves ('base-in reserves'), then
- distance positive fusional reserves ('base-out reserves'), then
- distance vertical fusional reserves – right infravergence ('base-up reserves'), and distance right supravergence ('base-down reserves').

These measurements may be repeated for a near target at 40 cm. The subject is directed to look at a vertical column of letters that can be resolved by the eye with the lesser acuity; alternatively, a single letter may be used. The horizontal prism bar is held vertically in front of either eye, and the prism strength increased stepwise until the subject reports that the target is blurred, then breaks into two targets, and then the prism strength is decreased until the recovery point is reached when fusion and single vision is regained. The results are recorded as blur/break/recovery. A vertical prism bar, also held vertically, is used for the two vertical reserves, but the target is a horizontal row of letters.

The near target is again a vertical column of letters for horizontal reserves and a horizontal row for vertical reserves, usually at 40 cm from the eyes.

- The blur point may not occur for distance negative reserves, or for vertical reserves, but otherwise it is an indication of **relative vergence**. This indicates the extent of fusional vergence that is available without involving accommodation. The use of distance positive fusional reserves initiates accommodation, and near negative fusional reserves inhibit accommodation.
- Horizontal distance fusional reserves should be: abduction (base-in) 5–9 Δ, adduction (base-out) 15–23 Δ. Vertical vergences: 3 Δ for both supravergence and infravergence. Where reserves are inadequate, it may be useful to record the time of day of the test.

- Cyclovergence can be measured with a synoptophore, or by more sophisticated methods, and typical values are 12 degrees to the break point with recovery to single vision at 8 degrees of arc for both incyclovergence and excyclovergence (Sharma *et al.*, 1999). There are about 6 arc degrees of motor cyclofusion and a further 6 degrees of sensory cyclofusion giving 12 degrees of cyclodisparity before loss of binocular fusion. Ogle (1950) gave the example of a vertical line object in physical space being imaged on corresponding vertical retinal meridians, including each fovea of the subject (i.e. an individual looking at the line). If the top of the line object were inclined away from the subject, the retinal image of the right eye would rotate clockwise to the subject, and the left retinal image anticlockwise. This would produce two effects. First of all, there would be a stereoscopic effect, so that the subject became aware of the tilt (see section 1.7 in Chapter 1). Secondly, in order to maintain single binocular vision of the line, there would have to be a cyclofusional rotation of the eyes, or else a sensory cyclofusional adaptation or, more likely, both.

There are also computer programs that measure fusional reserves, some using random-dot stereoscopic targets. Haploscopes and variable prism stereoscopes can be used for measurements but may introduce artefacts. It is possible to prescribe prisms based on the fusional reserve findings.

- The middle third technique uses Percival's criterion (or rule). The positive and negative fusional reserve (PFR and NFR) to the break point are each quantified in prism dioptres. Suppose the PFR is a larger amount (of prism dioptres) than the NFR: the PFR minus twice the amount of the NFR, divided by three, gives the prism to prescribe. If the NFR is larger, then PFR and NFR are swapped in this formula.
- Using Sheard's criterion, the heterophoria and the opposing fusional reserve to the blur point are quantified in prism dioptres. The opposing fusional reserve for exophoria is the PFR, and NFR for esophoria. The prism strength needed is twice the heterophoria amount, less the opposing fusional reserve to blur, and the result is divided by three. There is some evidence that Sheard's criterion (or rule) is best for exophoria. Only positive prism amounts need be prescribed for both these criteria. A decompensated heterophoria will not necessarily produce symptoms, particularly in children, but may have an adverse effect upon visual performance.

12.11   Sensory tests

Monocular sensory tests

Monocular sensory tests are needed because binocular vision depends on adequate monocular vision in each eye.

- **Visual acuity** requires different methods for infants, children and adults. From birth onwards preferential looking tests such as the Teller and Keeler acuity cards, and from 1 year old the Cardiff acuity cards, give a fair estimate of acuity, although often coupled with an assessment of the child's positive reaction in each eye to a fixation target. From 2 years old tests that allow for consideration of the crowding phenomenon can be used; the Kay linear acuity test presents a row of four child-identifiable targets, and for older children letter symbols with crowding features are available. Single symbol acuity tests may give a misleadingly higher level of acuity. Electrophysiological testing is also possible where simpler methods are unsatisfactory. For clinical testing of both schoolchildren and adults a logarithmic minimum angle of resolution (logMAR) test is preferable.
- Monocular loss of foveal visual direction can occur in **eccentric fixation**. More commonly, although an eccentric retinal area is used to fixate the object of regard, a strong stimulus such as a pen torch will produce past-pointing, where on being directed to point to the pen torch, the subject points to one side of it: the innate principal visual direction of the fovea and the correct local sign for non-foveal points is being tested. Eccentric fixation is associated with amblyopia in unilateral constant heterotropia, and is described in clinical texts. Although it is a monocular condition, it may be associated with anomalous correspondence, a binocular anomaly. The phenomenon of past-pointing is also associated with oculomotor paresis (see section 12.3).
- New **contrast sensitivity** tests are becoming available that have improved ease of use and will confirm sensory normality in this regard. The Vistech chart (Lighthouse International) is a forced choice preferential looking test, and the Pelli–Robson chart and the Rabin contrast sensitivity test (Precision Vision) are useful. An essential part of monocular sensory assessment is the **visual field** test, and this can be estimated in infants using the fixation reflex, and in cooperative preschool and older children using appropriate standard field screener equipment.

Binocular sensory tests

Binocular sensory tests include assessment of binocular summation ratio (BSR), visually evoked potential (VEP), simultaneous normal binocular single vision, sensory fusion (with good fusional reserves), stereopsis, retinal correspondence and pathological binocular suppression.

- The BSR is described in section 3.6, Chapter 3. It is basically a comparison of binocular contrast sensitivity against the unilateral contrast sensitivity of the better eye.
- VEP binocular summation testing: a larger VEP response is found for a chequer-board viewed binocularly, than for monocular viewing, or for binocular viewing in the absence of binocular summation (Harter *et al.*, 1973).

- **Simultaneous normal binocular single vision**: this relatively low grade of binocularity is most easily assessed with the appropriate (simultaneous vision) plate in the TNO stereotest, or by using simultaneous vision slides in a haploscope. A bar test may be used, in which a 20–30 mm wide vertical bar is held halfway between the subject's eyes and some reading material. If one eye is suppressed, the bar acts as an occluder. A diploscope may also be used to assess simultaneous normal binocular single vision. These instruments are described in Appendix 1 (sections A2 and A6, respectively).
- **Fusion with good fusional reserves**: this is a higher level of binocularity than simultaneous normal binocular single vision. Worth's historical classification was fusion with fusional amplitudes. 'Amplitude' implies that in addition to sensory fusion, the motor fusional reserves are adequate (the entire range of maximum abduction to maximum adduction): 'fusional amplitude' is a synonym for fusional reserves (see section 12.10).
- **Stereopsis measurement** is described in Measurement of stereopsis, Chapter 11. For children around 1 year old, the Lang I stereotest may often be used successfully, as may the modified Frisby stereotest (Holmes and Fawcett, 2005). Neither requires the use of analysing spectacles. From 3 years old the E-Randot and the Butterfly Randot stereotests give a gross assessment of stereopsis; also the Lang II test and the Vectograph tests may be used, and from 5 years old the TNO test gives a 'gold standard' level of stereopsis measurement. There are also computer-based random-dot stereopsis programs.
- **Retinal correspondence** is best assessed, as described below, with Bagolini striated lenses, or the near Mallett unit; using a neutral density filter bar (graduated in logarithmic units) to measure the depth of any anomalous correspondence. In the absence of a manufactured Bagolini striated lens, an approximation to its function may be made by lightly smearing a low power sight test trial lens.
- In orthotropia, orthophoria and heterophoria, the presence of a high level of stereopsis is compatible only with normal correspondence. If global stereopsis is better than 2000 seconds (i.e. 33 minutes) of arc by the TNO stereotest, then anomalous retinal correspondence (ARC) is not present. This therefore confirms the absence of (constant) heterotropia.
- It may, however, be difficult to distinguish between orthotropia and a small heterotropia – microtropia – using a cover test. In microtropia, there is amblyopia, eccentric retinal fixation, a central suppression area and anomalous retinal correspondence, which may be determined using the Cüppers foveal test, as described in clinical texts. These tests will therefore establish the presence of microtropia.
- For heterotropia, Bagolini striated lenses are placed before each eye, so that the light streaks they produce are located at 90 degrees to each other and at 45 degrees to the heterotropia direction. The subject looks at a small light spot at the test distance required, usually 6 m.

Where the two light streaks form a cross intersecting the spotlight, thus simulating the result in orthotropia, ARC is demonstrated. The subjective impression is the same as in orthotropia, but one eye is deviated and not fixating the spotlight. Alternatively, for heterotropia binocular sensory status assessment, a near Mallet unit may be used, having cross-polarised monocular nonius markers adjacent to a binocular central fixation target, and with cross-polarised filters for each eye. Where both nonius markers are seen and are aligned with each other despite the presence of heterotropia, then ARC is present. Placing a graduated neutral density filter in front of the deviated eye, and increasing the filter depth until the image seen by the deviated eye disappears, measures the depth of the ARC for both Bagolini and Mallett methods.

- **Pathological binocular suppression** is also best assessed with Bagolini striated lenses, or the near Mallett unit. In either case the graduated neutral density filter bar is placed before the fixating eye. The subject looks at the spotlight, or the OXO target of the near Mallett unit. The absorption depth of the neutral density filter is increased until the image received by the fixating eye is so faded that the previously suppressing eye now stops suppressing and sees the previously suppressed target; a light streak or a nonius bar, respectively. The value of the graduation in log units at this point indicates the **depth** of the (central) suppression area. The **size and shape** of the central suppression area may be estimated with a Bagolini striated lens by replacing the single spotlight with a row of lights. The subject is directed to look just below the lights, and in ARC will normally report a circular, or oval, gap in the array of vertical streaks.

- Another test for pathological binocular suppression is the relatively unrefined **Worth four-dot test**. This has two green, one red and one white circular light disc(s), i.e. the 'dots'. The subject wearing a red filter in front of the right eye and a green filter in front of the left eye views the test. If the right eye is suppressed, only the single red light disc is seen, and the white disc is coloured red. If the left eye is suppressed, then the two green lights are seen, and the white light is coloured green. If there is no suppression, all four light discs are seen and the white disc is coloured pink. If a suppression area is small enough to fall between the discs it will not be evident. This test is also prone to report a rearrangement of the light disc positions indicating diplopia, so it should be used cautiously and in conjunction with other suppression tests. In particular, it will not report anomalous correspondence, which is present in some 80–90% of heterotropia subjects.

- The presence of a pathological central suppression area may be detected using a **four base-out test**. It is used as an objective test of suppression in children too young for subjective tests. It is difficult to perform, and as the Lang tests give better information even in very young children, it is infrequently used. The subject looks at a small near target such as an isolated letter on a reading chart, and a 4Δ prism is placed before each eye in turn. If no vergence movement results, the assumption is that the target image has been displaced within a suppression area. Movement of that eye would indicate that there was no suppression present. This test should be combined with other tests of pathological binocular suppression, such as the (Javal) bar test described in Appendix 1 (section **A2**).

- **Haploscopes** (see Measurement of stereopsis in Chapter 11) such as the synoptophore may be used to check pathological binocular suppression providing that most of the detail of the target for each eye is similar, and only a small identifying mark is used to differentiate the right and left eye targets. This will reduce the risk of inappropriately inducing binocular rivalry. The size of the suppression area is assessed by starting with foveal binocular targets, and then increasing the size of the targets until the images for both eyes are perceived. A more natural viewing condition is provided by the single mirror haploscope (also described in Measurement of stereopsis, Chapter 11).

- Other pathological binocular suppression tests such as the **Bagolini red filter bar** (the Sbisa bar) method are available. This test utilises a series of red filters of increasing light absorption mounted in a vertical bar, like the logarithmic neutral density filter bar. However, the red filter density does not follow a logarithmic series. The red filter bar is placed with the faintest tint in front of the eye without pathological binocular suppression, with the subject looking binocularly at a small spotlight at 6 m. The bar is moved vertically to increase the depth of red tint. When the colour of the fixated spot light changes from red to white – or in heterotropia, a white spotlight is seen in addition to the red light – the pathological binocular suppression has changed to binocular rivalry, or to pathological binocular diplopia. The depth of suppression is thereby measured. However, only the foveal suppression area is being assessed in orthotropia, and only the suppression area of the non-central retinal point receiving the straight-ahead image in heterotropia. The neutral density filter bar and Bagolini lens method gives a logarithmic value over the whole of the retinal meridian being investigated.

- **Anisoeikonia** may be assessed as described in section 6.13, Chapter 6, or by using an eikonometer such as the Hawkswell instrument (Fig. 12.4).

- **The Humphriss immediate contrast** test, and the **Turville infinity balance test** are clinical methods for binocularly balancing the prescribed lens strengths for each eye. These techniques will be found in clinical textbooks.

12.12 Future developments

Although the experimental investigation of binocular sensory status is fairly sensitive, the same is not true for current clinical techniques. Stereopsis

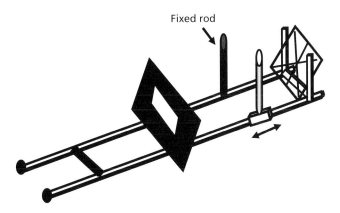

Fixed rod

Figure 12.4 The Hawkswell (1975) portable eikonometer. A universally tilting square frame with cross wires moves a gimbal mounting. Two vertical roads are used for overall size differences. Other types of size differences can be measured, involving rotations of the cross wires.

and binocular visual acuity tests are resilient to quite marked degradation of sensory input, whether by defocus or decreased light input. This is probably a result of **binocular summation**. Similarly increasing threats to binocular motor function may not be apparent immediately using current clinical methods, in this case as a result of fluctuating **fixation disparity** adaptation.

It must be expected that future advances in clinical investigation are likely to diagnose incipient hazards to normal binocular vision at an earlier stage, perhaps with the recognition of new types, or further subdivision of present binocular conditions.

Chapter 12: Revision quiz

Complete the missing words, perhaps in pencil.

The binocular motor status where both eyes are fixating the same object of regard is called _____ (1). If the eyes in this condition also do not deviate from the same direction of gaze even when each eye is occluded, the condition is known as _____ (2). If there is a deviation upon occlusion of one eye, the condition is known as _____ (3). Fixation disparity tests are used to check whether the motor function of heterophoria is within normal limits of control, and this is called _____ (4) heterophoria.

The clinical test using a pen torch and alternating cover test to check individual extra-ocular muscle function is called the _____ (5) test. This test also assesses an eye movement system called s_____ p_____ (6). Bagolini lenses are used to check the binocular fusion status called r_____ c_____ (7).

Answers
(1) orthotropia; (2) orthophoria; (3) heterophoria; (4) compensated; (5) motility; (6) smooth pursuit; (7) retinal correspondence.

Appendix 1

PRACTICAL EXPERIMENTS IN BINOCULAR VISION

Readers of the text presented in this book will have attended courses on the subject. These will have differed according to the institution involved, with regard to the amount and type of practical laboratory work involved. Here is a leisurely opportunity to experiment. This Appendix draws on well-tried features, allowing readers fresh approaches, which should reinforce some ideas on binocular vision. Colleagues can be involved, alternating the roles of subject and experimenter and engaging in stimulating discussion. Relatively simple materials are needed and a somewhat elementary approach should not be disdained. Many of the authors' students, in many lands, discovered the values of such practical work; some developed the procedures to their advantage.

Part A: Selected test methods

A1 Four dot test, section 12.12 (Fig. A1)

Cut four small apertures in an A4 sheet of cardboard, as in Fig. A1, backed by white diffusing material such as tissue paper. Cover the two circular middle holes with green transparent filters. Cover the top hole, a diamond shape, with transparent red filter material. Keep the lowest hole white. Hold the card in front of a window or lamp and have the subject (S) observe it through a red filter (right eye) and a green filter (left eye).

Note: filters can be from office suppliers, as coloured transparent files or sheets of acetate. Even wrappers of sweets might be used. Lee Filters (Central Way, Walworth Industrial Estate, Andover, SP10 5AN, UK; www.leefilters.com (accessed 26 May 2010)) supply sheets of excellent filters, in colours, neutrals and as diffusers, most with good transmission curves. The firm supplies sample swatches.

A2 Bar test, section 12.12

Use a ruler 20–30 mm wide, held at various distances from a book, between the text and the reader. The ruler ('bar') obscures part of the text from each eye but should enable normal binocular viewing to be used. Experiment with progressive reductions in monocular visibility, using layers of transparent polythene file folders in front of one eye.

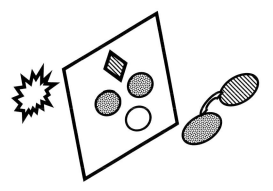

Figure A1 The four dot test, usually attributed to Claud Worth, circa 1903.

A3   Special type of diplopia, section 5.1

Extend the forefinger of each hand about 10 cm in front of the eyes, touching the tips together. Look just above the fingers at a distant wall then slowly separate the fingers about 1 cm and observe what appears to be a sausage, floating in the air.

A4   Different diplopias, section 5.1

Thread three beads at intervals on a string 50 cm long, holding one end at the bridge of the nose and extending the other end. Fixating each bead in turn, observe diplopias, crossed and uncrossed.

While investigating diplopia, try inducing diplopia on yourself, with gentle care. Look at an object with distinct vertical features. With a **clean** finger gently press one temporal canthus of one of your own eyes, moving the eye slightly to produce diplopia. Maintain the pressure and move the head horizontally, right and then left, to see any changes in the diplopia.

A5   Convergence and recovery from cover, section 8.1

Measure the near point of convergence by approaching a pencil point towards the nose until convergence fails. Discover the subject's subjective impressions. Note changes in pupil size during the approach and after the near point. Next cover one eye, with the subject fixating the pencil point at 30 cm. Swiftly remove the cover, noting the direction and rate of recovery of the freshly uncovered eye. Seek a description of the subject's impression as the cover is removed.

A6   Use of the hand diploscope, Chapter 5 (Fig. A2)

Use the following designs to construct your own hand instrument from strong card or plywood. Prompt the subject to observe DOG with fixation

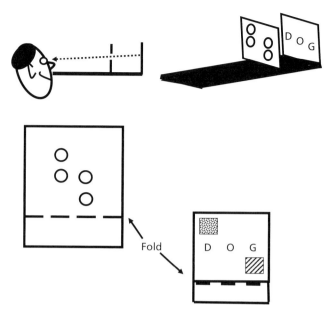

Figure A2 The hand diploscope (see sections 5.7 and 5.8 in Chapter 5). The front panel, made of cardboard, plywood or metal is 13 × 10 cm. It has 100 holes, edges 10 mm apart, and is mounted on a strong base 40 × 10 cm. The panels may be hinged for storage. The rear panel holds a red square at the top, and a green square. The central letter **O** is seen binocularly; the **D** and **G** are positioned for monocular viewing.

on the centre of the O. Then prompt more convergence, for a report of DG or OGDO. Relaxed convergence can induce the impression of DOOG. Obtain the subject's observations of the relative positions of the coloured areas at each stage. If no pathological binocular suppression is evident, induce this using a neutral filter (or an unnecessary lens) over one eye. Extemporise neutral density filters with several layers of transparent plastics film. A literature search should reveal the name of the originator of this instrument and of a larger type.

A7 Stereoscopes, see Measurement of stereopsis

(a) Pigeon–Cantonnet stereoscope (Fig. A3)

The Pigeon–Cantonnet stereoscope is made from thick cardboard. Plywood about 5 mm thick can be used. Several experiments are possible with this apparatus. Two 'leaves' (A and B) each 32 × 22 cm are hinged together, perhaps with glued fabric. On each a centimetre scale is fixed. A central triangular flap is also hinged, to carry a small mirror at the apex; the flap can be held in either of two positions when a string with a central ring is fitted over one of two small pegs, fixed to the flap. Suitable dimensions are shown in Fig. A3. One half of a complete stereogram is seen by reflection and fused with its counterpart placed on the other side of the flap. Relative

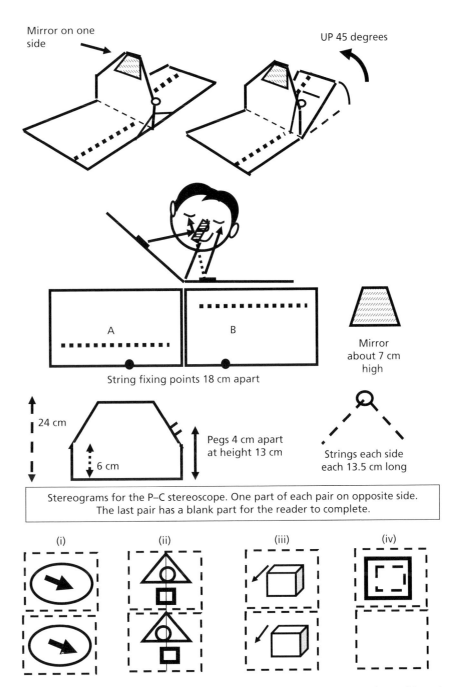

Figure A3 The Pigeon–Cantonnet stereoscope. Three strong boards are hinged together. One can be raised at 45 degrees by the string support. One stereogram in each pair can be moved along the scales **A** and **B**, one of the pair being a mirror image of the other. One pair has a blank for the reader to complete.

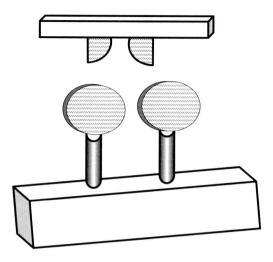

Figure A4 Holmes stereoscope. Two quadrants of a single hand magnifier lens are stuck to a bar, which can be held behind the lenses in a spectacle frame. Alternatively two identical hand magnifiers are mounted on a wooden base.

movement of the positions can be measured with the scales; thus relative convergence measurements and other features are possible.

(b) Holmes stereoscope, see Measurement of stereopsis (Fig. A4)

Although a common version of this stereoscope is made with two segments of positive spherical lenses, each +5.25 DS, with their optical centres separated by 85 mm, a practical substitute can be made from a single glass or plastics magnifier of similar strength. The lens must be cut into four quarters, two being cemented to a stick at a suitable separation. This can be held in the hand or supported by the sides of a spectacle frame.

Alternatively, two identical magnifiers can be mounted by their handles being stuck into holes in a piece of wood, suitably separated, allowing the subject's nose to fit between the rims.

A8 Convergence and accommodation, sections 9.3 and 9.4

Young subjects can monitor the interactions between these near vision functions, making measurements, which can develop various forms of accommodation-induced convergence to accommodation (A/CA) diagram.

(a) Accommodation induced by convergence, section 9.4 (Fig. A5)

The subject (S) fixates a vertical black line (F) on a white card, mounted on a small block of wood and increases convergence as F is moved nearer. The right eye looks through a small sheet of semi-transparent glass (M), which

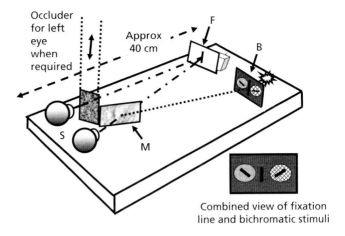

Combined view of fixation
line and bichromatic stimuli

Figure A5 Apparatus for accommodation and convergence studies. The subject views a fixation line **F** through a semi-reflecting mirror **M**. This line is superimposed on the reflected image of a red/green trans-illuminated display **B**. Moveable wooden blocks support **F** and **B**.

is fixed to a baseboard (a flat horizontal board on which equipment may be mounted).

Two small black marks on bright red and green areas are presented to the right eye. Coloured filters are illuminated by diffused light from behind. This 'bichromatic' unit (B) is mounted on a base, which can be moved over a board. S accommodates initially to see these two marks equally clear, by reflection from the glass mirror. Increasing accommodation causes the mark on the green areas to look more blurred than that on the red. Moving the unit towards the subject to equalise the marks locates the unit at the new accommodative position. The unit will need small lateral movements as convergence changes. The left eye is unable to see B because of a screen. Positions are arranged so that a combined view is seen, F being flanked by the images of the marks on the two coloured areas.

Procedure: Start with B and F at the same distance from the subject – say 33 cm – where all targets should look equally clear. Move F forward some 13 cm, adjusting the position of B, which should indicate the amount of accommodation induced by the new amount of convergence. Use other positions and plot the data.

(b)   Convergence induced by accommodation, section 9.3 (Fig. A6)

Here heterophoria is used as an index of the stimulus to convergence as accommodation is increased. Although a conventional clinical near vision device such as a Maddox wing test has some use, an improvised method works well. If a Maddox rod is not available, a horizontal transparent cylindrical lens can be made from a glass pharmaceutical eye solution

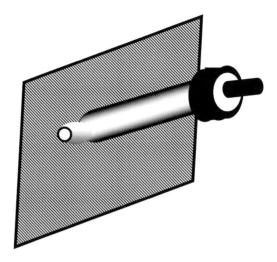

Figure A6 An improvised Maddox rod (an optical cylinder) made from a water-filled eye-solution dropper syringe, fixed over a thin slit in a card.

dropper filled with water. This should be mounted on a slit cut in a small background card, allowing the right eye to look only through the cylinder at a small bright light, set at various distances and seen by the left eye normally (Fig. A6). The vertical streak seen by the right eye is an image of the light and tends to be displaced as the eyes accommodate for nearer objects by the light, viewed by the left eye.

Procedure: The distance heterophoria is measured using a Maddox rod. Negative trial lenses are placed before each eye, and the heterophoria is measured again, using a prism bar. The change in heterophoria represents the amount of convergence induced by accommodation. Alternatively the same procedure can be used for near fixation using a Maddox wing test.

A9   Depth assessment, see Measurement of stereopsis (Fig. A7)

A useful piece of apparatus providing several experiments, using a wooden base about 50 cm square or a spare table. Measurements of stereoscopic acuity are a good start, followed by some interesting horopter work. Two people are involved, one a subject and one the experimenter. This portable apparatus has always been very popular!

The main dimensions listed here are lettered in relation to Fig. A7.

- A and B: front and back panels (plywood or similar) each 50×30 cm. The front is matt black; the back should be matt white. Fixing front and back with 'knock-down' 90 degree supports or pegs, which fit into the base, makes storage easy.
- A: aperture centrally cut in the front, 24×6 cm.

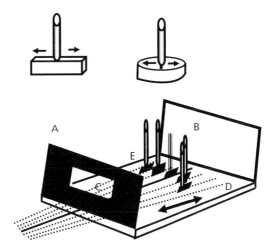

Figure A7 A depth perception and horopter assessment device. Converging lines are drawn on a table-mounted board. Sticks, supported on blocks, can slide to positions required for horopter plots. Three sticks suffice for stereoacuity measurement.

- B: 'track sides' each 35 cm long, about 1 × 1 cm in square section (these are tracks in which the wooden rods slide). Various alternatives are suitable.
- C: wooden rods, about 5 mm diameter in section, 35 cm long.

Each rod slides along one of (usually seven) tracks, all of which converge towards a point at the average distance likely to be used. This is usually 1 m from the front panel. One track lies along the centre line of the base and carries a differently coloured rod.

Different types of horopter are plotted using many rods. The central three rods (or two) are used to assess stereoscopic acuity, using a millimetre scale to measure relative positions of the rods. Different viewing distances are used. Calculate stereoacuity using the difference between the angles that the subject's interpupillary distance subtends at each rod. For example:

$$n = 2a.d/D^2$$

where n is the angular measure of stereoacuity, and is the angle subtended between the two rods from the centre of the entrance pupil. The stereoacuity is measured in radians, and the other measurements in metres. a is the distance between the centre of rotation of the eye and the median plane, so $2a$ is the interpupillary distance; d is the smallest resolvable distance in depth in an anteroposterior position in the median plane between two rods; D is the distance between the centre of the entrance pupils to the nearer object. To convert the stereoacuity in radians to stereoacuity in arc seconds, multiply by 206,256.

There should be good, even illumination on the rods. The subject's head must be stable, unless the effects of head movement are to be studied.

Binocular occlusion with a card is used to show any loss of acuity with brief exposure. Other variations can be explored, blurring one eye in some way or using a monocular neutral filter.

A10 Horopter experiments: the apparent fronto-parallel plane, section 6.4

Using the equipment described in section A9 (Fig. A7), with at least seven of the tracks with moveable rods, the apparent fronto-parallel plane can be investigated. Start with a viewing distance of 2 m and compare the effect of working at 4 m, then at about 40 cm, (a temporary reduction in the aperture size may be needed for short distances). The subject fixates the central rod, with the head still, moving the side rods until they appear to lie in the same plane through the fixation point, parallel to the plane of the subject's face. Using the main text, modify your methods, including the effects of any spectacles used by subjects. Try to establish Panum's area (Fig. 4.3 in Chapter 4).

A11 Horopter experiments: unequal retinal images, section 6.13

Using the equipment described in section **A9** (Fig. A7) and a pair of rods, attempt to increase the size of one of the subject's retinal images, as follows. If a case of 'trial lenses' is available, select a +11.00 DS flat lens and a −12.00 DS, placing them in contact. This resembles a nearly afocal 'thick' lens. If the lenses have Plano surfaces, these should be placed in contact. With this combination, or something close, a low-power Galilean telescope is imitated and can alter the size of one retinal image. Study the effects with and without this alteration when the subject adjusts the positions of the rods for the fronto-parallel plane.

A12 Optokinetic nystagmus, section 8.10 (Fig. A8)

Make a drum from cardboard or a large can, fitted with a central axle on which it can rotate, and paint with black-and-white stripes. Rotated in front of a subject at about 50 cm, with each stripe passing the eyes every 3 seconds, this should cause the eyes to follow with fairly slow lateral movements, tending to return rapidly. Ask the subject for any special sensation when the rotation stops abruptly.

Taking great care to prevent falling, ask the subject to look at a small object on the floor, close to and in front of their feet, with head bent forward. Then ask the subject to rotate around the object, maintaining fixation for four revolutions, then stop with the body and head straight up (*special care* against falling is needed at this point). Study any nystagmus/ after-nystagmus and consider the subject's reports of sensations.

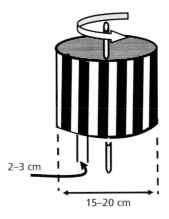

Figure A8 A drum to stimulate optokinetic nystagmus. The drum, made from a biscuit tin or card, should fit into a space that is cubical, with sides of 20 cm. Revolve the drum at a distance of 50 cm from the subject.

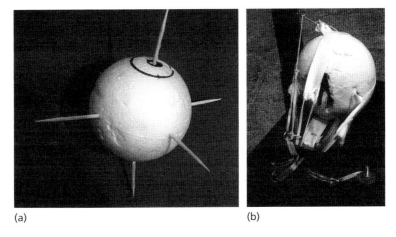

(a)   (b)

Figure A9 (a,b) An ophthalmotrope. This is a polystyrene sphere with elastic or ribbon 'extra-ocular muscles' attached. Different muscle actions can be studied.

A13 Ophthalmotrope, section 7.4 (Fig. A9)

Various models have been made to show the basic actions of the extra-ocular muscles, particularly when the eyes are converging or abducted. Simple models can be made from table tennis balls, using wooden toothpicks as rotational axes. Support during vertical movements about the y-axis is difficult, unless the 'inferior rectus muscle' is removed and the ball is poised on the open mouth of a bottle. A polystyrene ball may be used, with an embedded central wooden ball as 'rotation centrode'. This ball is supported horizontally by strong wire so that the model is raised from a baseboard, which has a suitably mounted trochlear pulley and an annulus of Zinn for the muscle origins.

A14   Panum's limiting case experiment, section 4.13 (Plate A1)

As stereopsis chiefly depends upon the disparity of retinal images between the two eyes, it is interesting to consider some special cases, among which is the Wheatstone–Panum 'limiting case'. Originally related to particular viewing of a cube as in Plate A1(a), it involves a subjective modification, even merging, of stimuli situated fairly close to a subject. Only the front face of the cube is seen by the left eye, while the right eye sees the adjacent side. The subjective binocular impression is of a decreased width of the face of the cube seen by the left eye, but the cube is seen in greater depth (than the impression seen monocularly by either eye).

The two foveas act as corresponding points, but the left fovea also has an affinity with one area of the right retina. Three separate stimuli are likely to be the lower limit of spatial locations regarded as capable of stimulating stereopsis, and Plate A1(b) shows such a case; here, normal eyes can use limited fixation disparity and some ocular movement. Viewed by the left eye alone, with three objects presented exactly on the same line of sight, results in the nearest object masking the further two. The two gaps between the three objects may start as equal, but experimentally the central object can be moved along the line of sight of the left eye. When the right eye is involved, it sees all three objects arranged in three dimensions, although only one object is viewed binocularly. Most subjects find that the central object must be moved to make the gaps appear equal. Hering's suggestion was that the right eye receiving the images of the two more distant objects might use either image for fixation. The right eye would then fuse either image with the single image received by the left eye, forming a disparate (and therefore stereoscopic) pair. Eye movements might enhance the impression of depth.

Note: movement of the central object may be required to equalise the two gaps, if the angles they subtend appear unequal. The gaps are adjusted first binocularly and then monocularly: often there is a difference. The effect may be varied using a monocular filter. Fixation disparity has been invoked as an explanation, but the cross sections of the three objects might be influential.

A15   Single mirror haploscope, see Measurement of stereopsis (Fig. A10)

In its simplest form, a small plane mirror is attached to a vertical ruler, and in the corner of a room the subject observes a target on one wall, and fuses a similar target on the adjacent wall, looking through the mirror. In Fig. A4 the mirror is attached to a vertical wooden rod, which is inserted into a hole in a wooden block. A protractor allows measurement of the angle of rotation of the vertical rod and mirror. The positive and negative horizontal fusional reserves can be measured. This can be repeated with different target sizes. Useful targets are a 10 cm high yellow letter 'U' on a black background

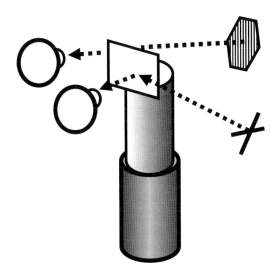

Figure A10 A single mirror haploscope. A handbag mirror stuck onto a rotating mount permits changes of ocular vergences. A pair of objects, generally set at 1 m away, may be fused.

for one eye, and a similar target, inverted, for the other eye. When fused, a vertically elongated letter 'O' is seen.

A16 Two-mirror haploscope, wooden construction, see Measurement of stereopsis (Fig. A11)

Two horizontal arms rotate around axes, here well in front of the rotation axes of the eyes, unless constructed to move on axes under the head. Plane mirrors reflect light from stereograms mounted at positions on the moving arms. A stable box is used as a mounting, with suitable protractor markings. Positive meniscus spherical lenses may be positioned on the apparatus, or worn as spectacles; in the latter case, stereogram image locations suffer from decentred lenses.

A17 Prism construction (Fig. A12)

Simple experiments often need low-power 'plano' prisms, with no focal power. These are found in refraction trial lens cases used by optometrists, and might be borrowed for a while. However, practical prisms are made by trapping water, oil or clear-setting resin between two glass or plastic rectangles. Polyester resin for glass fibre work is good. Lacking waterproof cement, use clay or putty made from flour and oil dough. A water prism is made from two thin glass slides used in microscopy, which are cut exactly as rectangles 75×25 mm, fixed as in Fig. A.12. A water prism of about 2.5 prism dioptres (Δ) needs a matchstick 2.3 mm thick as a temporary spacer 27 mm from the cemented acute angle. Prisms of 9.5Δ need the

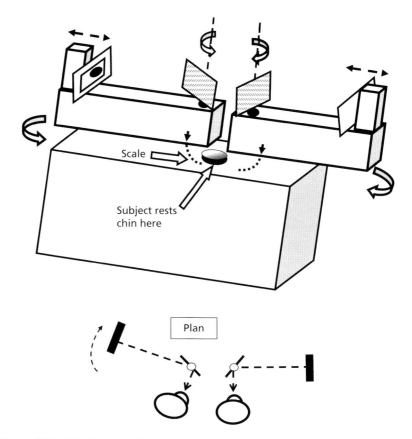

Figure A11   A basic two-mirror haploscope.

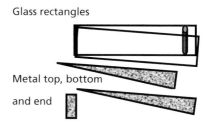

Figure A12   Prism construction.

greater spacing shown. Two of the prisms held base-out assist fusion of stereograms held at 40 cm. Outline the angle on paper, resting the microscope slides on edge as shown, sealing at the junction. Make two thin metal or plastic triangles to cover each side, sealing these in place. When each side is hardened, close the base with a rectangle of metal, having two holes. Insert water (with a trace of detergent) through one hole, and then seal both.

A18   Bagolini lenses

Slightly striated surfaces of plane glass or cheap low-power reading spectacles allow a small spot of light to appear as a streak but without obscuring the view of surrounding objects. Temporary unidirectional lightly greased smears do this. More permanent results are obtained by carefully scraping the surface across very fine abrasive paper or the rough 'ignition' edge of a matchbox.

A19   Locating the 'centre' of ocular rotation, section 7.1 (Fig. A13)

On a horizontal tray or board pin a large sheet of paper, at the level of the subject's eyes. Draw an initial line along the subject's right line of sight towards a pin **A** at the far end of the board; another pin **B** locates the line of sight. Ensure that the head moves as little as possible and cover the left eye. Place one pin **C** as far to the left as the subject can fixate it, still fixing the head, and another pin, **D**, nearer the subject, seen in line with **C**. Repeat with pins **E** and **F** over to the right. Note the distance of the subject's cornea from the near edge of the paper. Mark the three fixation lines on the paper and glue extra paper to cover their convergence. Assume that the centre of ocular rotation (the centrode) lies at that convergence and relate this to the corneal apex. Repetition should indicate the inaccuracy involved.

A20   Spectacle-induced binocular distortions in the fronto-parallel plane

Binocular vision with corrective spectacle lenses may be regarded as 'normal', yet spectacle magnification and prismatic effects should not be overlooked. Retinal images may be distorted by the optical properties of plano prisms

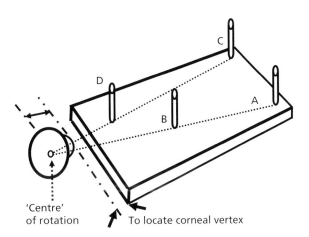

Figure A13   Centre of eye rotation apparatus.

and by decentration of spherical and astigmatic spectacles; such decentration may be on account of the visual point, where the line of sight intersects a lens. Some adaptation is often needed and hand–eye coordination restored by a learning process. A baby learns grasping skills by similar binocular experiences. A simple experiment is described that allows quantification of such learning. Using a pair of plano prisms is ideal, yet 'ready reading spectacles' may be substituted.

1. A small letter **x** serves as a fixation object, surrounded by centimetre scales, shown in Fig. A14(a).
2. With one eye covered, the subject first fixates the **x** and touches it lightly with the point of a pencil. Then a screen is fixed to hide the hand and all but the point of the pencil. The subject is asked to make repeated attempts to touch the **x**, with the hand hidden as in Fig. A14(b). Successive attempts are noted, including improvements, using the scale for scores.

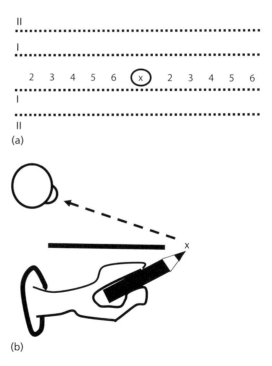

(a)

(b)

Figure A14 (a) Scale with a central 'x' point with which a simple experiment can quantify 'hand–eye' learning, with comparison of monocular and binocular skills. (b) Hand-held pencil beneath a horizontal screen. Fixate the central 'x' with one eye covered, holding the pencil beneath a screen to conceal your hand and all but the pencil point. Touch the 'x' with the pencil point, noting misjudgements on the scale. Successive attempts should yield an obvious 'plateau of learning'. Repeat binocularly, ideally wearing a pair of weak plano prisms, some 3–6△. Possibly a 'ready reader' spectacle may be used instead. Finally remove the prisms and rapidly discover how the learning has to be reversed. Changing hands may also be used.

3. Procedure 2 is repeated with both eyes uncovered, first with and then without a **base-in** prism in front of one eye. Errors and learning stages are noted.

4. The prism is removed, procedure 2 is continued, showing how a new learning plateau has to develop. Next, change the hand used, and note the effect.

5. Two prisms can be used, placed base-in in front of each eye. Monocularly, observe the distortion of the shape of the circle when viewed obliquely in a circular decentration around the prisms. Fig. A15 shows the effect of varying magnification across the prism, with less magnification at the base than at the apex. Then binocularly, note the curvature of the fronto-parallel plane in this situation. Fig. A16 illustrates the perception of the fronto-parallel plane as being distorted to be concave towards the observer with bilateral base-in prisms, and convex for base-out prisms. The horopter is curved in the opposite way to the visual perception.

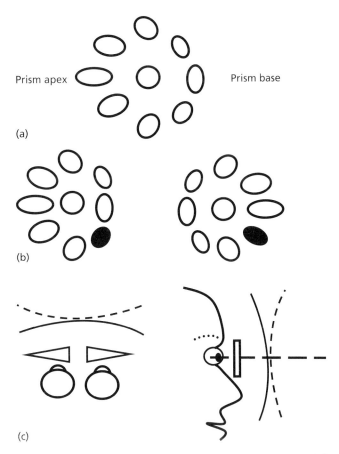

Figure A15 (a) Circles seen centrally and obliquely through a prism (after Remole 1981). (b) Circles as seen through base-in prisms, for each eye. Those down and to the right are dark. Fusion might be difficult. (c) Distortions of the fronto-parallel plane by base-in (solid line) and base-out prisms.

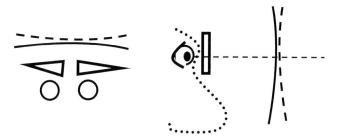

Figure A16 Apparent changes in the fronto-parallel plane with binocular base-out and base-in prisms.

Part B: Assessment of eye movements

Although methods of tracing ocular excursions (eye movements) are not considered in this book, readers may find it helpful to gain some background on the subject. Many experimental techniques have been used, including photography, moving pictures, mechanical systems and electronic means. For example, light and infrared radiation reflections from the ocular surface have been used. The electro-oculogram can be employed, even with closed eyes, while the combined 'search coil' and many contact lens designs have proved useful. After-images have some use. Excellent sources of information include the following:

Ditchburn, R.W. (1973) *Eye-movements and Visual Perception*. Clarendon Press, Oxford.
Eggert, T. (2007) Eye movement recordings: methods. In: *Neuro-Ophthalmology: Developments in Ophthalmology* (ed. A. Straube and U. Büttner). Karger, Basel.
Heckenlively, J.R. and Arden, G.B. (eds) (2006) *Principles and Practice of Clinical Electrophysiology of Vision*. MIT Press, Cambridge, Massachusetts.
Phillips, A.J. and Stone, J. (1972) *Contact Lenses*, 3rd edn. Butterworths, London.

Appendix 2

SUMMARY OF CORTICAL ORGANISATION IN RELATION TO VISION

1. The visual cortex (Brodmann areas 17, 18 and 19).
2. The auditory cortex (temporal lobe).
3. The somatosensory cortex (Brodmann areas 1, 3 and 4).
4. The motor cortex (Brodmann area 4).
5. The unimodal association cortex (adjacent to each primary sensory cortex).
6. Polymodal and supramodal cortex: these structures connect with the unimodal association cortex, and with higher-order association areas – language, vision and distributed networks.
7. The pre-frontal cortex lies anteriorly to motor and pre-motor areas. It is responsible for activities of the mind: planning behaviour; decision making and judgement, e.g. of the future effects of ongoing actions; expression of personality; and the relationship between thinking and acting.

Note: the left hemisphere is dominant for language, and the right hemisphere for some visuospatial faculties, including stereopsis. 'Attention' is mainly related to the right hemisphere.

Appendix 3
FURTHER READING

Blakemore, C., Adler, K. and Pointon, M. (1993) *Vision Coding and Efficiency*. Cambridge University Press, Cambridge.

Howard, I.P. and Rogers, B.J. (1996) *Binocular Vision and Stereopsis*. Oxford University Press, Oxford.

Leigh, R.J. and Zee, D.S. (2006) *The Neurology of Eye Movements*, 4th edn. Oxford University Press, Oxford.

Reading, R.W. (1983) *Binocular Vision: Foundations and Applications*. Butterworth-Heinemann, Boston.

Regan, D. (ed) (1991) *Binocular Vision, Vol. 9 of Vision and Visual Dysfunction* (ed. J.R. Cronly-Dillon). Macmillan, London.

Schwartz, S.H. (1999) *Visual Perception*, 2nd edn, Appleton and Lange, Connecticut.

Solomons, H. (1978) *Binocular Vision: a Programmed Text*. Heinemann, London.

Steinman, S.B, Steinman, B.A. and Garzia, R.P. (2000) *Foundations of Binocular Vision: a Clinical Perspective*. McGraw-Hill, New York.

von Noorden, G.K. and Campos, E.C. (2001) *Binocular Vision and Ocular Motility: Theory and Management of Strabismus*, 6th edn. Mosby, St Louis.

Useful websites

schorlab.berkeley.edu/vilis/QuaternionLL.htm (Listing's law) (accessed 26 May 2010).

webvision.med.utah.edu/space_perception.html (retinal disparity, the horopter, anisoeikonia) (accessed 26 May 2010).

Appendix 4
NORMS FOR BINOCULAR VISUAL FUNCTIONS

	Mean	Standard deviation	Normal range
Fusional reserves for distance fixation (6 m)			
Positive fusional reserve			
Blur	9Δ base-out	5Δ	7–11Δ
Break	19Δ base-out	8Δ	15–23Δ
Recovery	10Δ base-out	4Δ	8–12Δ
Negative fusional reserve			
Blur	(No blur)		
Break	7Δ base-in	3Δ	5–9Δ
Recovery	4Δ base-in	2Δ	3–5Δ
Vertical fusional reserves	3Δ up or down		
Mean heterophoria			
At 6 m	1Δ exophoria	2Δ	
At 40 cm	5Δ exophoria	5Δ	
Convergence	Convergence near point: 8 cm to break (diplopia) and 11 cm to recover single vision		
Vergence facility	Using a prism flipper with 1.5Δ base-out and 6Δ base-in, 12 cycles per minute should be possible while retaining binocular fixation		
AC/A ratio			
Gradient method	4/1Δ	2Δ	3–5Δ
Stereoacuity	Under experimental conditions human stereoacuity levels of 2 to 8 arc seconds have been recorded. Clinically, a value of 30 arc seconds for local stereopsis and 60 arc seconds for global stereopsis may regarded as normal. Dynamic stereoacuity levels of 50 arc seconds are normal		

AC/A ratio, accommodative convergence to accommodation ratio.

The norms for fusional reserves, mean heterophoria and AC/A ratio are quoted by Goss (1995) and derived from Morgan (1964) using different terminology (with acknowledgement to Blackwell-Heineman and David A. Goss). More recently, Jackson and Arnoldi (2004) found for the AC/A ratio: the gradient method to give a value of 2Δ/1 D and the clinical method to give a value of 5Δ/1 D.

Appendix 5
TERMINOLOGY

Alternative terminology

The literature of binocular vision is adorned by alternative terminology: for example, medical Latin, scientific and colloquial terms. One example is the situation in which the right line of sight/visual axis is deviated nasally, i.e. to the left of the object fixated by the left eye. Of course it does not then conform to the definition of either 'line of sight' or 'visual axis'! This anomalous condition is known as 'right convergent strabismus', 'right esotropia' or' right convergent squint', respectively. There is also a tendency in clinical practice for the persistence of older terminology. A pathological (partial, or complete) underaction of an extra-ocular muscle may be written using the scientific terms 'paresis' or 'paralysis', respectively, but may also be spoken of colloquially using the very old term 'palsy' in the same way that 'colon' and 'gut' are alternatives to each other. The use of the alternative terms 'line of sight' and 'visual axis' is explained in section 1.3, Chapter 1. Retinal rivalry is now called 'binocular rivalry', but the term relating to how the eyes work together, 'binocular', is still preferred in clinical practice to the scientific term 'interocular'. However, it is understood that 'binocular suppression' does not mean that both eyes are suppressed at the same time. It is also convenient to abbreviate the full technical description of a condition after it is first defined. Thus, 'binocular suppression' might initially ideally be described as (physiological or pathological) interocular sensory suppression, but as 'suppression' thereafter.

Terminology and future binocular vision developments

Amusingly, the 'half-life' of a medical fact has been suggested to be seven years. Generally, changes of understanding may either be completely innovative, such as stem-cell research, or may be a refinement of existing knowledge, where an existing category is divided into new subdivisions. A notable example in binocular vision is the concept of anomalous retinal correspondence (ARC) (see section 4.5 in Chapter 4). Because the equipment for analysis of binocular sensory function was originally quite unrefined, ARC was only infrequently detected in clinical practice. It was even thought by some to be the result of inappropriate treatment of strabismus. With more delicate sensory tests, ARC is currently found in 80–90% of constant heterotropias. The term 'retinal' in this context is misleading, as the change in interocular correspondence takes place in the visual cortex. And so the condition is sometimes referred to as 'anomalous correspondence'. However, the term 'anomalous' is normally used to describe an unusual finding, or one that is not explained by the current theory. This happened in quantum mechanics with the original term 'anomalous Zeeman effect', but as the theory now explains the effect, it is no longer anomalous. ARC appears to be a normal (physiological) constituent of constant heterotropia. So perhaps in the future the two subdivisions of ARC may change from HARC and UARC to HMC and UMC: **h**armonious and **u**nharmonious strabismus-**m**odified interocular sensory and motor **c**orrespondence, respectively.

Appendix 6
GLOSSARY

Abathic distance The distance from the subject's eyes at which physical and visual space occupy the same plane.

Abduction Lateral (temporal) rotation of one eye from the primary position.

Absolute depth The distance between a subject and an object in physical space.

Absolute disparity The difference between the external longitudinal angles.

AC/A ratio The stimulus AC/A ratio is the amount of accommodative convergence in prism dioptres for each unit of stimulus to accommodation (dioptres of accommodation). The response AC/A ratio is the amount of accommodative convergence in prism dioptres for each unit of accommodation (dioptres of accommodation) as measured, e.g., by an infrared optometer.

Accommodative convergence (AC) Convergence stimulated by accommodation.

Active position Bi-foveal fixation resulting from fusion of right and left images.

Adduction Medial (nasal) rotation of one eye from the primary position.

Aerial perspective A cue to depth perception related to the reduced contrast, and blue tint of distant objects.

Agonist A muscle receiving primary innervation to contract, and change the direction of gaze.

Aligning prism The amount of prism needed to bring the fixation disparity test nonius bars into alignment, i.e. to remove the fixation disparity.

Anatomical position of rest The position that the eyes take up in the absence of innervation.

Angle lambda The angle between the line of sight and the pupillary axis.

Angle of elevation The angle between the primary position and an elevated position of gaze.

Anisoeikonia The two ocular (or cortical) images of the same object differ in size.

Antagonist A muscle receiving primary innervation to relax, as the agonist receives innervation to contract.

Apparent depth perception The use by artists of red (or blue) to advance (or recede) objects.

Asthenopia Symptomatic weakness of the visual system.

Autostereopsis Interlacing images for each eye in a single test card.

Bielschowsky head tilt test A test for paresis of vertically acting extraocular muscles.

Binocular confusion Different images from each eye are seen in the same direction. It is due to misalignment of the right and left lines of sight, e.g. in heterotropia.

Binocular disparity For a particular object, the angle between the principal visual direction and the secondary visual direction in which the object seen is called the subtense angle. The angular difference between the subtense angles of the right and left eyes is called the retinal (receptive field) binocular disparity (usually abbreviated to 'disparity').

Binocular instability Unstable alignment of the lines of sight.

Binocular lock Any visual input that is common to both eyes, and thereby stabilises binocular fusion.

Binocular summation The result of adding visual information from each eye at the threshold level.

Binocular suppression Inhibition of binocular summation. May be physiological (e.g. to avoid awareness of physiological diplopia) or pathological (e.g. in heterotropia), when the early stages may be facultative, and the later stages obligatory.

Cardinal eye rotation Rotation of the eye about a vertical or horizontal axis.

Cervico-ocular reflex (COR) (synonym: tonic neck reflex) A non-visual proprioceptive reflex contributing to the stabilisation of gaze.

Common subjective principal visual direction The shared straight-ahead direction for the two foveas.

Common subjective visual direction Any shared direction of the two foveas.

Convergence A vergence eye movement in which the lines of sight are directed towards a closer object of regard.

Convergence amplitude The measurement of convergence function.

Convergence excess A binocular anomaly in which the esophoria or esotropia is larger for near, than for distance, fixation.

Convergence-induced accommodation (CA) Accommodation stimulated by convergence.

Convergence insufficiency A more remote near point of convergence than normal.

Convergence weakness A binocular anomaly in which the exophoria or exotropia is larger for near, than for distance, fixation.

Corresponding retinal points The points on each retina that receive images of the same object (in normal binocular vision).

Cover/uncover test A test to establish the presence and amount of any actual or potential misalignment of the lines of sight.

Critical period of development A well-defined period of development of a visual function. See also *Sensitive period*.

Crossed disparity The difference in local sign between a fixated object and one situated closer.

Crowding effect Reduced acuity due to the masking effect of adjacent symbols.

Cyclopean eye effect The visual direction associated with the common subjective principal visual direction.

Cyclopean vision   The absence of monocular clues in global stereopsis.

Cyclophoria   Tendency to rotation of the eyes around the line of sight.

Cyclotropia   Rotation of the eyes around the line of sight.

Da Vinci stereopsis   Depth perception resulting from overlap of objects seen.

Depth averaging   The pooling of a group of adjacent image depths.

Depth constancy   Judgement of the distance of an object independently from the actual distance at which it is located, biased by familiarity with the test object.

Dichoptic visual masking   A reduction in sensitivity to a visual stimulus associated with dissimilar stimuli being presented to each eye.

Diplopia   Two images of the same object are seen because they fall on non-corresponding retinal points.

Disjunctive fusional reflexes   Maintenance of fusion for approaching or receding objects of interest.

Disparity vergence system   The fast motor binocular fusional system.

Dissociated heterophoria   The measurement of the heterophoria amount by dissociating the eyes.

Divergence excess   An esophoria or esotropia that is larger for distance, than for near, fixation.

Divergence weakness   An exophoria or exotropia that is larger for distance, than for near, fixation.

Duction   Monocular movement of one eye, in, out, up or down. 'Ductions' is sometimes the plural of duction, and sometimes used to mean 'vergence'.

Dynamic stereopsis   The ability to recognise the position in depth of a moving target.

Eccentric fixation   Monocular loss of foveal visual direction.

Efference copy   A memory of eye position that is used to facilitate oculomotor movements, and to recognise the location of visual percepts. It is mediated by extra-ocular muscle proprioception. It is present for willed movements of the eyes, and also reflex movements such as saccadic, smooth pursuit and the rapid element of optokinetic nystagmus.

Egocentric localisation   Localisation by reference to the cyclopean eye.

Esophoria   Tendency for the eyes to deviate medially.

Exophoria   Tendency for the eyes to deviate temporally.

External longitudinal angles   Angle between binocular fixation at infinity, and the horizontal angle subtended by an object of regard.

Extorsion   Rotation of the upper eye temporally around the line of sight.

Extra-ocular muscles   The muscles external to the eye that control the direction of the line of sight.

Extra-retinal eccentricity   The lateral displacement of a (stereoscopic) target from fixation.

Facilitation   A subtype of binocular summation showing more than twice the sum of the monocular stimuli.

Figure–ground separation   The ability to identify important data within a confusing background.

Fixation disparity   A minimal misalignment of the lines of sight within Panum's fusional area.

Fusion   Motor fusion is the alignment of the lines of sight with the object of regard. Sensory fusion is the sensory integration of the right and left images into a single percept.

Fusional convergence   The increase in convergence from the passive to the active position.

Fusional reserves   The ability of the binocular fusional system to vary the horizontal, vertical or cyclorotational angle between the right and left eyes in maintaining fusion.

Geometric effect   The effect of a horizontal magnification of one ocular image, stretching the binocular disparities from their previous size, and creating an artificial stereoscopic effect that rotates the horopter away from the eye with the horizontal magnification and the objects perceived towards that eye.

Global stereopsis   Stereopsis appreciated without using monocular clues.

Gradient test   Measurement of heterophoria with varying accommodative demand allowing the AC/A ratio to be found.

Graphical analysis of AC/A ratio   A graph relating accommodation and convergence.

Haploscope   Any instrument that allows sensory fusion of separate right and left eye images.

Hering's law of equal innervation   This states (1) that the equal movement of each eye during saccades occurs because of innate equal nerve stimulation to muscles acting together, and (2) that the explanation for apparently monocular eye movements, in asymmetrical convergence for example, is explained by the mathematical combination of version and vergence movements.

Hering–Hillebrand deviation   The difference between the shape of the Vieth–Müller circle and the measured horopter.

Heterophoria   Controlled tendency for the eyes to deviate from fixation.

Heterophoria, uncompensated   Poorly controlled tendency for the eyes to deviate from fixation.

Heterotropia   The scientific term for deviation of one eye from the object of regard ('*strabismus*' in medical Latin).

Heterotropia, alternating   Deviation of either eye from the object of regard.

Horopter   The surface in visual space perceived by stimulation of corresponding points in each eye.

Hyperphoria   A potential vertical misalignment of the lines of sight.

Hypertropia   A vertical misalignment of the lines of sight.

Induced depth perception   Apparent changes in depth caused by reduction in visual stimulus of one eye.

Induced effect   A vertical magnification of one retinal image, which produces the same binocular effect as a horizontal magnification of the other eye, a horopter tilt away from the eye with the apparent horizontal magnification, and the objects perceived tilting towards that eye.

Infraduction   A movement of one eye downwards.

Intorsion   Rotation of the upper eye medially around the line of sight.

Law of oculocentric direction   All objects situated on the same line of sight (primary or secondary), will be seen in the same direction, even if at different distances. This law applies to one eye (i.e. either eye).

Leaf room   A room with monocular clues to depth removed, demonstrating the effects of uniocular magnification in binocular vision.

Line of sight   The line passing through the entrance pupil that connects the object to the retinal image.

Listing's law   Any cardinal or tertiary eye position can be reached from the primary eye position by rotation about any given single axis lying in the equatorial (Listing's) plane of the eye.

Listing's plane   The plane relating to the eye, which contains the transverse, or x-axis, and the vertical, or z-axis, of eye rotation.

Local sign   The unique direction associated with each retinal receptor.

Local stereopsis   Local or contour stereopsis is demonstrated by stereoscopic targets containing monocularly identifiable contours or lines, having different disparities for each eye.

Localisation   Oculocentric localisation is the awareness of the direction of an object in physical space with reference to one eye. Egocentric localisation: with reference to both eyes in the primary position. Headcentric localisation: with reference to the head, allowing for any movement of the eyes using extra-ocular muscle feedback.

LogMAR   A visual acuity measuring optotype chart from which the visual acuity of an individual may be written as the logarithmic value of the subtense of the smallest optotypes letter that can be resolved. It is a scientifically graduated replacement for the unequally spaced Snellen chart.

Masking stimulus   A method of modifying perception of a test stimulus by adding a second visual stimulus, before, with or after the test stimulus.

Middle third technique   The measurement of the middle third of the range of positive and negative relative convergence, for a specified fixation distance.

Motion in depth   A combination of depth and movement perception.

Motion parallax   Assessment of depth by comparison of differential movement of nearer and further objects.

Motion smear   The appearance of smeared vision during a saccade, when the normal saccadic monocular suppression mechanism is inoperative.

Nasal packing   The close arrangement of nasal retinal elements.

Near point of convergence   The closest point at which the lines of sight can be directed to obtain normal binocular single vision.

Nonius lines   Measuring stimuli for right and left eye binocular assessment. Nonius lines are used in other scientific areas also.

Optokinetic nystagmus (OKN)   The eye movement response to large moving visual fields when the head is stationary. It consists of a combination of a slow compensatory eye movement followed by a fast resetting saccadic movement. It produces the subjective impression of self-motion, rotating in a direction opposite to the visual field movement.

Optic axis   The optic axis of the eye is taken to be the average axis of alignment of the optical components of the eye, such that the images formed by each optical surface of the eye are in approximate alignment. Its assumed position may be found by reference to the anterior corneal reflection being in the centre of the pupil (unlike the visual axis).

Optic flow   Where peripheral images surrounding a fixation target move on the retina as the subject moves towards the target; also called 'visual flow'.

Orthophoria   The eyes remain fixating the object of regard, even when one is occluded.

Panum's fusional area   The locus of all objects on a surface, with retinal images that either fall on corresponding points in each eye, or are derived from objects close enough in depth from this surface to allow fusion and the perception of stereopsis.

Passive position   The direction of gaze of the eyes, under the effects of the physiological position of rest, when one eye is occluded.

Past-pointing   Defective localisation in recent paresis, or eccentric fixation.

Phoria line   The plot of the angles in prism dioptres between the dissociated lines of sight (visual axes) for increasing amounts of accommodation.

Physiological diplopia   The expected diplopia of objects outside Panum's fusional area.

Physiological position of rest   The direction of the right and left lines of sight when under the effect of the postural reflexes, but without the effects of fusion.

Postural reflexes   The cervico-ocular reflex (COR) and the vestibulo-ocular reflex (VOR).

Primary position of gaze   The direction of the right and left lines of sight when under the effects of the fusional reflexes, looking in the median plane horizontally towards optical infinity.

Principal visual direction   When the line of sight (the visual axis) from the fovea to the object of regard is aligned with the object of regard.

Prism adaptation text   This has several different meanings – see section 4.8 in Chapter 4.

Prism   A lens that deviates light, rather than focusing it.

Prism dioptre   A unit of deviation of a light ray of wavelength 587.6 nm, on a surface normal to the light ray, that forms the angle subtended by 1 cm at 1 m, and has the Greek symbol delta (Δ). It is approximately 0.57 of an arc degree.

Probability binocular summation   A summation of the input of both eyes, which is enhanced by the statistical chance of receiving additional stimulation from at least one eye.

Psycho-optical reflexes   The fixation, re-fixation, version, vergence and fusion reflexes.

Pulfrich phenomenon   An apparent stereoscopic effect associated with diminishing the luminance of the stimulus received by one eye.

Pulley sleeves   Orbital structures that lie between the origin and insertion of extra-ocular muscles, and thereby modify their actions.

Qualitative stereopsis The uncertain perception of depth for non-fixated objects beyond or closer than Panum's fusional area.

Rotational vestibulo-ocular reflex (r-VOR) The reflex that moves the eyes to correct for head rotations in pitch, yaw and roll.

Receptive field The retinal area producing stimuli affecting a single ganglion cell, and later structures in the visual pathway.

Receptive field disparity The cortical faculty of detecting binocular disparity.

Re-fixation reflex The reflex that moves the eyes to a new target.

Relative depth The depth difference between the fixated object and another object, as detected by stereopsis (rather than their exact location in depth).

Relative disparity The difference in depth of two or more objects in physical space is assessed (using binocular information) by their relative disparity, which is the difference between their two absolute disparities.

Relative magnification The difference in magnification between the right and left eye images.

Retinal correspondence The ability of the visual system to associate and integrate visual information from a point (or small area) of one eye with a point (or small area) of the other eye. The correspondence is normal when the lines of sight intersect on the object of regard, and anomalous when they do not.

Retinal disparity If the same object is imaged on retinal elements with a different local sign in right and left eyes, retinal disparity will be produced.

Retinal element A retinal element is a retinal–cerebral unit that produces a visual sensation in response to light falling upon a retinal unit-area.

Retinal rivalry Alternating suppression due to dissimilar images, better described as binocular rivalry.

Retinotopic mapping The mapping of the retina is maintained through the optic nerves, the chiasm, the dorsal lateral geniculate nucleus and the visual cortex.

Saccade A step-wise movement of both lines of sight: versions initiated by the fixation or the re-fixation reflexes.

Secondary common subjective visual direction The object seen by the two corresponding non-foveal points lies in a secondary common subjective visual direction.

Sensitive period A period of visual development that begins and ends gradually. See also *Critical period*.

Sheard's criterion A compensated heterophoria will have a fusional reserve twice the amount of the heterophoria (both measured in the same units, e.g. prism dioptres).

Sherrington's law of reciprocal innervation When a neural impulse to contract is received by an agonist muscle, an equivalent impulse to relax is received by the ipsilateral antagonist: i.e. reciprocal innervation.

Sine-wave stimulation A light source, which is gradually brightening and darkening, so that a graph of light intensity against time would undulate, or show a sine wave.

Smooth pursuit eye movements   An eye movement that will maintain the image of a moving object on the fovea.

Square-wave stimulation   A light source, which is effectively switching abruptly on and off, so that a graph of light intensity against time would look like a series of blocks, or square waves.

Stato-kinetic reflex   An innate reflex system, including COR and VOR, which stimulates appropriate eye and limb movements in response to a head movement.

Stereo blindness   Absence of any stereopsis, or absence of stereopsis for crossed, uncrossed or either crossed or uncrossed binocular disparity.

Stereogram   Separate right and left images that are similar enough for motor fusion, and dissimilar enough to present binocular disparity-producing stereopsis. Stereograms may be used for measurement and therapeutically.

Stereomotion   The perception of movement of any object towards or away from the subject.

Stereopsis   The perception of depth, usually by binocular disparity detection.

Strabismus   This is the medical Latin synonym of 'heterotropia'.

Supraduction   A movement of one eye upwards.

Suppression   See *Binocular suppression*.

Suspension   Previously a synonym for 'suppression', and better used for monocular visual phenomena (see section 5.4 in Chapter 5).

Tonic convergence   The element of convergence taking the eyes from the anatomical (without innervation) to the physiological (with active postural reflexes) position of rest.

Torsional movement   A rotational movement of an eye around the line of sight.

Translational vestibulo-ocular reflex (t-VOR)   The reflex that moves the eyes to correct for bobbing, heaving or surging head movements.

Triplopia   The object of regard is located in three separate visual directions.

Uncrossed disparity   The difference in local sign between a fixated object and one situated further away.

Varying relative magnification   A varying relative magnification of one retinal image compared with the other can be produced by the non-uniform arrangement of retinal elements, and therefore of local signs. One example is that an image may fall on the temporal retina of one eye, and the nasal retina of the other eye. Nasal retinal elements tend to be arranged closer than temporal elements: see also *Nasal packing*.

Vergence eye movements   Disjunctive movements of the eyes in opposite directions.

Vergence reflex   A reflex enabling bi-foveal fixation on an approaching or receding target.

Vestibulo-ocular reflex (VOR)   A non-visual gaze-stabilising reflex mediated by stimulation of the vestibular system.

Vieth–Müller Circle   The theoretical locus of points in visual space associated with corresponding points in each retina. It assumes that there is complete ocular symmetry of each eye and so successive corresponding points have equal angular displacement – from the fovea towards the retinal periphery and in both temporal and nasal directions – and also that the eyes rotate about their nodal points and not their centres of rotation.

Visual axis A clinical term for the line of sight (see section 1.3 in Chapter 1).

Visual direction The visual position of an object in a two-dimensional plane, i.e. its vertical and horizontal location.

Visual flow Where peripheral images surrounding a fixation target move on the retina as the subject moves towards the target; best called 'optic flow'.

Visual maturation The development of visual functions after birth.

Visuum The visual system.

Yoke muscles Where one or more muscles in each eye work together with one or more muscles in the other eye to produce a change in eye movements. Different muscles may be yoked together for different eye movements.

Zero disparity Where the local sign for a (fixated) object is the same for each eye, and no stereoscopic effect is produced.

Zone of comfort When the eyes are within the middle third of the fusional reserves, for a specific fixation distance.

REFERENCES

Abadi, R.V. and Scallan, C.J. (2001) Ocular oscillations on eccentric gaze. *Vision Research*, **41**, 2895–2907.

Adrian, E.D. (1947) *The Physical Background of Perception*. Clarendon Press, Oxford, p. 53.

Albright, T.D., Desimone, R. and Gross, C.G. (1984) Columnar organization of directionally selective cells in visual area MT of the macaque. *Journal of Neurophysiology*, **51**, 16–31.

Alpern, M. (1969) Specification of the direction of regard. In: *The Eye*, Vol. **3** (ed. H. Davson). Academic Press, New York.

Ames Jr, A. and Gliddon, G.H. (1928) Ocular measurements. *Transactions of the American Medical Association Ophthalmology Section*, 102–175.

Ames, A., Ogle, K.N. and Gliddon, G.H. (1932) Corresponding retinal points, the horopter, and the size and shape of ocular images. *Journal of the Optical Society of America*, **22**, 575–631.

Angelaki, D.E. and Dickman, J.D. (2003) Gravity or translation: central processing of vestibular signals to detect motion or tilt. *Journal of Vestibular Research*, **13**, 245–253.

Anzai, A., Ohzawa, I. and Freeman, R.D. (1997) Neural mechanisms underlying binocular fusion and stereopsis: position vs. phase. *Proceedings of the National Academy of Sciences USA*, **94**, 5348–5443.

Asher, H. and Law, F.W. (1952) Stereoscopy and a new stereoscope. *British Journal of Ophthalmology*, **36**, 225–238.

Aslin, R.N. (1977) Development of binocular fixation in human infants. *Journal of Experimental Child Psychology*, **23**, 133–150.

Aslin, R.N. and Jackson, R.W. (1979) Accommodative-convergence in young infants: development of a synergistic sensory-motor system. *Canadian Journal of Psychology*, **33**, 222–231.

Atkinson, J. (1984) Human visual development over the first six months of life: a review and a hypothesis. *Human Neurobiology*, **3**, 61–74.

Atkinson, J., Braddick, O. and Moar. K. (1977) Development of contrast sensitivity over the first three months of life in the human infant. *Vision Research*, **17**, 1037–1044.

Baitch, L.W. and Levi, D.M. (1988) Evidence for non-linear binocular interactions in human visual cortex. *Vision Research*, **28**, 1139–1143.

Bagolini, B. (1967) Anomalous correspondence: definition and diagnostic methods. *Documenta Ophthalmologica*, **23**, 346–398.

Baker, D.H. and Meese, T.S. (2007) Binocular contrast interactions: Dichoptic masking is not a single process. *Vision Research*, **47**, 3096–3107.

Baker, D.H., Meese T.S., Mansouri, B. and Hess, R.F. (2007) Binocular summation of contrast remains intact in strabismic amblyopia. *Investigative Ophthalmology and Visual Science*, **48**, 5332–5338.

Barlow, D. and Freedman, W. (1980) Cervico-ocular reflex in the normal adult. *Acta Otolaryngologica (Stockholm)*, **89**, 487–496.

Barlow, H.B., Blakemore, C. and Pettigrew, J.D. (1967) The neural mechanisms of binocular depth discrimination. *Journal of Neuroscience*, **193**, 327–342.

Benedek, G., Benedek, K., Deri, S., *et al.* (2003) The scotopic low frequency contrast sensitivity develops in children between the ages of 5 and 14 years. *Neuroscience Letters*, **345**, 161–164.

Birch, E.E., Shimojo, S. and Held, R. (1985) Preferential looking assessment of fusion and stereopsis in infants aged 1–6 months. *Investigative Ophthalmology and Visual Science*, **26**, 366–370.

Bishop P.O. and Pettigrew J.D. (1986) Neural mechanisms of binocular vision. *Vision Research*, **26**, 1587–1600.

Blake, R. and Camisa, J.C. (1979) On the inhibitory nature of binocular rivalry suppression. *Journal of Experimental Psychology: Human Perception and Performance*, **5**, 315–323.

Blake, R. and Fox, R. (1974) Adaptation to invisible gratings and the site of binocular rivalry suppression. *Nature*, **249**, 488–490.

Blake, R., Fox, R. and McIntyre, C. (1971) Stochastic properties of stabilised image binocular rivalry alternations. *Journal of Experimental Psychology*, **88**, 337–332.

Blake, R., O'Shea, R.P. and Mueller, R.P. (1992) Spatial zones of binocular rivalry in central and peripheral vision. *Visual Neuroscience*, **8**, 469–478.

Blakemore, C. (1969) Binocular depth discrimination and the nasotemporal division. *Journal of Physiology*, **205**, 471–497.

Blakemore, C. (1970) The range and scope of binocular depth perception in man. *Journal of Physiology*, **211**, 599–622.

Blakemore, C. and Julesz, B. (1971) Stereoscopic depth aftereffect produced without monocular clues. *Science*, **171**, 286–288.

Blitz, D.M. and Regehr, W.G. (2005) Timing and specificity of feed-forward inhibition within the LGN. *Neuron*, **45**, 917–928.

Boeder, P. (1952) Translation of Armin von Tschermak-Seysenegg. In: *Introduction to Physiological Optics*, 2nd edn. Charles C. Thomas, Springfield, Illinois. Blackwell Scientific Publications, Oxford.

Braddick, O.J., Atkinson, J., French. J. and Howland, H.C. (1979) A photorefraction study of infant accommodation. *Vision Research*, **19**, 1319–1330.

Bradley, D.C., Chang, G.C. and Andersen, R.A. (1998) Encoding of three-dimensional structure-from-motion by primate area MT neurons. *Nature*, **392**, 714–717.

Brautaset, R.L. and Jennings, J.A.M. (2005) Horizontal and vertical prism adaptation are different mechanisms. *Ophthalmic and Physiological Optics*, **25**, 215–218.

Brecher, G.A. (1951) A new method for measuring anisoeikonia. *American Journal of Ophthalmology*, **34**, 1016–1021.

Brewster, D. (1856) *The Stereoscope: its History, Theory and Construction, with its Application to the Fine and Useful Arts and to Education*. J. Murray, London.

Bron, A.J., Tripathi, R.C. and Tripathi, B.J. (1997) *Wolff's Anatomy of the Eye and Orbit*. Chapman & Hall Medical, London.

Bruce C.J., Goldberg, M.E., Bushnell, M.C. and Stanton, G.B. (1985). Primate frontal eye fields. II. Physiological and anatomical correlates of electrically evoked eye movements. *Journal of Neurophysiology*, **54**, 714–734.

Bruenech, J.R. (1996) Neuroanatomical studies of human extraocular muscles. Ph.D. thesis, City University, London.

Bruenech, J.R. and Ruskell, G.L. (2001) Muscle spindles in extraocular muscles of human infants. *Cells Tissues Organs*, **169**, 388–394.

Bucci, M.P., Kapoula, Z., Yang, Q., Bremond-Gignac, D. and Wiener-Vacher, S. (1997) Deficiency of adaptive control of the binocular coordination of saccades in strabismus. *Vision Research*, **37**, 2767–2777.

Büttner-Ennever, J.A. (2007) Anatomy of the oculomotor system. In: *Developmental Ophthalmology*, **40**, 1–14. Karger, Basel.

Campbell, F.W. and Green, D.G. (1965) Monocular versus binocular visual acuity. *Nature*, **208**, 191–192.

Carpenter, R.H.S. (1977) *Movements of the Eyes*, pp. 236–237. Pion, London.

Catz, N. and Their, P. (2007) Neural control of saccadic eye movements. In: *Neuro-ophthalmology, Developments in Ophthalmology*, Vol. **40**, (eds A. Straube and U. Büttner), pp. 52–75. Karger, Basel.

Cavonius, C.R. (1979) Binocular interactions in flicker. *Quarterly Journal of Experimental Psychology*, **31**, 273–280.

Chalupa, L.M. and Werner, J.S. (eds) (2004) *The Visual Neurosciences*. The MIT Press, Cambridge, Massachusetts.

Charnwood, J. (Lord) (1951) *Retinal slip. Transactions of the International Optical Congress*, pp. 165–172. British Optical Association, London.

Charnwood, J. (Lord) (1952) A new test for aniseikonia. *Optician*, Dec 26, 1952.

Chen, G, Lu, H.D. and Roe, A.W. (2006) Functional architecture of macaque cortical area V2 for depth surfaces revealed by optical imaging. In: *Society for Neuroscience Abstract*, Vol. **114**, p. 6. Atlanta, GA.

Ciuffreda, K.J., and Tannen, B. (1995) *Eye Movement Basics for the Clinician*. Mosby, St Louis.

Cline, D., Hofstetter, H.W. and Griffin, J.R. (1980) *Dictionary of Visual Science*, 3rd edn (eds D. Cline and M. Schapero). Chilton Book Company, Michigan.

Cohen, B. (1984) Erasmus Darwin's observations on rotation and vertigo. *Human Neurobiology*, **3**, 121–128.

Colby, C.L., Duhamel, J.R. and Goldberg, M.E. (1993) Ventral intraparietal area of the macaque: anatomic location and visual response properties. *Journal of Neurophysiology*, **69**, 902–914.

Collewijn, H., Steinman, R.M., Erkelens, C.J. and Regan, D. (1991) Binocular fusion, stereopsis and stereoacuity with a moving head. In: *Vision and Visual Dysfunction, Vol. 10A: Binocular Vision* (ed. D. Regan). MacMillan, London, pp. 121–136.

Cooper, S., Daniel, P.M. and Whitteridge, D. (1955) Muscle spindles and other sensory endings in the extrinsic eye muscles: the physiology and anatomy of these receptors and of their connections with the brain-stem. *Brain*, **78**, 564–583.

Corcoran, R.A., and Roth, N. (1983) Comparative monocular brightness contributions in normal binocular observers. *American Journal of Optometry and Physiological Optics*, **60**, 813–816.

Cormack, L.K., Stevenson, S.B. and Schor, C.M. (1991) Interocular correlation, luminance contrast and cyclopean processing. *Vision Research*, **31**, 2195–2207.

Coulter, R.A. and Shallo-Hoffman, J. (2000) The presumed influence of attention on accuracy in the developmental eye movement (DEM) test. *Optometry and Visual Science*, **77**, 428–432.

Crozier, W.J. and Wolf, E. (1941) The wavelength sensitivity function for the zebra finch. *Journal of General Physiology*, **24**, 625–633.

Cumming, B.G. and Parker, A.J. (1997) Responses of primary visual cortical neurons to binocular disparity without depth perception. *Nature*, **389**, 280–283.

Cumming, B.G. and Parker, A.J. (1999) Binocular neurons in V1 of awake monkeys are selective for absolute, not relative, disparity. *Journal of Neuroscience*, **19**, 5602–5618.

Currie, J.N., Goldberg, M.E, Matsuo, V. and Fizgibbon, E. (1986) Dyslexia with saccadic intrusions: a treatable reading disorder. *Neurology*, **36** (suppl.), 134.

Daum, K.M, Rutstein, K.P, Houston, G, Clore K.A. and Corliss, D.A. (1989). Evaluation of a new criterion of binocularity. *Optometry and Visual Science*, **66**, 218–228.

Davson, H. (1990a) *Physiology of the Eye*, 5th edn, pp. 279–300. Macmillan, London.

Davson, H. (1990b) *Physiology of the Eye*, 5th edn, pp. 486–597. Macmillan, London.

DeAngelis, G.C. and Newsome, W.T. (1999) Organization of disparity-selective neurons in macaque area MT. *Journal of Neuroscience*, **19**, 1398–1415.

Demer, J.L. (2007) The orbital pulley system: a revolution in concepts of orbital anatomy. *Journal of Applied Physiology*, **103**, 1706–1714.

de Wit, G.C. (2008) Clinical usefulness of the Aniseikonia Inspector: review. *Binocular Vision and Strabismus Quarterly*, **23**, 207–214.

Ditchburn, R.W. (1973) *Eye-movements and Visual Perception*. Clarendon Press, Oxford.

Donahue, S.P. (2005) The relationship between anisometropia, patient age, and the development of amblyopia. *Transactions of the American Ophthalmological Society*, **103**, 313–336.

Donders, F.C. (1864) *On the Anomalies of Accommodation and Refraction of the Eye: With a Preliminary Essay on Physiological Dioptrics*. The New Sydenham Society, London.

Dunne, M.C., Davies, L.N., Mallen, E.A., Kirschkamp, T. and Barry, J.C. (2005) Non-invasive phakometric measurement of corneal and crystalline lens alignment in human eyes. *Ophthalmic and Physiological Optics*, **25**, 143–152.

Earnshaw, J.R. (1962) The single mirror haploscope. *Transactions of the International Congress of the British Optical Association*, pp. 673–674. British Optical Association, London.

Eggert, T. (2007) Eye movement recordings: methods. In: *Neuro-ophthalmology: Developments in Ophthalmology* (eds A. Straube and U. Büttner), **40**, Karger, Basel, pp. 15–34.

Elliott, M.C. and Firth, A.Y. (2009) The logMAR Kay picture test and the logMAR acuity test: a comparative study. *Eye*, **23**, 85–88.

Erkelens, C.J. and Regan, D. (1986) Human ocular vergence movements induced by changing size and disparity. *Journal of Physiology*, **279**, 145–169.

Evans, B.F.W. (1998) The underachieving child. *Ophthalmic and Physiological Optics*, **18**, 153–159.

Evans, B.J.W. (2007) *Pickwell's Binocular Vision Anomalies*, 5th edn. Butterworth-Heineman, Oxford, pp. 195, 260.

Fawcett, S.F., Wang, Y.-Z., Birch, E.E. (2005) The critical period for susceptibility of human stereopsis. *Investigative Ophthalmology and Visual Science*, **46**, 521–525.

Ferraina, S., Pare, M., Wurtz, R.H. (1993) Disparity sensitivity of frontal eye field neurons. *Journal of Neurophysiology*, **83**, 625–629.

Fisher, S.K. and Ciuffreda, K.J. (1988) Accommodation and apparent distance. *Perception*, **17**, 609–621.

Fletcher, R.J. and Voke, J. A. (1985) Chapter 9: Assistance for colour vision defects. In: *Defective Colour Vision*. Adam Hilger, Bristol and Boston, pp. 417–434.

Fox, R. and Check, R. (1966) Binocular fusion: a test of the suppression theory. *Perception and Psychophysics*, **1**, 333–334.

Fox, R. Aslin, R.N., Shea, S.L. and Dumais, S.T. (1980) Stereopsis in human infants. *Science*, **207**, 323–324.

Freedman, K.A. and Brown, S.M. (2008) The effective corneal refractive surface as a function of a point in pace: a three-dimensional analysis. *Ophthalmic and Physiological Optics*, **28**, 584–594.

Gall, R., Wick, B. and Bedell, H. (1998) Vergence facility: establishing clinical utility. *Optometry and Visual Science*, **75**, 731–742.

Genovesio, A. and Ferraina, S. (2004) Integration of retinal disparity and fixation-distance related signals toward an egocentric coding of distance in the posterior parietal cortex of primates. *Journal of Neurophysiology*, **91**, 2670–2684.

Gibson, E. and Walk, R. (1960) The 'visual cliff'. *Scientific American*, **202**, 64–71.

Gilliland, K. and Hames, R.F. (1975) Binocular summation and peripheral visual response time. *American Journal of Optometry and Physiological Optics*, **52**, 834–839.

Gordon, G.E. and McCulloch, D.L. (1999). A VEP investigation of parallel visual pathway development in primary school age children. *Documenta ophthalmologica*, **99**, 1–10.

Goss, D.A. (1995) *Ocular Accommodation, Convergence, and Fixation Disparity: a Manual of Clinical Analysis*. Butterworth-Heinemann, Boston.

Gowen, E., Abadi. R.V. and Poliakoff, E. (2005) Paying attention to saccadic intrusions. *Cognitive Brain Research* **25**, 810–825.

Grounds, A. (1996) Child visual development. In: *Pediatric Eye Care* (eds S. Barnard and D. Edgar). Blackwell Science, Oxford, p. 61.

Han, S.J., Guo, Y., Granger-Donetti, B., Vicci, V.R. and Alvarez, T.L. (2010) Quantification of heterophoria and phoria adaptation using an automated objective system compared to clinical methods. *Ophthalmic and Physiological Optics*, **30**, 95–107.

Harris, W.F. (2010) Nodes and nodal points and lines in eyes and other optical systems. *Ophthalmic and Physiological Optics*, **30**, 24–42.

Harter, M.R., Seiple, W.H. and Salmon, L. (1973) Binocular summation of visually evoked responses to pattern stimuli in humans. *Vision Research*, **13**, 1433–1446.

Harwerth, R.S., Smith, E.L. and Levi, D.M. (1980) Suprathreshold binocular interactions for grating patterns. *Perception and Psychophysics*, **27**, 43–50.

Harwerth, R.S., Duncan, G.C., Smith, E.L., Crawford, M.I.J. and von Noorden, G.K. (1986) Multiple sensitive periods in the development of the primate visual system. *Science*, **232**, 235–238.

Hayes, G.J., Cohen, B.E., Rouse, M.W. and DeLand, P.N. (1998) Normative values for the nearpoint of convergence of elementary schoolchildren. *Optometry and Visual Science*, **75**, 506–512.

Heckenlively, J.R. and Arden, G.B. (eds) (2006) *Principles and Practice of Clinical Electrophysiology of Vision*. MIT Press. Cambridge, Massachusetts.

Held, R., Birch, E. and Gwiazda, J. (1980) *Stereoacuity of human infants*. Proceedings of the National Academy of Sciences USA, **77**, 5572–5574.

Helmchen, C. and Rambold, H. (2007) The eyelid and its contribution to eye movements. *Developments in Ophthalmology*, **40**, 110–131.

Helmholtz, H., von (1924) *Helmholtz's Treatise on Physiological Optics*. (English translation from 3rd German edn) (ed. P.C. Southall). The Optical Society of America, Ithaca.

Hering, E. (1868) *Die Lehre vom binokularen Sehen*. Engelmann, Leipzig.

Hering, E. (1879) *The Theory of Binocular Vision*. Translated by Bridgeman, B. (1977) (eds B. Bridgeman and L. Stark). Plenum Press, New York.

Hillis, J.M. and Banks, M.S. (2001) Are corresponding points fixed? *Vision Research*, **41**, 2457–2473.

Holmes, G. (1945) The organization of the visual cortex in man. *Proceedings of the Royal Society of London, Series B*, **132**, 348–361.

Holmes, J.M. and Fawcett, S.L. (2005) Testing distances stereoacuity with the Frisby–Davis 2 (FD2) test. *American Journal of Ophthalmology*, **139**, 193–195.

Holopigian, K., Blake, R. and Greenwald, M.J. (1988) Clinical suppression and amblyopia. *Investigative Ophthalmology and Visual Science*, **29**, 444–451.

Horowitz, M.W. (1949) An analysis of the superiority of binocular over monocular visual acuity. *Journal of Experimental Psychology*, **39**, 581–596.

Hubel, D.H. and Wiesel, T.N. (1962) Receptive fields, binocular interaction and functional architecture in the cat's visual cortex. *Journal of Physiology*, **160**, 106–154.

Hubel, D.H. and Wiesel, T.N. (1965) Extent of recovery from the effects of visual deprivation in kittens. *Journal of Neurophysiology*, **28**, 1060–1072.

Hubel, D.H. and Wiesel, T.N. (1970) Cells sensitive to binocular depth in area 18 of macaque monkey cortex. *Nature*, **225**, 41–42.

Jackson, J.H. and Arnoldi, K. (2004) The gradient AC/A ratio: what's really normal? *American Orthoptic Journal*, **54**, 125–132.

Jenkins, T.C.A, Pickwell, L.D. and Yekta, A.A. (1989) Criteria for decompensation in binocular vision. *Ophthalmic and Physiological Optics*, **9**, 121–125.

Jennings, J.A.M. (2001) Anomalies of convergence. In: *Binocular Vision and Orthoptics* (eds B.J.W. Evans and S. Doshi). Butterworth Heinemann, Oxford, pp 34–38.

Julesz, B. and Tyler, C.W. (1976) Neurontropy, an entropy–like measure of neural correlation, in binocular fusion and rivalry. *Biology Cybernet*, **22**, 107–119.

Kalarickal, G.J. and Marshall, J.A. (2000) Neural model of temporal and stochastic properties of binocular rivalry. *Neurocomputing*, **32–33**, 843–853.

Kapoula, Z., Bernotas, M. and Hashwanter, T. (1999) Listing's plane rotation with convergence: role of disparity, accommodation, and depth perception. *Experimental Brain Research*, **126**, 175–186.

Kerber, K.A, Ishiyama, G.P. and Baloh, R.W. (2006) A longitudinal study of oculomotor function in normal older people. *Neurobiology of Aging*, **27**, 1346–1353.

Kikuchi, E., Miyashita, M. and Tanaka, S. (2008) Influence of interocular inhibition in LGN on the formation of cortical receptive fields. *IEICE Technical Report 107*, **542**, 215–220.

Kintz, R.T. (1969) A comparison of monocular and binocular temporal resolution in human vision. Ph.D. thesis, University of Rochester.

Kjellevold-Haugen, I.-B. (2001) Comparison of proximal tendon receptors in extra-ocular muscles. M.Phil. thesis, The City University, London.

Larson, W.L. and Faubert, J. (1992) Stereolatency: a stereopsis test for everyday depth perception. *Optometry and Visual Science*, **69**, 926–930.

Le-Grand, Y. (1968) Light, Colour, and Vision. Chapman & Hall, London, pp. 305–307, 423.

Lehmkuhle, S. and Fox, R. (1975) The effects of binocular rivalry suppression on the motion after-effect. *Vision Research*, **15**, 855–860.

Leigh, R.J. and Zee, D.S. (2006) *The Neurology of Eye Movements*, 4th edn. Oxford University Press, Oxford.

Lemij, H.G. and Collewijn, H. (1991) Short-term nonconjugate adaptation of human saccades to anisometropic spectacles. *Brain Research*, **562**, 207–215.

LeVay, S, Wiesel, T.N. and Hubel, D.H. (1980) The development of ocular dominance columns in normal and visually deprived monkeys. *Journal of Comparative Neurology*, **179**, 233–244.

Levelt, W.J.M. (1965) Binocular brightness averaging and contour information. *British Journal of Psychology*, **56**, 1–13.

Lindblom, B. Westheimer, G. and Hoyt, W.F. (1997) Torsional diplopia and its perceptual consequences: a 'user–friendly' test for oblique muscle palsies. *NeuroOphthalmology*, **18**, 105–110.

Li, C.-Y. and Guo, K. (1995) Measurements of geometric illusions, illusory contours and stereo-depth at luminance and color contrast. *Vision Research*, **35**, 1713–1720.

Lit, A. (1978) Spatio-temporal aspects of binocular depth discrimination. In: *Frontiers in Visual Science* (eds S.J. Cool and E.L. Smith III). Springer-Verlag, New York, pp. 396–424.

Lotze, H. (1852) *Medicinische Psychologie oder Physiologie der Seele*. Weidmann, Leizig.

MacMillan, E.S., Gray, L.S. and Heron, G. (2007) Visual adaptation to interocular brightness differences induced by neutral-density filters. *Investigative Ophthalmology and Visual Science*, **48**, 935–942.

Maddox, E.E. (1907) *The Ocular Muscles*, 3rd edn. Keystone, Philadelphia.

Mallett, R.J.F. (1964) The investigation of heterophoria at near and a new fixation disparity technique. *The Optician*, **148**, 547–551.

Mallett, R.J.F. (1988) Techniques of investigation of binocular vision anomalies. In: *Optometry* (eds K. Edwards and R. Llewellyn). Butterworths, London, pp. 238–269.

Maples, W.C. and Hoenes, R. (2007) Near point of convergence norms measured in elementary school children. *Optometry and Visual Science*, **84**, 224–228.

Matin, L. (1962) Binocular summation at the absolute threshold for peripheral vision. *Journal of the Optical Society of America*, **52**, 1276–1286.

Maunsell, J.H.R. and Van Essen, D.C. (1983) Functional properties of neurons in middle temporal visual area of the macaque monkey. II. Binocular interactions and sensitivity to binocular disparity. *Journal of Neurophysiology*, **49**, 1148–1167.

Maxwell, G.F., Lemij, H.G. and Collewijn, H. (1995) Conjugacy of saccades in deep amblyopia. *Investigative Ophthalmology and Visual Science*, **36**, 2514–2522.

McComb, D.M., Tricas, T.C. and Kajiura, S.M. (2009) Enhanced visual fields in hammerhead sharks. *Journal of Experimental Biology*, **212**, 4010–4018.

Meissner, G. (1854) *Beitrage zur Physiologie des Sehorganes*. W. Engleman, Leipzig.

Merkel and Kallius (1901). Chapter 1. In: *Makroscopische Anatomie des Auges, Graefe–Saemisch Handbuch der Augenheil*, Vol. 1, 2nd edn. Cited by Whitnall, S.E. (1932) *The Anatomy of the Human Orbit*. Oxford University Press, Oxford, p. 271.

Mitchell, D.E. (1966) A review of the concept of 'Panum's fusional areas'. *American Journal of Optometry and Physiological Optics*, **43**, 387–401.

Mitchell, D.E. and Baker, A.G. (1973) Stereoscopic aftereffects: evidence for disparity–specific neurones in the human visual system. *Vision Research*, **13**, 2273–2288.

Mitchell, D.E. and Ware, C. (1974) Interocular transfer of a visual after-effect in normal and stereoblind humans. *Journal of Physiology*, **236**, 707–721.

Mitchell, D.E., Reardon, J. and Muir, D.W. (1975) Interocular transfer of the motion aftereffect in normal and stereoblind observers. *Experimental Brain Research*, **22**, 163–175.

Miyawaki, Y., Hayashi, R., Maeda, T. and Taci, S. (2002) The time course of stereopsis: the delayed VEP component correlate of figure–ground processes. IEICE Transactions on Information and Systems, Pt. 2 (Japanese edition). J85–D–2; No. 2, 337–350.

Montaser-Kouhsari, L., Lander, M.S., Heeger, D.J. and Larsson, J. (2007) Orientation-selective adaptation to illusory contours in human visual cortex. *Journal of Neuroscience*, **19**, 91–101.

Morgan, M.W. (1964) The analysis of clinical data. *Optometric Weekly*, 55, 23–25, 27–34.

Morgan, M.W. (1983) The Maddox analysis of vergence. In: *Vergence Eye Movements: Basic and Clinical Aspects* (eds C.M. Schor and K.J. Ciuffreda). Butterworth-Heinemann, Boston, pp 15–21.

Movshon, J.A., Chambers, B.E.I. and Blakemore, C. (1972) Interocular transfer in normal humans, and those who lack stereopsis. *Perception*, **1**, 483–490.

Müller, J. (1826). *Zur vergleichenden Physiologie des Gesichtssinnes des Menschen und der Thiere*. Cnobloch, Leipzig.

Nakayama, K. and Shimojo, S. (1990) Da Vinci stereopsis: depth and occluding subjective contours from unpaired image points. *Vision Research*, **30**, 1811–1825.

Nelson, J. (1988a) Amblyopia: the cortical basis of binocularity and vision loss in strabismus. In: *Optometry* (eds. K. Edwards and R. Llewellyn). Butterworths, London, pp. 199–200.

Nelson, J. (1988b) Binocular vision: disparity detection and anomalous correspondence. In: *Optometry* (eds. K. Edwards and R. Llewellyn). Butterworths, London, pp. 228–233.

Neri, P., Bridge, H., and Heeger, D.J. (2004) Stereoscopic processing of absolute and relative disparity in human visual cortex. *Journal of Neurophysiology*, **92**, 1880–1891.

Nguyenkim, J.D. and DeAngelis, G.C. (2003) Disparity-based coding of three-dimensional surface orientation by macaque middle temporal neurons. *Journal of Neuroscience*, **23**, 7117–7128.

Nolte, J. (2002) *The Human Brain: an Introduction to its Functional Anatomy*, 5th edn. Mosby, St Louis, pp. 410–447.

Norcia, A.M. and Tyler, C.W. (1985) Spatial frequency sweep VEP visual acuity during the first year of life. *Vision Research*, **25**, 1399–1408.

North, R. and Henson, D.B. (1992) The effect of orthoptic treatment upon the vergence adaptation mechanism. *Optometry and Visual Science*, **69**, 294–299.

Norton, T.T. and Siegwart, J.T. (1995) Animal models of emmetropisation: matching axial length to the focal plane. *Journal of the American Optometric Association*, **66**, 405–414.

Ogle, K.N. (1932) Analytical treatment of the longitudinal horopter. *Journal of the Optical Society of America*, **22**, 665–728.

Ogle, K.N. (1938). Induced size effect. *Archives of Ophthalmology*, **20**, 604–623.

Ogle, K.N. (1950) *Researches in Binocular Vision*. Saunders, Philadelphia.

Ogle, K.N. (1953) Precision and validity of stereoscopic depth perception from double images. *Journal of the Optical Society of America*, **43**, 906–913.

Ogle, K.N. (1954) Stereopsis and vertical disparity. *American Orthoptic Journal*, **4**, 35–39.

Ogle, K.N. (1963) *Physiology of the Eye* (ed. H. Davson), 4th edn. Churchill Livingstone, London, p. 333.

Ogle, K.N, Martens, G.G. and Dyer, J.A. (1967). *Oculomotor Imbalance in Binocular Vision and Fixation Disparity*. Lea and Febiger, Philadelphia.

Ohzawa, I, Freeman, R.D. (1986) The binocular organization of complex cells in the cat's visual cortex. *Journal of Neurophysiology*, **56**, 221–242.

Ohzawa, I. and Freeman, R.D. (1986) The binocular organization of simple cells in the cat's visual cortex. *Journal of Neurophysiology*, **56**, 243–259.

Ohzawa, I., DeAngelis, G.C.and Freeman, R.D. (1996) Encoding of binocular disparity by simple cells in the cat's visual cortex. *Journal of Neurophysiology*, **75**, 1779–1805.

Ooi, T.L. and Loop, M.S. (1994) Visual suppression and its effect upon color and luminance sensitivity. *Vision Research*, **34**, 2997–3003.

Ono, H. and Barbeito, R. (1982) The cyclopean eye versus the sighting dominant eye as the center of visual direction. *Perception and Psychophysics*, **32**, 201–210.

O'Shea, R.P., Sims, A.J.H. and Govan, D.G. (1997) The effect of spatial frequency and field size on the spread of exclusive visibility in binocular rivalry. *Vision Research*, **37**, 175–183.

Panum, P.L. (1858) *Physiologische Untersuchungen uber das Sehen mit zwei Augen*. Schwers, Kiel, p. 18.

Paradiso, M.A., Shimojo, S. and Nakayama, K. (1989) Subjective contours, tilt after-effects and visual cortical organisation. *Vision Research*, **29**, 1205–1213.

Pardhan, S. and Whittaker, A. (2000) Binocular summation in the fovea and peripheral field of anisometropic amblyopes. *Current Eye Research*, **20**, 35–44.

Park, R.S. and Park, G.E. (1933) The centre of ocular rotation in the horizontal plane. *American Journal of Physiology*, **104**, 545–552.

Parks, M.M. and Eustis, A.T. (1961) Monofixational phoria. *American Orthoptic Journal*, **11**, 38–45.

Perkins, E.S., Hammond, B. and Milliken, A.B. (1976) Simple method of determining the axial length of the eye. *British Journal of Ophthalmology*, **60**, 266–270.

Perlmutter, A.L. and Kertesz, A.E. (1978) Measurement of human vertical fusional response. *Vision Research*, **18**, 219–223.

Phillips, A.J. and Stone, J. (1972) *Contact Lenses*, 3rd edn. Butterworths, London.

Phillips, J.O., Finocchio, D.V., Ong, L., and Fuchs, A.F. (1997) Smooth pursuit in 1- to 4-month-old infants. *Vision Research*, **37**, 3009–3020.

Pirenne, M.H. (1943) Binocular and uniocular threshold of vision. *Nature*, **152**, 698–699.

Pobuda, M. and Erkelens, C.J. (1993) The relationship between absolute disparity and ocular vergence. *Biological Cybernetics* **68**, 221–228.

Poggio, G.F. and Fischer, B. (1977) Binocular interaction and depth sensitivity in striate and prestriate cortex of behaving rhesus monkey. *Journal of Neurophysiology*, **40**, 1392–1405.

Poggio, G.F. and Talbot, W.H. (1981) Mechanisms of static and dynamic stereopsis in the foveal cortex of the Rhesus monkey. *Journal of Physiology*, **315**, 469–492.

Porrill, A., Ivins, J.P. and Frisby, J.P. (1999) The variation of torsion with vergence and elevation. *Vision Research*, **39**, 3934–3950.

Quaia, C. and Optican, L.M. (2003) Three-dimensional rotations of the eye. In: *Adler's Physiology of the Eye: Clinical Application*, 10th edn (eds P.L. Kaufman and M.D. Alm). Mosby, New York, pp. 818–829.

Qiu, F.T. and von der Heydt, R. (2005) Figure and ground in the visual cortex: v2 combines stereoscopic cues with gestalt rules. *Neuron*, **47**, 155–166.

Rabbetts, R.B. (1972) A comparison of astigmatism and cyclophoria in distance and near vision. *British Journal of Physiological Optics*, **27**, 161–190.

Rabbetts, R.B. (2007) Convergence. In: *Bennetts and Rabbetts Clinical Visual Optics*, 4th edn (ed. R. Rabbetts). Butterworth Heinemann, London.

Rabbetts, R.B. (2009) Cataract and the nodal point fallacy. *Optometry in Practice*, **10**, 167–170.

Rainey, B.B., Schroeder, T.L., Goss, D.A. and Grosvenor, T.P. (1998) Inter-examiner repeatability of heterophoria tests. *Optometry and Visual Science*, **75**, 719–726.

Ramachandran, V.S. and Braddick O. (1973) Orientation-specific learning in stereopsis. *Perception*, **2**, 371–376.

Rashbass, C. and Westheimer, G. (1961) Disjunctive eye movements. *Journal of Physiology*, **159**, 339–360.

Raymond, J.E. (1993) Complete interocular transfer of motion adaptation effects on motion coherence thresholds. *Vision Research*, **33**, 1865–1870.

Read, J.C.A. and Cumming, B.G. (2006) Does depth perception require vertical-disparity detectors? *Journal of Vision*, **6**, 1323–1355.

Reading, R.W. (1983) *Binocular Vision: Foundations and Applications*. Butterworth-Heinemann, Boston, p. 48.

Regan, D. and Cyanader, M. (1979) Neurons in area 18 of cat visual cortex selectively sensitive to changing size: nonlinear interactions between responses to two edges. *Vision Research*, **19**, 699–711.

Regan, D., Erkelens, C.J. and Collewijn, H. (1986) Visual field effects for vergence eye movements and for stereo motion perception. *Investigative Ophthalmology and Visual Science*, **27**, 806–819.

Remole, A. (1981) Application of the aniseikonic ellipse to prisms. *American Journal of Optometry and Physiological Optics*, **58**, 378–385.

Richards, W. (1971) Anomalous stereoscopic depth perception. *Journal of the Optical Society of America*, **61**, 410–414.

Robinson, D.A. (1965) The mechanics of human smooth pursuit eye movements. *Journal of Physiology*, **180**, 569–591.

Robinson, D.A. (1972) Eye movements evoked by collicular stimulation in the alert monkey. *Vision Research*, **12**, 1795–1808.

Robinson, D.L. and McClurkin, J.W. (1989) The visual superior colliculus and pulvinar. In: *The Neurobiology of Saccadic Eye Movements* (eds. R.H. Wurtz and M.E. Goldberg), pp. 337–360. Elsevier, Amsterdam.

Rockland, K.S. (1995) Morphology of individual axons projecting from area V2 to MT in the macaque. *Journal of Comparative Neurology*, **355**, 15–26.

Roumbouts, S.A.R.B., Barkhof. F., Sprenger, M., Valk, J. and Scheltens, P. (1996) The functional basis of ocular dominance: functional MRI (fMRI) findings. *Neuroscience Letters*, **221**, 1–4.

Rowe, F. (2003) Supranuclear and internuclear control of eye movements: a review. *British Orthoptic Journal*, **60**, 2–9.

Rowe, F. (2004) *Clinical Orthoptics*. Blackwell Publishing, Oxford, p. 28.

Ruskell, G.L. (1978) The fine structure of innervated myotendinous cylinders in extraocular muscles of rhesus monkeys. *Journal of Neurocytology*, 7, 693–708.

Ruskell, G.L. (1989) The fine structure of human extraocular muscle spindles and their potential proprioceptive capacity. *Journal of Anatomy*, **167**, 199–214.

Ruskell, G.L. (1999). Extraocular muscle proprioceptors and proprioception. *Progress In Retinal and Eye Research*, **18**, 269–291.

Ruskell, G.L., Kjellevold Haugen, I.-B. Bruenech, J.R. and van der Werf, F. (2005) Double insertions of extraocular rectus muscles in humans and the pulley theory. *Journal of Anatomy*, **206**, 295–306.

Sakata, H., Tsutsui, K. and Taira, M. (2005) Toward an understanding of the neural processing for 3D shape perception. *Neuropsychologia*. **43**, 151–161.

Salzmann, M. (1912) *The Anatomy and Histology of the Human Eyeball*. University Press, Chicago, IL, p. 7.

Saude, T. (1993) *Ocular Anatomy and Physiology*. Blackwell Scientific Publications, Oxford.

Saunders, K.J., Woodhouse, M. and Westall, C.A. (1995) Emmetropisation in human infancy: rate of change is related to initial refractive error. *Vision Research*, **35**, 1325–1328.

Schectman, D., Shallo-Hoffmann, J., Rumsey, J., Riordan-Eva, P. and Hardigan, P. (2005) Maximum angle of ocular duction during visual fixation as a function of age. *Strabismus*, **13**, 21–26.

Schor, C.M. (1979) The relationship between fusional vergence eye movements and fixation disparity. *Vision Research*, **19**, 1359–1367.

Schor, C.M., Terrell, M. and Peterson, D. (1976) Contour interaction and temporal masking in strabismus and amblyopia. *American Journal of Physiological Optics*, **53**, 217–223.

Schreiber, K.M., Tweed, D.B. and Schor, C.M. (2006) The extended horopter: quantifying retinal correspondence across changes of 3D eye position. *Journal of Vision*, **16**, 64–74.

Schumer, R.A. and Ganz, L. (1979) Independent stereoscopic channels for different extents of spatial pooling. *Vision Research*, **19**, 1303–1314.

Sengpiel, F. and Blakemore, C. (1994) Interocular control of neuronal responsiveness in cat visual cortex. *Nature*, **368**, 847–850.

Sharma, P., Prasad, K. and Khokhar, S. (1999) Cyclofusion in normal and superior oblique palsy subjects. *Journal of Pediatric Ophthalmology and Strabismus*, **35**, 264–270.

Sheedy, J.E. and Fry, G.A. (1997) The perceived direction of the binocular image. *Vision Research*, **19**, 201–211.

Sheedy, J.E. and Saladin, J.J. (1978) Association of symptoms with measurements of oculomotor deficiencies. *American Journal of Optometry*, **55**, 670–676.

Sherrington, C.S. (1894) Experimental note on two movements of the eye. *Journal of Physiology (London)*, **17**, 27–29.

Sherrington, CS. (1904) On Binocular Flicker and the Correlation of Activity of Corresponding Retinal Points. *British Journal of Psychology*, I, (1904–5), 26–60.

Sherrington, C.S. (1906) The integrative action of the nervous system. Charles Scribner's Sons, New York. Reprinted by Cambridge University Press 1947 (with a new preface and full bibliography), and by Yale University Press 1961 (paperback).

Sherrington, C.S. (1918) Observations on the sensual role of the proprioceptive nerve-supply of the extrinsic ocular muscles. *Brain* **41**, 332–343.

Shikata, E., Tanaka, Y., Nakamura, H., Taira, M. and Sakata H. (1996) Selectivity of the parietal visual neurones in 3D orientation of surface of stereoscopic stimuli. *Neuroreport*, **7**, 2389–2394.

Shimojo, S. and Nakajima, Y. (1981) Adaptation to the reversal of binocular depth clues: effects of wearing left–right reversing spectacles. *Perception*, **10**, 391–402.

Shin, H.S., Park, S.C. and Park, C.M. (2009) Relationships between accommodative and vergence dysfunctions and academic achievement for primary school children. *Ophthalmic and Physiological Optics*, **29**, 615–624.

Shipp, S., and Zeki, S. (1985) Segregation of pathways leading from Area V2 to Areas V4 and V5 of macaque monkey visual-cortex. *Nature*, **315**, 322–325.

Siderov, J. (1999) Stereopsis, cyclovergence and the backward tilt of the vertical horopter. *Vision Research*, **39**, 1347–1357.

Simons, B. and Büttner, U. (1985) The influence of age on optokinetic nystagmus. *European Archives of Psychiatry and Neurological Science*, **234**, 369–373.

Spooner, J.D. (1957) *Ocular Anatomy*. Hatton Press. London, p. 76.

Steinman, S.B, Steinman, B.A. and Garzia, R.P. (2000) *Foundations of Binocular Vision: a Clinical Perspective*. McGraw-Hill, New York, p. 224.

Stidwill, D.B. (1990) *Orthoptic Assessment and Management*, 1st edn. Blackwell Scientific Publications, Oxford, p. 25.

Stidwill, D.B. (1997) Epidemiology of strabismus. *Ophthalmic and Physiological Optics*, **17**, 536–539.

Stidwill, D.B. (1998) *Orthoptic Assessment and Management*, 2nd edn. Blackwell Science, Oxford, p. 41.

Stidwill, D.B. (2009) The objective line of sight heterotropia test. *The Orthoptic and Binocular Vision Association Newsletter*, **45**, 1:1.

Straube, A. and Büttner, U. (2007) *Neuro-Ophthalmology: Neuronal Control of Eye Movements*. Karger, Basel.

Sundet, J.M. (1976) Two theories of colour stereoscopy. *Vision Research*, **16**, 469–472.

Sylvestre, P.A. and Cullen, K.E. (2002). Dynamics of abducens nucleus neuron discharges during disjunctive saccades. *Journal of Neurophysiology*, **88**, 3452–3468.

Thomas, O.M., Cumming, B.G. and Parker, A.J. (2002) A specialization for relative disparity in V2. *Nature Neuroscience*, **5**, 472–478.

Tokoro, T. and Suzuki, K. (1968) Significance of changes of refractive components to development of myopia during seven years. *Nippon Geka Gakkai*, **72**, 1472.

Tschermak, A. (1900) Beitrage zur Lehre vom Langshoropter. *Pflüger's Archiv*, **81**, 328–348.

Tsuetaki, T.K. and Schor, C.M. (1987) Clinical method for measuring adaptation of tonic accommodation and vergence accommodation. *American Journal of Optometry and Physiological Optics*, **64**, 437–449.

Tyler, C.W. and Clarke, M.B. (1990) *The Autostereogram*. SPIE Stereoscopic Displays and Application, pp. 182–196.

Uka, T. and DeAngelis, G.C. (2003) Contribution of middle temporal area to coarse depth discrimination: comparison of neuronal and psychophysical sensitivity. *Journal of Neuroscience*, **23**, 3515–3530.

Uka, T. and DeAngelis, G.C. (2006) Linking neural representation to function in stereoscopic depth perception: roles of the middle temporal area in coarse versus fine disparity discrimination. *Journal of Neuroscience*, **26**, 6791–6802.

Uka, T., Tanabe, S., Watanabe, M. and Fujita, I. (2005) Neural correlates of fine depth discrimination in monkey inferior temporal cortex. *Journal of Neuroscience*, **25**, 10796–10802.

Umeda, K., Tanabe, S. and Fujita, I. (2007) Representation of stereoscopic depth based on relative disparity in macaque area V4. *Journal of Neurophysiology*, **98**, 241–252.

Van der Meuklen (1873) cited by Boeder, P. (1952) In: *Tschermak's Introduction to Physiological Optics*. Charles Thomas, Springfield, IL, p. 179.

Varela, F. and Singer, W. (1987) Neuronal dynamics in the visual cortico-thalamic pathway as revealed through binocular rivalry. *Experimental Brain Research*, **66**, 10–20.

Vieth, G.U.A. (1818). Uber die Richtung der Augen. *Annalen der Physik*, **58**, 233–253.

Von Kries, J. (1925). In: *Helmholtz's Treatise on Physiological Optics*, Vol. 3 (ed. J.P.C. Southall), pp. 528–559 (particularly p. 537) and Appendix pp. 560–688 (particularly pp. 607–625). Dover, New York.

von Noorden, G.K. and Campos, E. (2002) *Binocular Vision and Ocular Motility*, 6th edn. Mosby, St Louis.

Vos, J.J. (1960) Some new aspects of color stereoscopy. *Journal of the Optical Society of America*, **50**, 785–790

Walker, P. and Powell, D.J. (1979) The sensitivity to binocular rivalry to changes in the non-dominant stimulus. *Vision Research*, **19**, 247–249.

Walls, G.L. (1942). *The Vertebrate Eye*. Cranbrook Institute, Bloom Fields, p. 295.

Walsh, F.N. and Hoyt, W.F. (2004) *Walsh and Hoyt's Clinical Neuro-ophthalmology*, 6th edn (eds N.R. Miller, N.J. Newnan, V. Biousse and J.B. Kerrison). Lippincott Williams & Wilkins, Philadelphia.

Warnking, J., Dojat, M., Guerin-Dugue, A., Delon-Martin, C., Olympieff, S. et al. (2002) fMRI retinotopic mapping – step by step. *Neuroimage*, **17**, 1665–1683.

Weale, R.A. (1954a) Theory of the Pulfrich effect. *Ophthalmologica*, **128**, 380–388.

Weale, R. A. (1954b) Variations in the latent period of vision. *Proceedings of the Royal Society of London, Series B*, 142–258.

Westendorf, O. and Fox, R. (1977) Binocular detection of disparate light flashes. *Vision Research*, **17**, 697–702.

Westheimer, G. (1979) Co-operative neural processes involved in stereoscopic acuity. *Experimental Brain Research*, **36**, 585–597.

Westheimer, G. and McKee, S.P. (1978) Stereoscopic acuity with defocussed and spatially filtered retinal images. *Journal of the Optical Society of America*, **70**, 772–778.

Westheimer. G. and Mitchell, D.E. (1969) The sensory stimulus for sensory eye movements. *Vision Research*, **9**, 749–755.

Wexler, M. (2005) Anticipating the three-dimensional consequences of eye movements. *Proceedings of the National Academy of Sciences USA*, **102**, 1246–1251.

Wheatstone, C. (1838) Contributions to the physiology of vision – part the first. On some remarkable, and hitherto unobserved, phenomena of binocular vision. *Philosophical Transactions of the Royal Society*, **128**, 371–394.

Wheatstone, C. (1852) Contributions to the physiology of vision – part the second. On some remarkable, and hitherto unobserved, phenomena of binocular vision. *Philosophical Transactions of the Royal Society*, **142**, 1–17.

Whitnall, S.E. (1932) *The Anatomy of the Human Orbit*. Oxford UK, Oxford University Press, p. 294.

Wolfe, J. and Blake, R. (1985) Monocular and binocular processes in human vision. In: *Models of Visual Cortex* (eds D. Rose and V. Dobson). Wiley, New York.

Worth, C. (1903) *Squint, its Causes, Pathology and Treatment*. Bathers, Tindal and Cox, London.

Ye, M., Bradley, A, Thibos, L.N. and Zhang, X. (1991) Interocular differences in transverse chromatic aberration determine chromostereopsis for small pupils. *Vision Research*, **31**, 1787–1796.

Yekta, A.A., Pickwell, L.D. and Jenkins, T.C.A. (1989) Binocular vision, age and symptoms. *Ophthalmic and Physiological Optics*, **9**, 115–120.

Young, B.J., Sueke, H., Wylie, J.M. and Kaye, S.B. (2009) Contribution of a real depth distance stereoacuity test to clinical management. *Journal of Ophthalmology*, Epub 2009 Jul 5, Article ID 343827, 10.1155/2009/343827.

Zeki, S. and Shipp, S. (1988) The functional logic of optical connections. *Nature*, **335**, 311–317.

INDEX

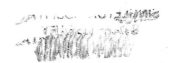